Skin Decontamination

Hanjiang Zhu • Howard I. Maibach
Editors

Skin Decontamination

A Comprehensive Clinical Research Guide

Springer

Editors
Hanjiang Zhu, PhD
Department of Dermatology
University of California
San Francisco, CA
USA

Howard I. Maibach, MD
Department of Dermatology
University of California San Francisco
School of Medicine
San Francisco, CA
USA

ISBN 978-3-030-24011-0 ISBN 978-3-030-24009-7 (eBook)
https://doi.org/10.1007/978-3-030-24009-7

This Springer imprint is published by the registered company Springer Nature Switzerland AG
The registered company address is: Gewerbestrasse 11, 6330 Cham, Switzerland

Preface

To general toxicologist and those involved in skin, hair and nail decontamination of chemical warfare and chemicals of mass destruction. The birth of this field occurred in Belgium – a century ago, when both government contenders utilized chemicals which produced marked lethality and/or incapacitation.

This led to many countries being involved in research in the field of chemical decontamination – mainly aimed at chemicals of mass destruction. Much of the experimental data remains buried in governmental archives such as the United States and the United Kingdom, and some remains classified until now.

Today there is wide acceptance, by many governments, of various Fuller's earth formulations (such as France) and the so-called RSDL – the United States. Combined with these highly specialized formulations, with deep research background, is another major approach to mass decontamination – the water wash approach. In addition, worldwide, material safety data sheets (MSDS) recommend water wash for acute skin decontamination. Recent data suggests that water wash may, at various time points, increase skin penetration and the potential for increasing acute general toxicity from highly toxic chemicals.

What appears to be a major paradigm shift is the apparent need to decontaminate millions of people from chemicals of nonacute lethality – such as the workers in the chemical industry who are exposed typically 5 days weekly for decades – to chemicals whose systemic toxicity (reproduction, carcinogenicity, and/or other internal organ toxicity) is often inadequately understood. This paradigm shift will require major new approaches to daily skin decontamination – not only for the acute event but for lifeline work, lifelong skin exposures. In addition, recently the American Food and Drug Administration (FDA) has suggested that maybe we have inadequate information on the chronic toxicity related to percutaneous penetration of sunscreens in man. Hence, even the cosmetic chemical ingredient domain may require a neo-evaluation of their long-term exposure and what can be done in daily skin decontamination.

The editors wish to thank Ms. Gina Kahn for her indispensable support and assistance throughout the book production.

The editors welcome your corrections and suggestions, which will be for the next edition.

San Francisco, CA, USA

Hanjiang Zhu
Howard I. Maibach

Contents

Contributors

Nahum Allon, PhD Department of Pharmacology, Israel Institute for Biological Research, Ness Ziona, Israel

Adina Amir, PhD Department of Pharmacology, Israel Institute for Biological Research, Ness Ziona, Israel

Richard Amlôt, BA (hons), MSc, PhD Emergency Response Department Science and Technology, Public Health England, Salisbury, UK

Izhak Barness, PhD Department of Pharmacology, Israel Institute for Biological Research, Ness Ziona, Israel

Christina Baxter, PhD Department of Defense, Combating Terrorism Technical Support Office, Virginia, CA, USA

Hillel Buch, BSc Agr. Department of Pharmacology, Israel Institute for Biological Research, Ness Ziona, Israel

Yachao Cao, PhD Department of Dermatology, University of California San Francisco, San Francisco, CA, USA

Holly Carter, BSc(hons), PhD Emergency Response Department Science and Technology, Public Health England, Salisbury, UK

Emmanuel Clavaud Service départemental d'incendie et de secours de la Savoie, Saint Alban-Leysse, France

Shlomit Dachir, PhD Department of Pharmacology, Israel Institute for Biological Research, Ness Ziona, Israel

Alison Director-Myska, PhD Defense Threat Reduction Agency, Ft. Belvoir, VA, USA

John Drury, BA(hons), MSc, PhD School of Psychology, University of Sussex, Brighton, UK

Arik Eisenkraft, MD Department of Pharmacology, Israel Institute for Biological Research, Ness Ziona, Israel

Akram Elmahdy, MD Department of Dermatology, University of California San Francisco, San Francisco, CA, USA

Françoise Falson, PhD, PharmD Université de lyon 1, UMR 5305-CNRS/ UCBL1; LBTI Lyon and Direction générale de la Sécurité civile et de la gestion des crises Ministère de l'interieur, Paris, France

Laboratoire de galénique industrielle ISPB UCBL1 Lyon, Lyon, France

Eliezer Fishbine, BSc Department of Pharmacology, Israel Institute for Biological Research, Ness Ziona, Israel

Sharyn Gaskin, BEH, BSc(Hons), PhD Department of Occupational & Environmental Health, School of Public Health, University of Adelaide, Adelaide, SA, Australia

Marie-Paule Gustin Université Lyon 1, CNRS UMR 5308,- Inserm U1111 / UCBL1, ENS Lyon, Lyon, France

Jill A. Harvilchuck, Ph.D., D.A.B .T. Battelle Memorial Institute, Columbus, OH, USA

Xiaoying Hui, MD Department of Dermatology, University of California San Francisco, San Francisco, CA, USA

Denis Josse, PhD, PharmD Colonel in the French Fire and Rescue Services, Alpes-Maritimes, Villeneuve-Loubet, France

Eui-Chang Jung, PhD Department of Dermatology, University of California San Francisco, San Francisco, CA, USA

Department of Dermatology, Gyeongsang National University Changwon Hospital, Changwon, South Korea

Tamar Kadar, DSc Department of Pharmacology, Israel Institute for Biological Research, Ness Ziona, Israel

Kelly Kyburz, PhD Office of the Assistant Secretary of the Army for Manpower and Reserve Affairs, Pentagon, Washington, DC, USA

Glenn Lawson, PhD Defense Threat Reduction Agency, Ft. Belvoir, VA, USA

Cong-Anh-Khanh Le, PhD, PharmD Université de lyon 1, UMR 5305-CNRS/ UCBL1; LBTI Lyon and Direction générale de la Sécurité civile et de la gestion des crises Ministère de l'interieur, Paris, France

Laboratoire de galénique industrielle ISPB UCBL1 Lyon, Lyon, France

Michael Logan, PhD Research and Scientific Branch, Queensland Fire and Emergency Services, Brisbane, QLD, Australia

Howard I. Maibach, MD Department of Dermatology, University of California San Francisco, San Francisco, CA, USA

Jacob Meshulam, MSc Department of Pharmacology, Israel Institute for Biological Research, Ness Ziona, Israel

Yakov Meshulam, MSc Department of Pharmacology, Israel Institute for Biological Research, Ness Ziona, Israel

Dan Noort, PhD TNO Defence, Security and Safety, Rijswijk, The Netherlands

Reyna N. Parker Bowdoin College, Brunswick, ME, USA

Christina Phuong, BS, MD Department of Dermatology, University of California San Francisco, San Francisco, CA, USA

Fabrice Pirot, PhD, PharmD Université de lyon 1, UMR 5305-CNRS/UCBL1; LBTI Lyon and Direction générale de la Sécurité civile et de la gestion des crises Ministère de l'interieur, Paris, France

Laboratoire de galénique industrielle ISPB UCBL1 Lyon, Lyon, France

Dino Pisaniello, BSc(Hons), MPH, PhD Adelaide Exposure Science and Health Laboratory, School of Public Health, University of Adelaide, Adelaide, SA, Australia

Annick Roul, PhD, PharmD Université de lyon 1, UMR 5305-CNRS/UCBL1; LBTI Lyon and Direction générale de la Sécurité civile et de la gestion des crises Ministère de l'interieur, Paris, France

Laboratoire de galénique industrielle ISPB UCBL1 Lyon, Lyon, France

Rita Sahar, BSc Department of Pharmacology, Israel Institute for Biological Research, Ness Ziona, Israel

Bernard Verrier, PhD Université de lyon 1, UMR 5305-CNRS/UCBL1; LBTI Lyon and Direction générale de la Sécurité civile et de la gestion des crises Ministère de l'interieur, Paris, France

Miranda Verschraagen, PhD, PharmD, Toxicologist-ERT Netherlands Forensic Institute, The Hague, The Netherlands

Hanjiang Zhu, PhD Department of Dermatology, University of California San Francisco, San Francisco, CA, USA

Chapter 1
Isolated Human and Animal Stratum Corneum As a Partial Model for the 15 Steps of Percutaneous Absorption: Emphasizing Decontamination, Part I

Xiaoying Hui and Howard I. Maibach

Introduction: 15 Steps of Percutaneous Absorption

The stratum corneum (SC) of humans and animals holds key insights to the development of an efficient protective barrier against contamination and to devising effective decontamination interventions. SC constitutes the main barrier to the absorption of molecules while participating in the homeostasis of the organism particularly by limiting outward movement of water.

Current understanding no longer considers the SC of the skin barrier as dead "brick and mortar", but rather a dynamic, living defense system. For instance, the acid mantle, a fine film with a slightly acidic pH on the surface of the skin, plays an integral role in making the skin less permeable to water and polar compounds and is formed in higher amounts with increased activity of enzyme phospholipase A2 [20, 57]. Additionally, acute perturbation of SC by organic solvents, detergents, or tape stripping resulting in lipid removal initiates a sequence of biological responses including epidermal lipid synthesis acceleration to rapidly restore the skin lipid content and barrier function [4].

Upon skin exposure, many chemical agents are locked into the SC within minutes [6]. For examples, many organic solvents including methyl chloroform, perchloroethylene and trichloroethylene can be found in expired air of humans subsequent hand exposures to contaminated water within as little as 6 min, proving rapid systemic absorption [32–34, 54]. The SC acts as a "reservoir" for topically applied molecules, and even rapid washing with water post-dermal exposure frequently fails to remove most chemicals [10]. Importantly, Rougier et al. [40, 41] discovered that SC sampling in vivo in humans and rats via tape stripping 30 min-

X. Hui (✉) · H. I. Maibach
Department of Dermatology, University of California San Francisco,
San Francisco, CA, USA
e-mail: Xiaoying.Hui@UCSF.edu

H. Zhu, H. I. Maibach (eds.), *Skin Decontamination*,
https://doi.org/10.1007/978-3-030-24009-7_1

utes post exposure accurately predicts and quantifies chemical penetration for up to 4 days with linear-type correlation. While percutaneous penetration is often considered a simplistic one-step diffusion process, it consists of at least 15 steps [51] related to absorption and excretion kinetics, extraction, vehicle characteristics, wash effects, etc. (Table 1.1). Examination of the chemical partitioning/diffusion of a wide array of compounds with differing physicochemical properties showed minimally differing lag times through the SC. Therefore, different compounds have approximately the same diffusion coefficients with regard to their percutaneous absorption in vivo. Thus, for a given thickness of SC and a specific anatomical site, the penetration flux value of a substance depends mainly on its SC/vehicle partition coefficient [42, 43].

The abovementioned observations offer us new insights for improving decontamination techniques. The recommended emergency treatment of many chemical sprays and splashes to the skin consist of rinsing or washing with water and/or soap. However, many topically applied chemicals are not easily removed by water washing. Skin decontamination is the primary required intervention for chemical, biological, and radiological exposures and involves immediate removal of the contaminant via the most effective manner. Such removal techniques include physi-

Table 1.1 15 Steps related to the process of percutaneous absorption[a]

Number	Factors determining percutaneous absorption
1	Release from vehicle[b] Varies with solubility in vehicle, concentration, pH, etc.
2	Kinetics of skin penetration[b] Influenced by anatomical site, degree of occlusion, intrinsic skin condition, animal age, concentration of dosing solution, surface area dosed, frequency of dosing, post absorption, etc.
3	Excretion kinetics[b]
4	Tissue disposition
5	Substantivity to skin[b]
6	Wash effects[b] Wash resistance Wash enhancement
7	Rub effects[b] Rub resistance Rub enhancement
8	Transfer—skin, clothing + inanimate surface[b]
9	Exfoliation[b]
10	Volatility[b]
11	Binding—all layers[b]
12	Anatomic pathways
13	Lateral spread[b]
14	Vascular perfusion[b]
15	Cutaneous metabolism[b]

[a]Modified with permission from Wester and Maibach [51]
[b]Metric developed

cal removal of the contaminant, solvating or emulsifying the contaminant in a liquid vehicle, transferring the contaminant to another medium through absorption/adsorption of the chemical, chemical alteration of the contaminant, and the use of friction to dislodge the contaminant.

Ideally, a decontaminant effectively and rapidly removes the contaminant of interest, easily removes itself without undesirable residue, does not cause enhancement or wash-in effect, and does not damage the skin. Additionally, it is readily available, affordable, and easily disposed of [7]. In the first part of this review, we explore the many steps involved in percutaneous penetration, the laboratory techniques that provided the background for this knowledge, and the insights advancing our knowledge of chemical exposure risk assessment, exposure prevention and barrier methods, and postexposure decontamination.

Stratum Corneum

Stratum Corneum and Barrier Function

SC is the outermost layer of the five layers of the epidermis and is largely responsible for barrier function. The biological and chemical activity of SC is both intricate and complex. As SC is vital to maintain healthy skin, a comprehensive understanding of its structure and function is essential [9] (Table 1.2).

The structure of SC is synonymous with that of "brick and mortar." The bricks are corneocytes, protein complexes of tiny keratin threads in an organized matrix, and keratin is capable of holding large amounts of water between the fibers. SC contains approximately 12–16 layers of corneocytes, each with a mean thickness of 1 micrometer that varies with age, anatomical location, and UV radiation exposure [27].

Corneocytes are surrounded by crystalline lamellar lipid regions. Lamellar bodies are formed in the keratinocytes of the stratum spinosum and stratum granulosum layers, and as keratinocytes mature and ascend, enzymes degrade the lamellar body envelopes, releasing free fatty acids and ceramides that fuse to form a continuous lamellar lipid bilayer. This lipid bilayer is analogous to a "mortar" and is essential in maintaining the barrier properties of the skin [28, 36].

Each corneocyte is surrounded by an insoluble protein envelope primarily composed of two proteins, loricrin and involucrin, that have extensive structural links with one another. Cell envelopes are either "rigid" or "fragile" depending on the envelope's interaction with the lamellar bilayer [28, 36].

Attached to the cell envelope is a layer of ceramide lipids that repel and trap water. This assembly prevents the absorption of water into the lower layers of the epidermis.

The corneocytes are held together by corneodesmosomes that function as "rivets" and are the primary structures that must be degraded for desquamation [28, 36].

Natural moisturizing factor (NMF), a collection of water-soluble compounds specific to the SC, represents approximately 20–30% of the dry weight of the cor-

Table 1.2 Stratum corneum structure and function

Name	Location—composition	Function
Corneocyte	Cornified envelope: outer surface of the corneocyte Keratin filaments; γ-glutamyl isopeptide bonds	Mechanical barrier (impact and shear resistance) Resiliency of stratum corneum
	Cytosol: filaggrin proteolytic product; glycerol	Hydration
	Cytosol: cis-urocanic acid (histidase activity)	Electromagnetic radiation barrier
	Cytosol: cytokine activation· Proteolytic activation of pro IL-1α/β	Initiation of inflammation
Extracellular matrix	Lamellar bilayers: ceramides, cholesterol, nonessential fatty acids, proper ratio	Permeability
	Corneodesmosomes Intercelluar DSG1/DSC1 homodimers	Cohesion (integrity)/ desquamation
	Lamellar bilayers: antimicrobial peptides, FFA, sph	Antimicrobial barrier (innate immunity)[a]
	Extracellular lacunae: hydrophilic products of corneodesmosomes	Toxic chemical/antigen exclusion
	Lamellar bilayers: cholesterol, FFA, secreted vit. E, redox gradient	Antioxidant
	Lamellar bilayers: barrier lipids	Psychosensory interface
Natural moisturizing factors	Within SC	Water holding capacity of SC
pH and calcium gradients	Within SC and all through epidermis	Provides differentiation signals and lamellar granule secretion signals
Specialized enzymes (lipases, glycosidase, proteases)	Within lamellar granules and all through epidermis	Processing and maturation of SC lipids, desquamation
Melanin granules and "dust"	Produced by melanocytes of basal layer, melanin "dust" in SC	UV protection of skin

[a]This lipid bilayer is analogous to 'mortar' and is essential in maintaining the barrier properties of the skin [28, 36].

neocyte. NMF components absorb water molecules from the atmosphere to maintain SC hydration, but their water solubility allows them to easily leach from the cells upon water contact. Repeated contact with water can dehydrate the skin; however, the lipid layer surrounding the corneocyte helps to form a seal to inhibit NMF loss [37].

The stratum basale consists of a single layer of columnar epidermal stem cells attached to the basal lamina via hemidesmosomes. The stratum spinosum just above is rich with progressively enlarging lamellar bodies with ongoing keratin synthesis and lipogenesis. The stratum granulosum is next with mature lamellar bodies capable of differentiating into corneocytes. Here, the intracellular organelles undergo self-destruction, and the packaged lipid in the lamellar granules (LG) is released to the intercellular space. SC forms the outermost seal with 18–21 cell layers of dead corneocytes and lipids that is 20–40 micrometers thick in humans.

Filaggrin, a key protein in the hydration and formation of the SC barrier, acts as a source of hygroscopic amino acids and their derivatives including NMF [28, 36, 37].

Stratum Corneum Hydration

Normal skin has a consistent water content of 5–15%, independent of variations in environmental humidity. The superficial SC plays a dual barrier role of minimizing transepidermal water loss (TEWL) and preventing the entrance of external molecules. Hydration fluctuations alter SC permeability, and percutaneous absorption may be enhanced with increasing SC water content. Water is an endogenous skin constituent with minimal irritants or toxic exposure effects that are quickly reversible. Skin hydration can be increased easily with an occlusive vehicle or more elegantly with vehicles containing specific NMFs or polymer patch delivery systems [61].

High SC water content is essential in sustaining its flexibility, and its water holding capacity correlates directly with its protein and lipid domains and water-soluble substances [18].

Table 1.3 shows the water holding capacities and lipid content of normal powdered versus delipidized powdered SC (the protein fraction) as determined by the amount of [^{3}H]-water (μg equivalent) per milligram (mg) powdered SC after equilibration [17]. No statistical differences ($p > 0.05$) were observed in the capacities of normal powdered SC, delipidized powdered SC, or the combination of delipidized powdered SC plus its lipid content. Powdered SC can absorb up to 49% of its dry weight in water, a value consistent in the literature. Middleton [26] found that the

Table 1.3 Lipid content and water holding capacity of powdered human stratum corneum[a]

		Water uptake (μg/mg dry powdered SC)			
	Lipid content		Delipidized SC		
Stratum corneum source	(% dry wt)	Normal SC	Lipid	Protein	Total
1	2.38	495.85	26.44	452.40	478.84
2	2.21	452.49	39.26	364.96	404.22
3	2.39	585.62	23.09	498.40	521.49
4	2.69	554.27	40.05	492.31	532.36
5	2.08	490.04	49.86	363.30	413.16
6	2.01	381.61	14.82	324.18	339.00
Mean	2.29	493.31	32.26	415.92	448.18
SD	0.25	72.66	12.97	74.50	75.47

[a]Modified with permission from Hui et al. [18]. The powdered SC absorbs up to 49% by weight of dry untreated, which is consistent with literature reports

amount of water bound to guinea-pig footpad SC intact, in small pieces, or powdered was 40%, 40%, and 43% of dry corneum weight, respectively. Leveque and Rasseneur [21] demonstrated that human SC absorbs up to 50% of its dry weight in water.

Powdered SC not in an intact sheet exhibits lower water retention capacity. Powdering ruptures the corneocyte walls, allowing water to extract the hydrophilic NMFs, a process normally requiring a solvent. The results obtained suggest the protein domain of the powdered SC plays an important role in water absorption. Furthermore, depletion of the powdered SC lipid content did not significantly affect water retention ($p > 0.05$, [17]).

Additionally, if powdered SC is pretreated with water and ethanol or the dosing vehicle contains an ethanol concentration of 40% (v/v) or higher, the water retention capacity of the powdered SC can be reduced significantly ($p < 0.05$) when compared to untreated powdered SC or when vehicles with lower concentrations of ethanol are used (<40%, [17]). The data suggest that NMF is removed by the ethanol solution during processing.

Regional Variation in Stratum Corneum

Percutaneous absorption in both humans and animals varies depending on the anatomical location to which the chemical is applied. This implies a regional deviation of the barrier structure. Because the effect of any chemical applied to the skin is limited by the amount absorbed, estimation of the human health hazard effects from the environmental contaminant exposure illustrates the need to understand this variation. For example, after skin exposure to pesticide residue, estimation of prognostic factors and treatment doses requires the pesticide mass absorbed, and accuracy of this measure is crucial.

We review regional variation in skin absorption and its application to assess human risk. Risk assessment is achieved by determining skin absorption and multiplying it by the skin area involved. Accuracy improves by factoring in clothing and anatomical regions [50].

Feldmann and Maibach [11] explored the potential for regional variation in percutaneous absorption of hydrocortisone and/or parathion in men *in vivo*. The anatomical site absorbing the highest proportion of steroid was the scrotum, providing insight to the causation of scrotal cancer in chimney sweeps. Absorption was lowest for the sole of the foot and higher for the head and face.

The percutaneous absorption of multiple pesticides in humans has been shown to vary by anatomical region [24]. Importantly, regional variation was confirmed with parathion and malathion, and the higher absorbing sites including the head and face are more likely exposed to pesticides or other environmental contaminants. Parathion shows absorption variability by site with time, and variation is evident early in exposure [52]. Even though it is completed within minutes after exposure, wash with soap and water is not a perfect decontaminant. Using the combined

Table 1.4 Penetration indices for five anatomical sites assessed using hydrocortisone skin penetration data and pesticides (malathion and parathion) absorption results[a]

Site	Penetration index based on	
	Hydrocortisone data	Pesticide data
Genitals	40	12
Arms	1	1
Legs	0.5	1
Trunk	2.5	3
Head	5	4

[a]Modified with permission from Guy and Maibach [12]

hydrocortisone and pesticide data, Guy and Maibach [12] constructed penetration indices for five anatomical sites (Table 1.4). Wester et al. [53] examined the percutaneous absorption of paraquat in humans and showed that absorptions for the leg (0.29 ± 0.02%), hand (0.23 ± 0.1%), and forearm (0.29 ± 0.1%) were similar. Interestingly, paraquat showed low absorption and negligible regional variation.

To examine how anatomical site affects chemical penetration and the amount remaining in the SC, Rougier et al. [40] applied benzoic acid (BA) to humans and performed tape stripping after 30 minutes. The total BA penetration varied by anatomical site with the forehead being three times more permeable than the back. Using the BA levels in the SC post 30-minute application and then its penetration over 4 days, additional correlations to anatomical sites were made (r = 0.97, p = 0.001). The forearm is commonly believed to be the best location to test for immediate contact irritation; however, Wertz et al. [49] showed the areas of greatest to least irritant response were the neck, the perioral region, the forehead, and the volar.

The face exhibits its own anatomical variation, and Marrakchi and Maibach [25] used noninvasive skin bioengineering technology to establish a map showing the six biophysical parameters: skin blood flow, transepidermal water loss (TEWL), SC hydration (capacitance), temperature, pH, and sebum content of the skin surface. Testing multiple locations on both young and old human volunteers, both age groups had the greatest skin blood flow on the nose, the chin was the most alkaline area, the neck had the highest capacitance value, and the perioral and nasolabial areas exhibited the highest TEWL. The highest skin temperature was on the neck in the young and the nasolabial area in the old. These values provide a framework for disease and intervention-related considerations.

Regional Stratum Corneum Variation: Application to Human Risk Assessment

Chemical warfare agents (CWAs) are easily produced and of significant threat to military forces and the public. Most well-known CWAs are organophosphorus compounds, a number of commonly used pesticides, including parathion. Investigating the in vitro percutaneous absorption of parathion through dry and sweated uniformed and naked human skin, the percentage absorbed through naked skin (1.78 ± 0.41) was greater than that through dry (0.29 ± 0.17; $p = 0.000$) and sweated uniformed skin (0.65 ± 0.16; $p = 0.000$). A difference was also noted between sweated and dry uniformed skin ($p = 0.007$). Applying the uniformed skin absorption to the skin permeability of the CWA VX for the head, neck, arms, and hands shows a 50% mortality within the first hour of exposure for a sweated soldier wearing a uniform. By 8 hours post-trunk exposure in either a dry or sweated uniform, mortality is predicted. 96 hours after, any uniformed region is exposed individually would be lethal [56].

Another example of human regional variation is exhibited by the bioavailability and body burden after permethrin exposure in the uniformed soldier. Permethrin, a toxic pesticide and repellent of potential disease-carrying insects, is imbedded in military uniform material and provided to soldiers in spray cans for protection. Table 1.5 summarizes the predicted permethrin human bioavailability of uniformed and exposed skin at 1.24 mg/kg body burden [56]. Animal studies generated a no observable effect level (NOEL) of approximately 5 mg/kg, thus estimating a five-fold safety margin.

In conclusion, review of current data shows important trends; however, regional variation of skin absorption has not been fully explored. Absorption disparities in all areas of animal skin have not been completely uncovered, but more importantly, many areas of human skin remain unstudied. The absorption differences of fingers, nails, eyelids, perirectal regions, and upper versus lower extremities need to be deciphered. While current data is sufficient to estimate human risk of percutaneous pen-

Table 1.5 Permethrin bioavailability and body burden for uniformed soldier[a]

Human part	Body surface area (cm^2)	Permethrin dose[b] ($\mu g/cm^2$)	Percutaneous absorption[c]	Body region index[d]	Uniform[e]	Total (μg)
Head	1180	4	0.087	X 4	1	1642.56
Neck	420	4	0.087	X 4	1	584.64
Trunk	5690	125	0.087	X 3	0.29	53834.51
Arms	2280	125	0.087	X 1	0.29	7190.55
Hands	840	4	0.087	X 1	1	292.32
Genitals	180	125	0.087	X 12	0.29	6812.10
Legs	5050	125	0.087	X 1	0.29	15926.44
Feet	1120	4	0.087	X 1	1	389.76
Total (μg)						86672.88
Total (mg)						86.67
Total body burden[f]						1.24 mg/kg

[a]Modified with permission from Wester et al. [56]
[b]Uniform = 125 $\mu g/cm^2$/spray open skin 4 $\mu g/cm^2$
[c]8.7% (0.087) permethrin dose absorbed/
[d]region body absorption index
[e]0.29 is 29% absorption from cloth relative to open skin (index)
[f]Total body burden (mg/70 kg soldier)

etration by exposure region, evidence of absorption from clothing must also be explored for real-life applications. With more comprehensive absorption maps for a broader range of chemical moieties, refining our knowledge of skin penetration within dermatopharmacology and dermatotoxicology would be possible.

Rougier Method: A Quick Stripping Method to Predict Systemic Absorption Following Short-Time Dermal Exposure

Stratum corneum (SC) is the main barrier against dehydration and xenobiotics. A relatively noninvasive technique, adhesive tape stripping, can partially or entirely remove this micrometer-thin skin layer for a more thorough examination. Initially employed by Pinkus [31], this methodology has become common practice to remove SC layers, to reveal susceptible skin for irritant or allergen application, to predictably disrupt the water barrier for efficacy evaluation of barrier restoring compounds, or to obtain cells for mycological culture or to investigate SC quality [2]. Additionally, bioengineering methods including TEWL measurement can be employed post tape stripping to measure changes in water barrier properties [48].

Tape stripping may also assess the uptake of topically administered compounds into the SC. Rougier et al. [40–43] used tape stripping 30 minutes post chemical application to quantify the amount present in the SC. The reservoir capacity of the SC was determined at different anatomical regions and correlated with systemic excretions to predict the total molecular penetration over 4 days in both humans and rats in vivo.

Rougier Method to Determine Regional Variation of Chemicals in Human Stratum Corneum Post Exposure

The rate of molecule absorption depends on the application conditions, partially explaining the wide absorption variations reported for the same substances. The factors significantly affecting the absorption rate of a compound include the animal species, vehicle, dose applied, and length of contact. Contradicting explanations for regional permeability differences are often stated in literature reviews.

Rougier et al. [40] used tape stripping in vivo to explore how anatomical site affected the relationship between total chemical penetration and the amount remaining in the SC post application. Four chemicals were studied, and 1000 nmol of ^{14}C-radiolabeled chemical was applied to 1 cm^2 of skin at various anatomical sites. For each molecule and site, total absorption was determined by measuring urine chemical excretion after an initial application on one side of the body. Another application to tape-stripped areas on the contralateral side 48 hours later measured the substance present in the SC at the end of application (30 minutes). The calculated skin permeabilities varied substantially, depending on both the physicochemical

Table 1.6 Percutaneous absorption of benzoic acid and anatomical site[a]

Anatomical site	Urinary extraction 0–24 hour (1) (nmol/cm^2)	Total penetration in 4 days (2) (nmol/cm^2)	Amounts in stratum corneum 30 minutes after application (nmol/cm^2)	Predicted penetrations in 4 days (nmol/cm^2)
Back	6.41 ± 0.99	8.55 ± 1.32	6.19 ± 1.27	10.80 ± 2.32
Arm	7.06 ± 0.77	9.41 ± 1.02	5.92 ± 0.62	10.31 ± 1.14
Chest	8.78 ± 0.98	11.70 ± 1.31	8.07 ± 1.19	14.25 ± 2.18
Thigh	9.38 ± 1.07	12.50 ± 1.43	6.80 ± 0.72	11.92 ± 1.31
Abdomen	11.44 ± 1.44	15.26 ± 1.93	8.20 ± 1.24	14.48 ± 2.18
Forehead	20.74 ± 2.71	27.65 ± 3.61	11.91 ± 2.28	21.24 ± 4.16

(2) Values calculated from (1), i.e., (2) = (1)/0.75. Urinary excretion data was expressed in nmol. cm^{-2} application area

The table gives the amounts of benzoic acid found in the urine over 24 hours and the total amounts having penetrated over a period of 4 days (calculated). Total benzoic acid penetration in relation to the anatomical sites treated is: back < arm < chest < thigh < abdomen < forehead

[a]Modified with permission from Rougier et al. [40]

nature of the molecule and on the anatomical location. The forehead was always twice as permeable as the arm or abdomen (Table 1.6). Importantly, the Rougier method provides a rapid means to determine flux in vivo in humans.

Rougier Method: Animal Model to Predict Human Percutaneous Absorption In Vivo

When interpreting comparative percutaneous absorption studies in humans and animals, it is essential to assess the influence the methodology and animal model had on the results, especially when comparing animal and human data. Ascertaining morphologic skin differences between species is difficult, and combining data generated in different species with varying techniques may be impossible.

A comparison study conducted by Rougier et al. [41] explored the percutaneous absorption of benzoic acid, benzoic acid sodium salt, caffeine, and acetylsalicylic acid, each administered in vivo to humans and hairless rats under identical conditions. Tape stripping was used to quantify the chemical in treated SC 30 minutes post application to determine SC reservoir function at different anatomical regions. This partially answered a controversial question: when can animals be used as relevant research models for humans?

Percutaneous absorption of four radiolabeled molecules through hairless rat back skin was compared to that through multiple human anatomical sites. The experimental conditions were similar for both species, and the results showed the variation in absorption by chemical was the same for both species: benzoic acid sodium salt < caffeine < benzoic acid < acetylsalicylic acid (Table 1.7). Additionally, both species displayed the same absolute difference between the most and the least absorbed molecules, and each permeability varied significantly with the physicochemical property and the anatomical site of application. Independent of the molecules stud-

Table 1.7 Percutaneous absorption of the tested molecules according to anatomical site[a]

Compound	Anatomical site	Number	Amount in urine samples after 24 hours	Total amount penetrated within 4 d	Amount in the stratum corneum 30 minutes after application	Predicted penetration within 4 d
		(*n*)	(nmol/cm^2)	(nmol/cm^2)	(nmol/cm^2)	(nmol/cm^2)
Benzoic acid sodium salt	Arm (upper, outer)	6	3.02 ± 0.34	4.02 ± 0.45	2.83 ± 0.58	4.67 ± 1.07
	Abdomen	6	5.73 ± 0.54	7.65 ± 0.72	4.04 ± 0.98	6.88 ± 1.80
	Postauricular	6	7.54 ± 0.62	10.06 ± 0.82	6.29 ± 0.93	11.02 ± 1.72
	Forehead	8	9.31 ± 1.76	12.32 ± 2.30	5.94 ± 0.99	10.34 ± 1.81
Caffeine	Arm (upper, outer)	7	6.04 ± 0.92	12.09 ± 1.84	6.75 ± 0.84	11.83 ± 1.53
	Abdomen	6	3.76 ± 0.67	7.53 ± 1.34	4.31 ± 0.60	7.36 ± 1.11
	Postauricular	7	5.87 ± 0.52	11.72 ± 1.05	7.46 ± 1.24	13.13 ± 2.26
	Forehead	6	11.17 ± 1.20	22.35 ± 2.39	11.60 ± 1.52	20.71 ± 2.79
Benzoic acid	Arm (upper, outer)	8	6.87 ± 0.75	9.15 ± 1.01	5.70 ± 0.58	9.90 ± 1.00
	Abdomen	7	10.88 ± 1.23	14.51 ± 1.64	7.89 ± 1.12	13.92 ± 1.97
	Postauricular	8	16.87 ± 3.85	22.49 ± 5.14	10.53 ± 0.63	18.75 ± 1.15
	Forehead	7	20.30 ± 2.39	26.80 ± 3.19	13.20 ± 2.70	23.63 ± 4.79
Acetyl salicylic acid	Arm (upper, outer)	7	5.27 ± 0.18	17.00 ± 0.37	11.99 ± 1.34	21.42 ± 2.45
	Abdomen	6	5.34 ± 1.03	17.20 ± 3.35	9.98 ± 1.34	17.74 ± 3.62
	Postauricular	6	11.04 ± 2.50	29.20 ± 5.37	14.56 ± 1.30	26.10 ± 2.38
	Forehead	6	10.89 ± 1.02	35.14 ± 3.29	21.97 ± 4.29	40.20 ± 7.75

The amount of molecules present in the 24-hour urine sample, and the total amount absorbed in 4 d (calculated from the amount in the 24-hour urine sample), for each anatomical site. There are appreciable differences in permeability among the sites

[a]Modified with permission from Rougier et al. [42]

ied, the permeability by human anatomical site was: arm ≤ abdomen< postauricular < forehead. Additionally, ratios were calculated for the total percutaneous absorption of human to hairless rat, and they were constant for any given anatomical site or molecule tested. This implies that careful control of conditions can allow prediction of chemical absorption in man based on values determined in animals.

Rougier Method to Predict Human Percutaneous Absorption Post Short Dermal Exposure

By correlating quantitative data from a tape-stripped SC 30 minutes post chemical application and systemic excretion in both humans and hairless rats, Rougier et al. [40–43] showed that the amount of chemical likely to penetrate over 4 days could be predicted. Furthermore, correlation of these two measurements proved the penetration was unrelated to the physiochemical nature of the molecule, the dose, the period of application, or the vehicle.

This relationship was confirmed again for different anatomical sites. A linear correlation exists ($r = 0.97$, $P < 0.001$) between the amount of substance present in the SC 30 minutes post application and the total amount penetrated over 4 days that is independent of the regional permeability variation.

Interestingly, the quantity of chemical present in the SC post application corresponds to the molecule affinity for the horny layer and indicates the level of partitioning between the vehicle and SC. The relationship in humans between the amount of substance present in the SC at 30 minutes post application and that absorbed over 4 days is confirmed for different anatomical sites. The correlation curve with the equation $y = 1.83x - 0.52$ corresponds to the curve first developed in benzoic acid absorption studies in humans, thus standardizing the proposed method. The close proximity of the experimental points to the curve correlates to a coefficient of variation of 0.97 and $p < 0.001$ (95% confidence interval). Consequently, by measuring the quantity (x) of substance present in the SC 30 minutes post application, prediction of the total absorption over 4 days is possible.

In conclusion, tape stripping method can be used to predict the total penetration for different chemicals, independent of the anatomical site, by measuring the quantity present in the SC post application. This adds a simple, robust tool to validate in vitro SC binding assays.

Important Factors in Tape Stripping

Tape stripping is a highly regarded technique to assess bioequivalence of topical drugs. To quantify the SC removed, the tape is weighed before and after stripping, and either spectroscopic analysis or protein extraction and quantification with a total protein assay is proposed.

Anatomical Regions

Tape stripping shows regional TEWL variation. A significantly higher TEWL was measured for the forehead and back as compared to the forearm. One reason may be that the SC of face and trunk is thinner with fewer corneocyte layers than that of the forearm. Additionally, tape striping removes a larger portion of SC from the face and trunk, leading to a faster increase in TEWL from these areas. Furthermore, site-dependent differences in spontaneous desquamation and SC cohesion may contribute to the reason that tape stripping does not result in the same TEWL change.

The mechanism of spontaneous desquamation is far from completely understood, but physiological and anatomical site-dependent mechanisms are suspected. Corneodesmosome physiology, proteolysis, and intercorneocyte lipid composition and structure are also likely factors. The pressure resistance during tape application may also contribute to the variation of the SC removed, being a function of visco-elasticity of the underlying tissue which varies regionally. For instance, the skull is just underneath the forehead surface, altering the overall pressure on this area during tape placement. The extent of how biomechanical properties and the underlying structure influence SC removal during tape stripping has yet to be defined. Consequently, results from different anatomical regions may not be comparable and should be adjusted by the fraction of SC removed [22, 23]. The Dreher method [8] is a means to quantify the protein mass retained in each strip.

Pressure and Contact Time

During tape stripping, longer pressure application led to increased TEWL with fewer strip applications, indicating that a larger fraction of SC had been removed. Pressure-sensitive adhesives form a strong bond with substrates with slight pressure over a short time. This property, known as "tack," increases with contact time and pressure until a plateau is reached that is dependent on the adhesive and substrate properties. Importantly, until the critical contact pressure and time are reached, the amount of SC removed increases with higher applied pressure and longer contact time. Furthermore, the type of pressure applied may influence the homogeneity of the SC layer removed. For example, skin furrows can affect tape-stripping outcomes, but Lademann et al. [19] showed this influence may be minimized by using a standardized roller to stretch and flatten the skin for a homogeneous tape application.

Velocity of Removal

The velocity of tape removal also impacts the SC mass extracted. With rapid tape removal, TEWL is less. When tape removal is performed slowly, corneocytes adherence is greater even with fewer strips. For any given adhesive, the force required for removal is influenced by the viscoelastic properties of the substrate. The skin may become extended during slow removal, resulting in more SC removed per tape strip, likely due to increased corneodesmosome "stress" during this removal procedure. This hypothesis warrants further investigation [22].

Types of Adhesives

Different tapes remove varying amounts of SC under standardized conditions secondary to their adhesive characteristics. Therefore, it is essential to define the adhesive used. As many parameters significantly affect SC removal during tape stripping, it is recommended that the relevant parameters such as adhesive type, pressure, contact time, and removal technique are explicitly defined and controlled when utilizing the method. Combining the different procedures in a single test protocol could represent a new dynamic SC stress test (DSCST). This would allow the capture of small differences in intrinsic SC cohesion, and DSCST may be a valuable means to investigate the effect of topically applied keratolytics or other agents capable of influencing SC cohesion [23].

Powdered Stratum Corneum Binding/Partitioning Assay: A Predictive Dermal Exposure Model

Stratum Corneum Sample Preparation and Assay Procedure

The human SC includes the callus, or horny pads of the palms and soles, and the membranous SC covering the remainder of the body [1]. Traversing this barrier represents the rate-limiting permeation step for most chemicals [5, 9, 44, 59]. Chemicals must first partition into the SC before they can penetrate the remaining epidermal layers, dermis, and vascular system. Partitioning is more expedient than complete diffusion through the SC and equilibrium is quickly achieved [45]. In partitioning, chemicals are either bound within the SC or retained in a reservoir [60], thus providing insights to the SC barrier properties and transport mechanisms.

To better understand and predict chemical partitioning into the SC, many in vitro experiments have been conducted. However, most studies utilized quantitative structure–activity relationships (QSAR) of related chemicals, and few have focused on structurally unrelated chemicals [13]. Since the range of molecular structure and physicochemical properties is broad, any predictive model must also address a broad scope of the partitioning behavior. The SC assay provides a tool to assess the variation between chemicals partitioning between water and either powdered or sheet SC.

The powdered SC binding/partitioning assay was first designed by Wester et al. [55] to determine how the powdered SC is affected by chemical concentration, incubation time, and chemical lipophilicity, along with other factors. These parameters were used to develop an in vitro model to predict the risk of dermal exposure to hazardous chemicals.

A Micro-Mill Grinder (Bel-Art Products, Pequannock, NJ) was used to grind adult foot callus, and a powder was formed with liquid nitrogen. SC particles passing through a 50-mesh sieve and not an 80-mesh sieve were used because this size range is favorable and powdered SC increases experimental accuracy [55]. Varying doses of radiolabeled chemicals in 4.0 ml of distilled deionized water vehicle were mixed with 10.0 mg of the powdered callus in a glass vial and incubated with moderate perturbation at 35 °C for differing lengths of time. Centrifugation at 1500 g for 15 minutes allowed for supernatant removal, and the powdered SC was resuspended three times. Radioactivity of the chemical bound to PHSC and that remaining in the vehicles was determined by scintillation counting.

The powdered human SC/water partition coefficient [16] is determined by the following equation:

$$\mathrm{PC}(\mathrm{SC}/\mathrm{w}) = C(\mathrm{SC})/C(\mathrm{water}) \tag{1.1}$$

where *C* PHSC is the amount (μg) of the chemical absorbed in 10 mg of the powdered SC and *C* (water) is the amount (μg) remaining in 4000 mg of water after removing the powdered SC pellet. Since the chemical amount in the powdered SC or water is proportional to the scintillation counts, partitioning of chemical into the powdered SC equaled the decrease of the chemical concentration in the vehicle. An alternative calculation method was also used:

$$\mathrm{PC}(\mathrm{SC}/\mathrm{w}) = \frac{\mathrm{dpm}(\mathrm{SC})/\mathrm{mg}(\mathrm{SC})}{\left[\mathrm{dpm}(i) - \mathrm{dpm}(\mathrm{SC})\right]/\mathrm{mg}(\mathrm{water})} \tag{1.2}$$

where dpm (*i*) is the initial chemical concentration in the vehicle. These two methods gave similar results. The reported experiments use the second method.

Chemical Partitioning and Binding to Stratum Corneum

Percutaneous absorption of a chemical in a vehicle depends on chemical solubility, concentration, pH, and its partitioning between the vehicle and the SC.

Chemical Concentration and Degree of Partitioning

Chemical partitioning from the vehicle into the SC also involves molecular binding. The equilibration of partitioning largely depends on the chemical binding site saturation in the SC [39, 46]. Tables 1.8 and 1.9 demonstrate that the maximum degree of partitioning is compound-specific. As the SC proteins, lipids, and other lower molecular weight substances have differing properties, the available binding sites have different chemical affinities. Thus, maximum binding and equilibration vary with molecular structure [39].

Limitation of the Stratum Corneum's Binding Sites

Drug concentration influences PC SC/W (Table 1.9). In all experiments, the PC values of SC P/W and SC S/W decreased as drug concentration increased. This may be due to saturation of the available "binding sites" in the skin layers. As partitioning increases, the binding sites become saturated, while the concentration of unbound compound increases. Therefore, this process continuously decreases the

Table 1.8 Effect of initial aqueous phase chemical concentration on partition coefficient of powdered human stratum corneum/water[a]

Chemical (log PC $_{O/W}$)	Concentration (g/100 ml)	Partition coefficient (Mean ± S.D.)
Dopamine	0.23	5.42 ± 0.22
(−3.40)	0.46	6.04 ± 0.28
	0.92	5.74 ± 0.28
Glycine	0.05	0.36 ± 0.01
(−3.20)	0.10	0.40 ± 0.02
Urea	0.03	0.26 ± 0.02
(−2.11)	0.06	0.15 ± 0.02
	0.12	0.17 ± 0.02
Glyphosate	0.02	0.79 ± 0.04
(−1.70)	0.04	0.68 ± 0.04
	0.08	0.70 ± 0.01
Theophylline	0.18	0.37 ± 0.02
(−0.76)	0.36	0.43 ± 0.03
	0.54	0.42 ± 0.02
Aminopyrine	0.07	0.44 ± 0.09
(0.84)	0.14	0.46 ± 0.03
Hydrocortisone	0.09	0.37 ± 0.01
(1.61)	0.18	0.34 ± 0.01
	0.36	0.29 ± 0.02
Malathion	0.47	0.50 ± 0.09
(2.36)	0.94	0.40 ± 0.03
	1.88	0.53 ± 0.04
Atrazine	0.09	0.53 ± 0.06
(2.75)	0.14	0.59 ± 0.07
	0.19	0.58 ± 0.03
2,4-D	0.27	7.52 ± 0.81
(2.81)	0.54	7.53 ± 1.01
	0.82	8.39 ± 1.67
Alachlor	0.32	1.11 ± 0.05
(3.52)	0.64	1.08 ± 0.04
	1.28	1.96 ± 0.15
PCB	0.04	1239 ± 146
(6.40)	0.08	1325 ± 167
	0.16	1443 ± 181

Results suggest that the degree of chemical partitioning from water to powdered stratum corneum was more related to available "binding sites" than its concentration

[a]Modified with permission from Hui et al. [16]. Test chemicals were mixed with powdered stratum corneum at 35 °C for a 2-hour incubation period

Table 1.9 Effect of aqueous phase chemical concentration on skin layers/water partition coefficient[a]

Chemical (log $P_{O/W}$)	Concentration (μg/cm³)	Partition coefficient (Mean ± S.D.)		
		SC S/W	SCE/W	D/W
Propranolol	0.1	804 ± 86	691 ± 76	224 ± 60
(3.09)	0.3	707 ± 88	433 ± 11	116 ± 59
	0.5	462 ± 103	321 ± 24	65 ± 11
	0.9	336 ± 21	235 ± 55	43 ± 6.3
	1.8[b]	271 ± 50	150 ± 17	22 ± 1.8
Atrazine	1.5	110 ± 39	74 ± 16	45 ± 17
(2.75)	2.9	111 ± 16	57 ± 17	12 ± 1.1
	5.8	70 ± 11	32 ± 1.8	16 ± 8.1
	12	59 ± 13	35 ± 1.8	10 ± 4.2
	23[b]	37 ± 4	29 ± 1.1	11 ± 1.1
8-MOP	1.1	69 ± 12	60 ± 0.2	15 ± 1.5
(2.53)	2.2	57 ± 14	56 ± 9.1	13 ± 3.8
	4.4	52 ± 11	40 ± 11	11 ± 1.4
	8.8	56 ± 3.2	46 ± 15	10 ± 1.7
	17[b]	56 ± 18	48 ± 19	11 ± 1.6
Salicylic acid	1.3×10^2	150 ± 62	16 ± 4.3	6.6 ± 0.5
(1.74)	2.6×10^2	194 ± 41	101 ± 32	7.0 ± 0.6
	5.8×10^2	182 ± 38	108 ± 31	9.8 ± 1.0
	12×10^2	91 ± 21	85 ± 41	16 ± 1.3
	24×10^2[b]	68 ± 10	60 ± 3.2	27 ± 0.8
Indolecetic acid	3.2	31 ± 0.7	14 ± 1.4	11 ± 1.5
(1.41)	6.3	16 ± 3.1	9.7 ± 0.4	5.8 ± 0.8
	13	11 ± 1.0	6.0 ± 1.4	5.6 ± 1.1
	25	8.2 ± 0.8	4.2 ± 0.4	3.2 ± 0.8
	50[b]	6.8 ± 0.3	4.4 ± 0.3	3.8 ± 0.6
Acetaminophen	1.1×10^2	27 ± 2.2	13 ± 1.5	13 ± 0.5
(0.32)	2.2×10^2	15 ± 0.5	8 ± 0.9	7.8 ± 3.1
	4.4×10^2	22 ± 8.6	8 ± 1.2	5.1 ± 0.7
	8.8×10^2	14 ± 2.8	4.7 ± 0.8	5.8 ± 1.9
	17×10^2[b]	17 ± 2.6	6.3 ± 0.9	6.4 ± 0.7
Theophylline	0.6×10^3	12 ± 0.9	11 ± 0.9	4.4 ± 0.7
(−0.78)	1.1×10^3	11 ± 0.3	9.4 ± 1.6	4.2 ± 0.6
	2.2×10^3	8.3 ± 0.3	7.1 ± 2.9	5.1 ± 0.6
	4.4×10^3	6.7 ± 1.3	8.1 ± 1.7	3.3 ± 0.5
	8.8×10^3[b]	4.6 ± 0.5	7.1 ± 2.4	3.0 ± 0.4

[a]Modified with permission from Gogoleva et al. [14]. Data demonstrate the influence of drug concentration on PC of the model compounds. As the concentration of the chemical increases, the PC values inversely decrease. Equilibration time was 24 hours. *SC S* sheet stratum corneum, *SCE* stratum corneum/epidermal layer, *D* dermal layer

[b]Saturation solubility concentrations (μg/cm³) are as follows: propranolol (1.8), atrazine (23), 8-MOP (17), salicylic acid (2.4×10^2), indoleacetic acid (50), acetaminophen (1.7×10^2), theophylline (8.8×10^3)

partition coefficient. Partitioning may include a protein domain and a "sponge domain" for both hydrophilic compounds and some lower lipophilic compounds. The sponge domain, named by Raykar et al. [38], is assumed to have properties of bulk water and to carry the same amount of solute into the SC as that in an equal volume of bathing solution.

The Importance of Chemical Solubility

As suggested by Potts and Guy [35], the compound solubility limit in the SC is important in determining the degree of partitioning (Tables 1.10 and 1.11). Based on this limit, the absorption of water- or lipid-soluble substances is controlled by the protein domain, the lipid domain, or a combination of the two [38]. The SC lipid

Table 1.10 Effect of SC hydration on chemical partitioning/binding

			Partition coefficient (log P $_{SC/W}$)		
Chemicals	Log P $_{O/W}$	Water solubility (mg/L)	Dry	Prewetted	*p*-value
Hydrocortisone	1.61	320	−0.16 ± 0.04	−0.24 ± 0.03	0.015
Malathion	2.36	143	1.15 ± 0.11	0.67 ± 0.06	0.001
Alachlor	3.52	240	0.84 ± 0.02	0.85 ± 0.04	0.841
Estradiol	4.01	3.6	1.23 ± 0.02	1.27 ± 0.05	0.160
Acitretin	6.40	0.073	2.69 ± 0.04	2.69 ± 0.03	0.815

Results suggest that partitioning of low lipophilic chemicals, hydrocortisone and malathion (expressed as low log Po/w values), to powdered stratum corneum was interrupted after the stratum corneum was prewetted with water for 30 minutes, whereas high lipophilic chemicals were not
[a]Modified with permission from Hui et al. [16]. Test chemicals were mixed with powdered stratum corneum at 35 °C for a 2-hour incubation period

Table 1.11 Effect of delipidization on chemical SC partitioning/binding[a]

			SC partition coefficient (log P $_{SCP/W}$)		
Chemicals	Log P $_{O/W}$	Water solubility (mg/L)	Normal	Delipidized	*p*-value
Glyphosate	−1.70		−0.03 ± 0.04	−0.03 ± 0.03	>0.05
Theophylline	−0.76		−0.86 ± 0.01	−0.09 ± 0.02	0.05
Hydrocortisone	1.61	320	−0.16 ± 0.04	−0.56 ± 0.05	0.001
Malathion	2.36	143	1.15 ± 0.11	0.98 ± 0.09	0.045
Atrazine	2.75		0.47 ± 0.05	0.35 ± 0.04	0.05
Alachlor	3.52	240	0.84 ± 0.02	0.99 ± 0.03	0.001
Estradiol	4.01	3.6	1.23 ± 0.02	1.29 ± 0.10	>0.05
Acitretin	6.40	0.073	2.69 ± 0.04	2.33 ± 0.10	0.001

Results suggest that the degree of partitioning from water into powdered stratum corneum is closely related to chemicals' log P o/w value for normal SC, but for delipidized SC, it seems individual-specific
[a]Modified with permission from Hui et al. [17]. Test chemicals were mixed with powdered stratum corneum at 35 °C for a 2-hour incubation period

domain is more lipophilic than water, so lipophilic compounds would partition into the SC more favorably than water. Therefore, when the vehicle is water, PC SCP/W increases with increasing solute lipophilicity [45]. Conversely, the SC protein domain is more polar than octanol, therefore dictating the absorption of hydrophilic chemicals [38]. Additionally, some chemicals may be taken into the SC secondary to sponge domain hydration. Table 1.9 presents the partition coefficient values for lipophilic compounds in the three skin layers, and the PCs of propranolol, salicylic acid, and atrazine are higher in the SC than in the epidermis or dermis, while the PC of theophylline is relatively constant in the three skin layers.

Delipidized Stratum Corneum

Table 1.9 shows the partitioning values of eight compounds with different lipophilicities described by their log PC (octanol/water) values into normal and delipidized powdered SC. Lipid depletion of powdered SC did not change the lipophilic compound partition coefficients equally. The partition coefficients of acitretin, atrazine, and hydrocortisone decreased significantly for delipidized SC versus normal skin ($p < 0.05$); however, alachlor had significantly increased partitioning into delipidized skin ($p < 0.01$). Glyphosate, a hydrophilic compound, or estradiol did not show partitioning differences between normal and delipidized powdered SC. However, theophylline showed lower partitioning into delipidized versus normal powdered SC ($p < 0.05$). Comparing the partition coefficients (SC/w) of chemicals with varying lipophilicities between normal and delipidized SC groups provides interesting insights. Raykar et al. [38] found that the partition coefficient (SC/w) of the lipophilic compound hydrocortisone 21-ester was reduced through delipidized SC, while Surber et al. [46] reported increasing of partition coefficients (SC/w) for hydrocortisone and four other lipophilic compounds. Table 1.6 shows that the lipophilic compounds atrazine, acitretin, and malathion decrease partitioning into delipidized powdered SC, while alachlor caused an increase and estradiol remained the same. A potential explanation for these differences by Surber et al. [47] was that the structure of the delipidized SC was damaged after treatment with organic solvent; therefore, solute partitioning into a delipidized membrane was different from that of an intact membrane.

Vehicle Effects

While alachlor, atrazine, and glyphosate have different lipophilicities, their partitioning patterns were similar and the coefficients decreased as ethanol concentration increased. When using an ethanol concentration of less than 40%, the lipophilic compounds atrazine and malathion partitioned more into powdered SC than delipidized powdered SC ($p < 0.05$), while glyphosate displayed no difference in partitioning ($p > 0.05$). Alachlor showed a significant difference in partitioning between the normal and delipidized powdered SC when water was the only solvent ($p < 0.05$), but none when ethanol was employed ($p > 0.05$).

Ethanol is a widely used skin penetration enhancer. Using an ethanol–water solvent system as a vehicle, Hatanaka et al. [15] found that SC permeability coefficients changed markedly for lipophilic but not hydrophilic compounds. This change was dependent on the compound's lipophilicity and the solvent's ethanol fraction. The partition coefficients of atrazine, alachlor, and glyphosate decreased for powdered SC/water when an ethanol–water solvent vehicle was used. The partition coefficient of malathion for powdered SC/water was increased at a low concentration of ethanol (<40%) and decreased at a high concentration (>40%). The effect of low ethanol concentrations on a compound's SC permeability could result from ethanol physically perturbing the lipid region in the SC barrier [15]. At high concentrations of ethanol, it may cause dehydration or shrinkage of the protein domain and partial extraction of the SC lipid [3, 15].

pH Effects on Chemical Partitioning and Stratum Corneum Binding

Human SC has a pH from acidic to neutral that is important for barrier function and viability of the pH-dependent enzymes [29, 30, 58].

The percent binding rates of saturated solutions of compounds of differing pH ranges to powdered stratum corneum (SC P) is shown with the compound solubility regardless of molecular weight or pKa value in Table 1.12. Lower pH values increase the binding rate for chemicals with a positive log P, and higher pH values favor chemicals with negative log P. pH did not affect the binding rate for chemicals with neutral log P values [14].

Salicylic acid with vehicles at differing pH values showed similar partitioning into the three layers of human skin. At a pH of 2.4, the PC for salicylic acid was

Table 1.12 Effect of pH change on chemical binding powdered human stratum corneum in saturated concentration[a]

Chemicals	Parameters				Percent dose bound mean (S.D)		
	MW	Solubility	Log $P_{O/W}$	pKa	pH: 1~3	pH: 6~8	pH: 10~14
Salicylic acid	138	2240	2.26, 1.74	2.97	17.67 (1.38)	3.75 (0.21)	0.42 (0.12)
Hydroquinone	110	7200	0.59	10.9	2.45 (0.38)	1.33 (0.26)	0.71 (0.12)
Urea	60	545,000	−2.11	0.1	0.66 (0.37)	0.41 (0.39)	2.47 (1.86)
Glycerol	92	1,000,000	−1.76	14.4	0.08 (0.03)	0.08 (0.02)	0.35 (0.07)
Propylene glycol	76	1,000,000	−0.92	14.9	0.11 (0.04)	0.17 (0.07)	0.11 (0.01)
Caffeine	194	21,600	−0.07	10.4	11.69 (1.84)	13.03 (1.90)	10.47 (4.11)

Results show that optimum pH range for maximum chemical binding to powdered stratum corneum is related to chemical lipophilicity (expressed as log P o/w)

[a]Modified with permission from Hui et al. [18]

higher than that at pH 5.0 in any skin layer. According to the Henderson–Hasselbalch equation, the solvent pH dictates the degree of ionization. The pKa of salicylic acid is 3.0, so at pH 2.4, 80% of salicylic acid molecules are unionized and their lipid membrane permeation occurs more readily. At pH 5.0, 99% of the drug is unprotonated and poorly lipid soluble, and the skin PC decreases. The partitioning behavior of unionized and ionized salicylic acid between octanol and water is similar to that of the compounds in the skin layers studied in the model [14].

Acknowledgments This publication was supported by Skin Disease Research Foundation—The San Francisco Foundation.

References

1. Barry BW. Structure, function, diseases, and topical treatment of human skin. In: Barry BW, editor. Dermatological formulations: percutaneous absorption. New York: Marcel Dekker; 1983. p. 1–48.
2. Bashir SJ, Chew AL, Anigbogu A, Dreher F, Maibach HI. Physical and physiological effects of stratum corneum tape stripping. Skin Res Technol. 2001;7(1):40–8.
3. Berner B, Juang RH, Mazzenga GC. Ethanol and water sorption into stratum corneum and model systems. J Pharm Sci. 1989;78:472–6.
4. Bhandari KH, Lee DX, Newa M, Yoon SI, Kim JS, Kim DD, Kim JA, Yoo BK, Woo JS, Lyoo WS, Lee JH, Choi HG, Yong CS. Evaluation of skin permeation and accumulation profiles of ketorolac fatty esters. J Pharm Pharmaceut Sci. 2007;10(3):278–87.
5. Blank IH. Cutaneous barriers. J Invest Dermatol. 1965;45:249–56.
6. Bronaugh RL, Maibach HI. Percutaneous absorption: drugs, cosmetics, mechanisms, methods. 4th ed. Boca Raton, FL: Informa Healthcare; 2005.
7. Chan HP, Zhai H, Hui X, Maibach HI. Skin decontamination: principles and practices. Toxicol Ind Health. 2012; https://doi.org/10.1177/0748233712448112.
8. Dreher F, Modjtahedi BS, Modjtahedi SP, Maibach HI. Quantification of stratum corneum removal by adhesive tape stripping by total protein assay in 96-well microplates. Skin Res Technol. 2005;11(2):97–101.
9. Elias PM. Lipids and epidermal permeability barrier. Arch Dermatol Res. 1981;270: 95–117.
10. Federal Working Group on Pest Management. Occupational exposure to pesticides – report to the Federal Working Group on Pest Management from the Task Group on Occupational Exposure to Pesticides. Washington, D.C.: Federa Working Group on Pest Management; 1974.
11. Feldmann RJ, Maibach HI. Regional variation in percutaneous penetration of (^{14}C) cortisol in man. J Invest Dermatol. 1967;48:181–3.
12. Guy RH, Maibach HI. Calculations of body exposure from percutaneous absorption data. In: Bronaugh RL, Maibach HI, editors. Percutaneous absorption. New York: Marcel Dekker; 1985. p. 461–6.
13. Guy RH, Hadgraft J. Principles of skin permeability relevant to chemical exposure. In: Hobson DW, editor. Dermal and ocular toxicology. Boston: CPC Press; 1991. p. 221–46.
14. Gogoleva TE, Ademola JI, Wester RC, Magee PS, Maibach HI. Relative contributions of human skin layers to partitioning of chemicals with varying lipophilicity. In: Bronaugh R, Maibach HI, editors. Percutaneous absorption- drugs- cosmetics- mechanism- methodology. 3rd ed. New York; Chapter 26.: Marcel Dekker; 1999. p. 451–62.

15. Hatanakaa T, Shimoyama M, Sugibayashia K, Morimotoa Y. Effect of vehicle on the skin permeability of drugs: polyethylene glycol400-water and ethanol-water binary solvents. J Control Release. 1993;23:247–60.
16. Hui X, Wester RC, Magee P, Maibach HI. Partitioning of chemicals from water into powdered human stratum corneum (callus): a model study. Vitro Toxicol. 1995;8(2):159–67.
17. Hui X, Wester RC, Magee P, Maibach HI. Partitioning of chemicals from water into powdered human stratum corneum (callus). In: Hayes A, Thomas J, Maibach HI, editors. Toxicology of skin. Philadelphia: Taylor & Francis; 2001. p. 159–78.
18. Hui X, Wester RC, Zhai H, Cashmore AK, Barbadillo S, Maibach HI. Chemical partitioning into powdered human stratum corneum: a useful in vitro model for studying interactions of chemicals and human skin. In: Zhai H, Wilhelm KP, Maibach HI, editors. Marzulli and Maibach's dermatotoxicology. 7th ed. Boca Raton: CRC Press, Taylor and Francis Group; 2008. p. 87–94.
19. Lademann J, Weigmann HJ, Schanzer S, Richter H, Audring H, Antoniou C, Tsikrikas G, Gers-Barlag H, Sterry W. Optical investigations to avoid the disturbing influences of furrows and wrinkles quantifying penetration of drugs and cosmetics into the skin by tape stripping. J Biomed Opt. 2005;10(5):054015.
20. Levin CY, Maibach HI. Exogenous ochronosis: update. In: Zhai H, Wilhelm KP, Maibach HI, editors. Dermatotoxicology. 7th ed. Boca Raton: CRC Press, Taylor and Francis Group; 2008. p. 669–72.
21. Leveque JL, Rasseeneur L. Mechanical properties of stratum corneum: influence of water and lipids. In: Marks RM, Barton SP, Edwards C, editors. The physical nature of the skin. Norwell: MTP Press Limited; 1988; Chapter 17.
22. Loffler H, Dreher F, Maibach HI. Stratum corneum adhesive tape stripping: influence of anatomical site, application pressure, duration and removal. Br J Dermatol. 2004;151(4):746–52.
23. Loffler H, Weimer C, Dreher F, Maibach HI. Parameters influencing stratum corneum removal by tape stripping. In: Zhai H, Wilhelm KP, Maibach HI, editors. Dermatotoxicology. 7th ed. Boca Raton: CRC Press, Taylor and Francis Group; 2008. p. 339–42.
24. Maibach HI, Feldmann RJ, Milby TH, Sert WF. Regional variation in percutaneous penetration in man. Arch Environ Health. 1971;23:208–11.
25. Marrakchi S, Maibach HI. Functional map and age-related differences in the human face: nonimmunologic contact urticaria induced by hexyl nicotinate. In: Barel AO, Paye M, Maibach HI, editors. Handbook of cosmetic science and technology. 3rd ed. New York: Informa Healthcare USA, Inc; 2009. p. 25–8.
26. Middleton JD. The mechanism of water binding in stratum corneum. Brit J Derm. 1968;80:437–50.
27. Nemes Z, Steinert PM. Bricks and mortar of the epidermal barrier. Exp Mol Med. 1999;31(1):5–19.
28. Norlen L. Stratum corneum keratin structure, function and formation – a comprehensive review. Int J Cosmet Sci. 2006;28:397–425.
29. Öhman H, Vahlquist A. In vivo studies concerning a pH gradient in human stratum corneum and upper epidermis. Acta Derm Venereol. 1994;74:375–9.
30. Öhman H, Vahlquist A. The pH gradient over the stratum corneum differs in X-linked recessive and autosomal dominant ichthyosis: a clue to the molecular origin of the "acid skin mantle"? J Invest Dermat. 1998;111:674–7.
31. Pinkus H. Examination of the epidermis by the strip method of removing horny layers. J Invest Dermatol. 1951;16:383–6.
32. Poet TS, Thrall KD, Corley RA, Hui X, Edwards JA, Weitz KK, Maibach HI, Wester RC. Utility of real time breath analysis and physiologically based pharmacokinetic modeling to determine the percutaneous absorption of methyl chloroform in rats and humans. Toxicol Sci. 2000a;54:42–51.
33. Poet TS, Thrall KD, Corley RA, Hui X, Edwards JA, Weitz KK, Maibach HI, Wester RC. Assessment of the percutaneous absorption of trichloroethylene in rats and humans

using MS/MS real-time breath analysis and physiologically based pharmacokinetic modeling. Toxicol Sci. 2000b;56:61–72.
34. Poet TS, Thrall KD, Corley RA, Hui X, Edwards JA, Weitz KK, Maibach HI, Wester RC. PBPK modeling of the percutaneous absorption of perchloroethylene from a solid matrix in rats and humans. Toxicol Sci. 2002;67:17–31.
35. Potts RO, Guy RH. Predicting skin permeability. Pharm Res. 1992;9(5):663–9.
36. Proksch E, Brandner JM, Jensen JM. The skin: an indispensable barrier. Exp Dermatol. 2008;17(12):1063–72.
37. Rawlings AV, Harding CR. Moisturization and skin barrier function. Dermatol Ther. 2004;17(Suppl 1):43–8.
38. Raykar PV, Fung MC, Anderson BD. The role of protein and lipid domains in the uptake of solutes of human stratum corneum. Pharm Res. 1988;5(3):140–50.
39. Rieger M. Factors affecting sorption of topically applied substances. In: Zatz L, editor. Skin permeation fundamentals and application. Wheaton: Allured Publishing Co; 1993. p. 33–72.
40. Rougier A, Dupuis D, Lotte C, Roguet R, Wester RC, Maibach HI. Regional variation in percutaneous absorption in man: measurement by the stripping method. Arch Dermatol Res. 1986;278:465–9.
41. Rougier A, Lotte C, Maibach HI. The hairless rat: a relevant animal model to predict in vivo percutaneous absorption in human? J Invest Dermatol. 1987a;88:577–81.
42. Rougier A, Lotte C, Maibach HI. In vivo percutaneous penetration of some organic compounds related to anatomic site in humans: predictive assessment by the stripping method. J Pharm Sci. 1987b;76(6):451–545.
43. Rougier A, Rallis M, Krien P, Lotte C. In vivo percutaneous absorption: a key role for stratum corneum/vehicle partitioning. Arch Dermatol Res. 1990;282:498–505.
44. Scheuplein RJ, Blank IH. Mechanisms in percutaneous absorption. IV. Penetration of nonelectrolytes (alcohols) from aqueous solutions and from pure liquids. J Invest Dermatol. 1973;60(5):286–96.
45. Scheuplein RJ, Bronaugh RL. Percutaneous absorption. In: Goldsmith LA, editor. Biochemistry and physiology of the skin, vol. 1. Oxford: Oxford University Press; 1983. p. 1255–94.
46. Surber C, Wilhelm KP, Hori M, Maibach HI, Guy RH. Optimization of topical therapy: partitioning of drug into stratum corneum. Pharm Res. 1990a;7(12):1320–4.
47. Surber C, Wilhelm KP, Hori M, Maibach HI, Guy RH. Partitioning of chemicals into human stratum corneum: implications for risk assessment following dermal exposure. Fundam Appl Toxicol. 1990b;15:99–107.
48. van der Valk PG, Maibach HI. A functional study of the skin barrier to evaporative water loss by means of repeated cellophane-tape stripping. Clin Exp Dermatol. 1990;15(3): 180–2.
49. Wertz PW, Swartzendruber DC, Squier CA. Regional variation in the structure and permeability of oral mucosa and skin. Adv Drug Deliv Rev. 1993;12:1–12.
50. Wester RC. Twenty absorbing years. In: Surber C, Elsner P, Bircher AJ, editors. Exogenous dermatology. Basel: Karger; 1995. p. 112–23.
51. Wester RC, Maibach HI. Cutaneous pharmacokinetics: 10 steps to percutaneous absorption. Drug Metab Rev. 1983;14(2):169–205.
52. Wester RC, Maibach HI. In vivo percutaneous absorption and decontamination of pesticides in humans. J Toxicol Environ Health. 1985;16:25–37.
53. Wester RC, Maibach HI, Bucks DAW, Aufrere MB. In vivo percutaneous absorption of paraquat from hand, leg and forearm of humans. J Toxicol Environ Health. 1984;14: 759–62.
54. Wester RC, Maibach HI, Hui X, and Tanojo H. 1999. Progress Report of Environmental Management Science Program (DOE grant #DE-FG07-97ER62509): Bioavailability of organic solvents in soils: input into biologically-based dose-response models for human risk assessment. http://www.osti.gov/em52/1999projsum/59828.pdf.

55. Wester RC, Mobayen M, Maibach HI. In vivo and in vitro absorption and binding to powdered stratum corneum as methods to evaluate skin absorption of environmental chemical contaminants from ground and surface water. J Toxicol Environ Health. 1987;21:367–74.
56. Wester RM, Tanjo H, Maibach HI, Wester RC. Predicted chemical warfare agent VX toxicity to uniformed soldier using parathion in vitro human exposure and absorption. Toxicol Appl Pharmacol. 2000;168:149–52.
57. Yosipovitch G, Maibach HI. Significance of skin surface pH. Harefuah. 1996;130(7): 478–80.
58. Yosipovitch G, Xiong GL, Haus E, Sackett-Lundeen L, Ashkenazi I, Maibach HI. Time dependent variations of the skin barrier function in humans: transepidermal water loss, stratum corneum hydration, skin surface pH, and skin temperature. J Invest Dermatol. 1998;110:20–3.
59. Yardley AJ. Epidermal lipids. Int J Cosmet. 1987;59:13–9.
60. Zatz JL. Scratching the surface: rational approaches to skin permeation. In: Zatz JL, editor. Skin permeation fundamentals and application. Wheaten: Allured Publishing Co; 1993. p. 11–32.
61. Zhang J, Purdon CH, Smith EW, Maibach HI, Surber C. Penetration enhancement by skin hydration. In: Smith EW, Maibach HI, editors. Percutaneous penetration enhancers. 2nd ed. Boca Raton: CRC Press, Taylor and Francis Group; 2006. p. 67–71.

Chapter 2
Isolated Human and Animal Stratum Corneum as a Partial Model for the 15 Steps of Percutaneous Absorption: Emphasizing Decontamination Part II

Xiaoying Hui and Howard I. Maibach

The stratum corneum (SC) of humans and animals holds key insights to the development of an efficient protective barrier against contamination and to devising effective decontamination interventions. Advancing knowledge of this ever-changing defense layer with respect to the percutaneous penetration of chemicals provides many opportunities to optimize chemical-specific decontamination protocols. The SC acts as a "reservoir" for topically applied molecules, and even rapid washing with water post dermal exposure frequently fails to remove most chemicals [11]. Importantly, Rougier et al. [28, 29] discovered that SC sampling in vivo in humans and rats via tape stripping 30 minutes post exposure accurately predicts and quantifies chemical penetration for up to 4 days with linear-type correlation. While percutaneous penetration is often considered a simplistic one-step diffusion process, it consists of at least 15 steps [37] related to absorption and excretion kinetics, extraction, vehicle characteristics, wash effects, etc. (Table 2.1) Additionally, the chemical partitioning/diffusion behavior of a wide array of compounds with differing physicochemical properties has approximately the same diffusion coefficients with regard to their percutaneous absorption in vivo. Thus, for a given thickness of SC and a specific anatomical site, the penetration flux value of a substance depends mainly on its SC/vehicle partition coefficient [30, 31].

The abovementioned observations provide novel insights for improving decontamination techniques. Despite many emergency treatment protocols, numerous topically applied chemicals are not easily removed by water washing. Skin decontamination is the primary required intervention for chemical, biological, and radiological exposures and involves immediate removal of the contaminant via the

X. Hui (✉)
Department of Dermatology, University of California San Francisco, San Francisco, CA, USA
e-mail: Xiaoying.Hui@UCSF.edu

H. I. Maibach
Department of Dermatology, University of California San Francisco, San Francisco, CA, USA

H. Zhu, H. I. Maibach (eds.), *Skin Decontamination*,
https://doi.org/10.1007/978-3-030-24009-7_2

Table 2.1 15 steps related to the process of percutaneous absorption[a]

Number	Factors determining percutaneous absorption
1	Release from vehicle[b] Varies with solubility in vehicle, concentration, pH, etc.
2	Kinetics of skin penetration[b] Influenced by anatomical site, degree of occlusion, intrinsic skin condition, animal age, concentration of dosing solution, surface area dosed, frequency of dosing, post absorption, etc.
3	Excretion kinetics[b]
4	Tissue disposition
5	Substantivity to skin[b]
6	Wash effects[b] Wash resistance Wash enhancement
7	Rub effects[b] Rub resistance Rub enhancement
8	Transfer—skin, clothing + inanimate surface[b]
9	Exfoliation[b]
10	Volatility[b]
11	Binding—all layers[b]
12	Anatomic pathways
13	Lateral spread[b]
14	Vascular perfusion[b]
15	Cutaneous metabolism[b]

[a]Modified with permission from Wester and Maibach [37]
[b]Metric developed

most effective manner. Contaminant removal techniques can consist of physical removal including the use of friction, use of a liquid vehicle to solvate or emulsify the contaminant, contaminant transfer to another medium through absorption/adsorption, and chemical alteration of the contaminant. Decontaminants should effectively and rapidly remove contaminants without causing enhancement, wash-in effect, or skin damage while easily removing itself without undesirable residue. It should additionally be readily available, affordable, and easily disposed of [8]. In the second part of this review, we continue to explore the many steps involved in percutaneous penetration, the laboratory techniques providing the background for this knowledge, and the insights advancing our knowledge of chemical exposure risk assessment, exposure prevention and barrier methods, and postexposure decontamination. We address knowledge gaps to guide future research to guide our ability to minimize the harmful effects of hazardous dermal chemical exposure.

Tissue Disposition and Binding: All Layers

The skin is an organized, heterogeneous, and multilayered organ. The SC, epidermis, dermis, appendages, and vasculature constitute the outer living protective system. Percutaneous absorption of topically applied agents is the sum of the penetration and permeation of a chemical through the SC, epidermis, and part of the dermis [10, 22, 32]. The effect of the skin layers on percutaneous absorption was evaluated by quantifying the partitioning of compounds in water and isopropyl myristate (IPM) between skin layers. The influence of vehicle drug concentration, equilibration time, hydrophilicity, lipophilicity, and pH on the partitioning behavior of compounds was examined [13].

Chemical Binding and Dispersion to Different Skin Layers

Chemical partitioning occurs in human SC, epidermis, and dermis, and partitioning in the SC as a function of equilibration time is shown in Fig. 2.1. The lipophilic chemicals propranolol, atrazine, and salicylic acid reached equilibrium in 3–6 hours in the SC and epidermis. Theophylline, the most hydrophilic compound, required 12 hours to achieve equilibrium; however, in the dermis, equilibrium was reached in 3 hours secondary to the ease of dermal hydration. MOP exhibited a different PC time profile with the skin layers not reaching saturation until 24 hours post

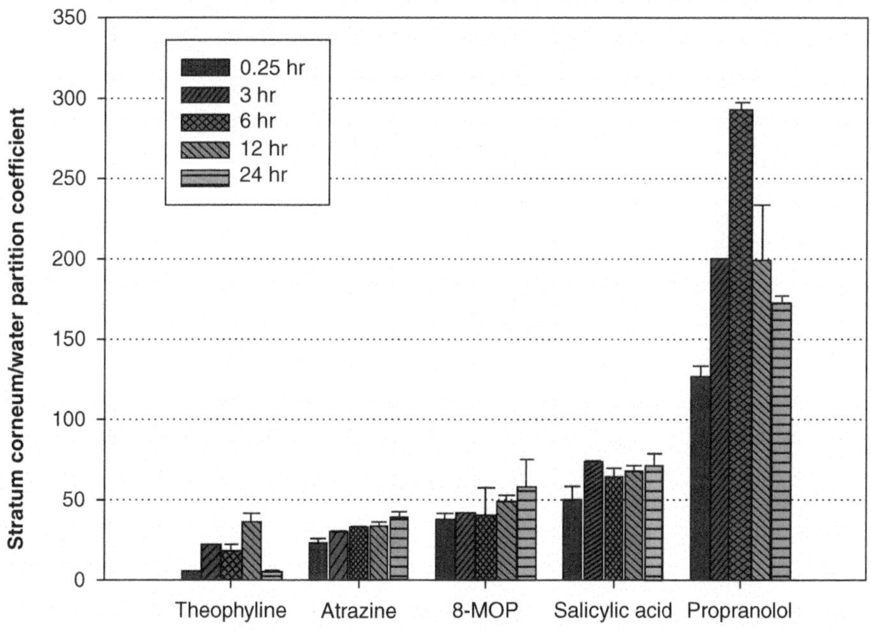

Fig. 2.1 The graph is modified with permission from Gogoleva et al. [13]. Stratum corneum (sheet)/water partition coefficient (mean ± SD, $n = 3$) of model compounds as a function of equilibrium time. In the stratum corneum, the lipophilic chemicals propranolol, atrazine, and salicylic acid reached equilibrium in 3–6 hours. The hydrophilic compound theophylline required 12 hours to achieve equilibrium. Solutions of chemicals used were at saturation solubility concentrations. The lipophilic chemicals, propranolol, atrazine, and salicylic acid, reached equilibrium in 3–6 hours. The most hydrophilic compound, theophylline, required 12 hours to achieve equilibrium

exposure, although the PC continued to increase with contact time. Lipophilic compounds including propranolol, salicylic acid, and atrazine exhibit higher PCs in the SC than in the epidermis or dermis; however, the PC values of theophylline remained relatively constant in the three skin layers.

The data presented here corroborates that in previous literature reports. The calculated partition coefficients for the compounds as a function of equilibration time, chemical concentration, and solvent nature may be valuable in predicting the in vivo and in vitro transport of drugs and environmental agents through human skin.

Raykar et al. [26] suggested that a lipid and protein domain exist in the SC. The uptake of highly lipophilic compounds (log P values near 3.0) may be governed by the lipid domain of SC, and hydrophilic solutes are taken up in the protein domain. Because theophylline partitions equally into the skin layers, the retention could be secondary to its binding to the protein domain. The data presented here verify earlier observations [5, 7, 17].

Wash Effects and Skin Decontamination

The Powdered Stratum Corneum Model to Rapidly Evaluate Wash Resistance and Decontamination Efficiency

Most material safety data sheets (MSDS) recommend soap and water to remove chemicals from the skin surface. Because of the varying physical-chemical properties, each chemical has different SC binding sites with diverse affinities. Therefore, understanding a chemical's wash resistance can help to identify optimal decontaminants.

The powdered SC model provides a tool to rapidly evaluate the chemical's potential skin binding and partitioning behavior and to determine washing solution efficacy. A radiolabeled contaminant chemical was mixed with powdered SC and incubated in a 37 °C water bath for 0.5–2 hours. The chemical and SC mixture was washed multiple times with the selected solution and centrifuged to separate the washing solution from the SC pellet, and then the radioactivity of each sample was measured. Using this protocol, the decontaminant effects of multiple decontaminants could be compared [16].

Decontamination Efficiency Related to Chemical Dose-Exposure Time

Table 2.2 shows that [^{14}C]-2,4-D was easily washed from the bound SC particles with water alone, and five washings five times removed more than 90% of the bound compound. Most bound compounds (50% or more) are removed after the first

Table 2.2 Water decontaminates environmental hazardous chemicals (2,4-d) from human skin[a]

	Radioactivity recovery as percent dose of [^{14}C]-2,4-D (%) applied						
		Powdered stratum corneum					
Dose (μCi)	Supernatant	Before washing	After first washing	After second washing	After third washing	After fourth washing	After last washing
0.22	87.4 ± 0.5	12.6 ± 0.5	4.8 ± 0.8	4.5 ± 0.8	2.2 ± 0.2	0.9 ± 0.1	0.9 ± 0.1
0.44	84.6 ± 1.9	15.4 ± 1.9	6.8 ± 1.6	4.4 ± 0.5	2.6 ± 0.4	1.1 ± 0.2	1.1 ± 0.1
0.88	82.9 ± 1.9	17.1 ± 1.9	8.3 ± 2.0	4.9 ± 0.7	2.3 ± 0.5	1.1 ± 0.2	1.1 ± 0.1
1.76	86.1 ± 1.2	13.9 ± 1.2	5.5 ± 0.7	4.2 ± 0.7	2.5 ± 0.6	1.2 ± 0.2	1.1 ± 0.2
2.20	78.9 ± 1.8	20.1 ± 1.8	10.9 ± 2.9	4.6 ± 1.2	2.4 ± 0.3	1.4 ± 0.3	1.2 ± 0.3
3.52	81.7 ± 4.1	18.3 ± 4.1	8.7 ± 4.0	5.0 ± 0.6	2.0 ± 0.2	1.6 ± 0.5	1.5 ± 0.5

Water washing five times removed more than 90% of bound [^{14}C]-2,4-D from the powdered SC. Most bound compounds (50% or more) were washed off after the first washing

[a]Modified with permission from Wester RC et al. [43] and [44]. Results indicate that most radioactive residues were washed off within first two washes. After a 2-hour incubation/equilibration period, the test sample was centrifuged and then separated to the supernatant and pellet parts. The pellet sample was further washed by water for five times to remove unbound test chemicals. Each time after washing, the sample was centrifuged again to separate the supernatant and pellet parts

washing [27, 43, 44]. Alachlor readily binds powdered SC without dependence on contact duration; thus, water washing alone removes only about 2% of the compound regardless of dose, concentration, or contact duration. Using 10% soap washing solution, about 77% of the alachlor was removed and 50% washing solution removed 90% of bound alachlor from the powdered SC [6, 42]. This elegantly shows the effectiveness of soapy water for washing hands and how powdered SC can be used to determine the effectiveness of skin decontaminants [33].

Comparison of Decontamination Efficiency Post Short-Time Exposure

Potential environmental exposures may happen during manufacturing, distribution, application, deliberate exposure, or by residual presence. The concentrations of chemical agents and the contact duration are primary determinants of the degree of skin destruction and systemic poisoning. To prevent and diminish chemical absorption, immediate washing with appropriate decontaminating agents is essential to reduce damage and percutaneous penetration.

Glyphosate is a broad-spectrum, postemergence, translocated herbicide. Human exposure can occur through production or general use. The extent of glyphosate binding, systemic absorption, and removal post exposure was studied.

A powdered SC model examined the skin binding affinity. Table 2.3 shows glyphosate is easily removed from SC with water, regardless of time exposure or dose concentration. After three water washes, less than 0.1% of the chemical remained bound to the powdered SC [41].

Table 2.3 Glyphosate partition from roundup vehicle to powdered stratum corneum[a]

	Radioactivity recovery as percent dose of [^{14}C]-glyphosate applied		
	Undiluted	Diluted 1:20	Diluted 1:32
30 minutes exposure			
Vehicle	96 ± 0.9	102 ± 1.2	96 ± 1.6
Water washing	2.4 ± 0.2	1.2 ± 0.07	1.1 ± 0.2
Stratum corneum	0.04 ± 0.04	0.03 ± 0.03	0.02 ± 0.01
4 hour exposure			
Vehicle	96 ± 2.4	104 ± 1.3	91 ± 2.9
Water washing	3.3 ± 0.8	1.2 ± 0.2	5.0 ± 2.2
Stratum corneum	0.01 ± 0.01	0.02 ± 0.03	0.05 ± 0.04
8 hour exposure			
Vehicle	96 ± 0.4	98 ± 6.6	95 ± 1.4
Water washing	3.0 ± 0.2	2.2 ± 0.5	2.3 ± 1.2
Stratum corneum	0.02 ± 0.0	0.01 ± 0.01	0.02 ± 0.01

Results show that glyphosate was weakly bound with powdered stratum corneum. In all cases, the amount remaining with the powdered stratum corneum pellet after the water washing was less than or equal to 0.05%

[a]Modified with permission from Wester et al. [41]. Undiluted, 1.1 mg glyphosate/ml/mg SC; 1:20, 0.059 mg; 1:32, 0.037 mg. Data expressed as mean ± S.D

Washing with water or water with soap is traditionally used to reduce potential damage and percutaneous penetration of chemicals topically applied, but may not be effective for decontamination of lipophilic compounds. For instance, the removal of alachlor with water is less effective than soap with water. In contrast, both soap-and-water wash and emergency water shower are relatively ineffective at removing the potent contact sensitizer methylene bisphenyl isocyanate from the skin [45]. Residual chemical on the skin post standard washing procedures can have toxic consequences [19]. Additionally, the "wash-in" effect can potentially enhance percutaneous penetration and systemic absorption of chemicals [21].

Skin decontamination is often emergent. A human skin in vitro model was used to compare the decontamination capacity of three decontaminant solutions: tap water, isotonic saline, and hypertonic saline mixed with radiolabeled [^{14}C]-glyphosate (Table 2.4). After a defined exposure time, the skin surface was washed three times with 4 mL of each solution. Tape stripping was then employed to collect an SC sample, and all collected samples were analyzed by a liquid scintillation counter to determine radioactivity. This in vitro model is economical, rapid, and provides quantitative data to aid screening for optimal decontaminants.

For glyphosate, no statistical differences between decontaminants were found. The total mass recovered and the wash-off rates at the three exposure times ranged from 94.8% to 102.4% and 79% to 101.2%, respectively. Therefore, the decontaminants were similarly effective [50].

Table 2.4 Human skin decontamination of glyphosate in vitro[a]

	Radioactivity recovery as percent dose of [^{14}C]-glyphosate applied		
	1 minutes exposure	3 minutes exposure	30 minutes exposure
Water washing			
Wash solution	93.52 ± 16.42	94.60 ± 26.39	85.09 ± 14.06
Stratum corneum	0.10 ± 0.10	0.14 ± 0.10	1.78 ± 0.84
Skin residue	2.21 ± 1.99	0.70 ± 0.44	7.50 ± 3.82
Systemic absorption	0.04 ± 0.05	0.05 ± 0.10	2.26 ± 2.19
Hypertonic saline			
Wash solution	101.23 ± 14.20	98.69 ± 21.16	85.04 ± 14.62
Stratum corneum	0.12 ± 0.07	0.14 ± 0.09	1.54 ± 1.06
Skin residue	1.02 ± 1.27	1.45 ± 1.69	5.06 ± 3.29
Systemic absorption	0.04 ± 0.04	0.54 ± 0.84	3.17 ± 6.66
Isotonic saline			
Wash solution	98.72 ± 18.34	95.56 ± 28.08	78.95 ± 9.38
Stratum corneum	0.08 ± 0.05	0.14 ± 0.11	2.23 ± 2.10
Skin residue	0.74 ± 0.90	3.53 ± 5.15	9.84 ± 12.58
Systemic absorption	0.07 ± 0.10	0.32 ± 0.39	5.42 ± 7.07

[a]Modified with permission from Zhai et al. [50]. Three decontamination agents were compared

In the rhesus monkey, soap-water versus tap water washing was significantly more effective 5 minutes post topical exposure of glyphosate ($p < 0.05$, [41]).These models provide a simple, robust means to enhance our knowledge of decontamination mechanisms.

Comparison Vehicle: Washing Agent Effects on Decontamination

To assess multiple vehicles for decontamination, an in vitro decontamination technique for removing Aroclor 1242 and polychlorinated biphenyls (PCBs) was used. Interestingly, PCBs would not partition from the SC into water (<1%). Soap and water led to an average of 33% of partitioned PCBs, mineral oil removed 66.7% of PCBs, and ethanol removed approximately 85% [38, 40–42].

In vivo skin decontamination of Aroclor 1242 from the rhesus monkey post topical application is shown in Table 2.5. Using a trichlorobenzene vehicle, no differences in decontamination were seen through 1 hour, but from 3 to 24 hours, the amount removed by decontamination decreased. By 24 hours, only about 25% of the PCBs could be recovered from the skin's surface. With a mineral oil vehicle, soap and water removed about 70% of the PCBs over 3 hours, 50% at 6 hours, and 30% at 24 hours and was more efficient in removing the PCBs in the initial 15 minutes with its decontamination ability dissipating in 10 minutes. However, in vitro

Table 2.5 In vivo skin decontamination of Aroclor 1242 as percent dose removed[a]

Time interval of washing post application	Percent dose partitioned removed					
	Trichlorobenzene vehicle				Mineral oil vehicle	
	Soap and water	Trichlorobenzene	Mineral oil	Ethanol	Soap and water	Mineral oil
0 minutes	93 ± 7	102 ± 7	63 ± 4	102 ± 9	71 ± 18	90 ± 10
10 minutes	87 ± 10	86 ± 9	68 ± 5	95 ± 6	71 ± 27	68 ± 19
1 hour	81 ± 11	92 ± 8	72 ± 8	79 ± 11	71 ± 33	63 ± 28
3 hour	63 ± 17	74 ± 12	49 ± 3	74 ± 8	68 ± 13	64 ± 15
6 hour	57 ± 26	58 ± 15	52 ± 7	56 ± 12	51 ± 33	65 ± 22
24 hour	26 ± 13	25 ± 19	26 ± 7	36 ± 8	30 ± 14	45 ± 40

Removal efficacies of both decontaminants were reduced from 3 hours to the end (24 hours)
[a]Modified with permission from Wester et al. [40]. In early stage—the initial 15-minute period, mineral oil was more efficient in removing the PCBs

Table 2.6 Aroclor 1242 removal from rhesus monkey skin with successive washes following initial 15-minute application time[a]

Wash number	Percent dose removed[b]			
	Soap/water	Trichlorobenzene	Mineral oil	Ethanol
1	62 ± 13	79 ± 12	64 ± 5	51 ± 7
2	19 ± 9	14 ± 4	21 ± 6	8 ± 2
3	7 ± 2	5 ± 1	10 ± 2	2 ± 1
4	3 ± 1	3 ± 1	5 ± 1	1 ± 0
5	2 ± 1	1 ± 1	3 ± 2	1 ± 1
Total	93 ± 7	102 ± 7	102 ± 9	63 ± 4

[a]Modified with permission from Wester et al. [40]
[b]Application vehicle is trichlorobenzene

partitioning suggested that ethanol, not soap and water, would be effective, the opposite seen in vivo.

In vivo skin decontamination involves a "rubbing" component and a "solvent" component. The soap-and-water detergent helps to wash cells and the absorbed PCBs away. As a solvent, ethanol may facilitate penetration of PCBs. Soap, water, and rubbing for PCB removal in vivo are shown in Table 2.6.

Rubbing and Transferring Effects on Skin

Rubbing off, rubbing on, and transfer are terms used to describe the ability of a compound to be removed from an object's surface, to penetrate deeper, or to be transferred from one surface to another. All three represent tangential movements between two surfaces such as skin and fabric.

Rubbing Effects: Animal Model

Traditional belief holds that rubbing of topically applied drugs is necessary for penetration. McMaster et al. [20] examined whether rubbing enhances dermal absorption in animals. In a crossover experiment, they applied [^{14}C]-cortisone cream (4 μg/cm^2) to the naked retroauricular area of a guinea pig and abdomen of a rhesus monkey. In the guinea pig, 20.1 ± 4.3% of the nonrubbed dose was absorbed versus 20.0 ± 3.7% of the rubbed dose ($p > 0.05$), while 5.3 ± 3.3% of the nonrubbed dose and 6.2 ± 2.7% of the rubbed dose was absorbed in the rhesus monkey ($p > 0.05$) (Table 2.7). These results suggest that application with rubbing may have no effect on dermal absorption of topical formulations. This implies the spreading application technique for patients with damaged skin could be more efficacious and beneficial. This finding may have significant clinical importance for the administration of topical treatments.

Rubbing and Transferring Effects: Human Evaluation

Rubbing effects on the percutaneous penetration of [^{14}C]-estradiol gel were examined in human subjects in vivo. Topical application of 0.17 g (22 μCi) [^{14}C]-estradiol gel formulation was applied to a 14.3 × 3.5 cm^2 skin area on a ventral forearm; group B received topical doses on both sides of the forearm; and group C received a topical dose on the left forearm only. Group B allowed the application to air-dry before being covered with a Tyvek paper sleeve. Group C subjects' dosed skin was placed in contact for 15 minutes with the ventral forearm of Group D subjects,

Table 2.7 Effect of rubbing and spreading on dermal absorption of cortisone[a]

	Percent dose excreted			
	Rhesus monkey		Guinea pig	
Time(days)	Rub	Spread	Rub	Spread
1	2.2 ± 1.7	1.2 ± 1.0	15.7 ± 4.3	15.6 ± 5.0
2	1.9 ± 0.9	1.7 ± 1.5	2.0 ± 0.6	2.1 ± 0.4
3	0.8 ± 0.3	0.9 ± 0.5	0.8 ± 0.2	0.9 ± 0.2
4	0.4 ± 0.2	0.6 ± 0.2	0.5 ± 0.2	0.5 ± 0.2
5	0.2 ± 0.1	0.4 ± 0.0	0.3 ± 0.1	0.4 ± 0.1
6	0.3 ± 0.0	0.3 ± 0.1	0.4 ± 0.2	0.4 ± 0.1
7	0.4 ± 0.3	0.2 ± 0.0	0.4 ± 0.2	0.3 ± 0.1
Total	6.2 ± 2.7	5.3 ± 3.3	20.0 ± 3.7	20.1 ± 4.3

Data suggest that application by rubbing compared to simply spreading an ointment had no obvious effect on the dermal absorption, at least for cortisone cream
[a]Modified with permission from McMaster et al. [20]

Table 2.8 Rubbing effect on dose transferring of estradiol

	Radioactivity recovery as percent dose			
	Group B		Group C	Group D
	Dosed left forearm	Dosed right forearm	Dosed forearm	Nondosed forearm
Skin wash (24 hours)	27.2 ± 4.0	29.0 ± 4.0	36.1 ± 14.4	2.3 ± 2.0
Sleeve	24.2 ± 14.4	13.7 ± 3.8	12.9 ± 6.6	4.1 ± 3.6
Urinary ^{14}C excretion (0–168 hours)	4.2 ± 3.2		3.4 ± 4.0	2.2 ± 2.0
Dose accountability	56.9 ± 11.0		56.9 ± 7.0	10.8 ± 7.9
Topical bioavailability	8.2 ± 6.3		6.6 ± 7.6	4.3 ± 3.8

In Group B, the majority of the topical dose resided on the surface of the skin during the 24-hour dosing period. The amount of radioactivity of the sleeve sample was from the dosed skin due to the process of chemical rubbing off

The dose was available for skin transfer (Group C) and that skin-transferred dose was absorbed by the recipient person (Group D). Group C wash recovery was 36%, and 13% was recovered from the sleeve. Group D wash recovery was 2.3 and 4.1% recovered from the sleeve

[a]Modified with permission from Wester et al. [46]

who did not receive other topical application or treatment. Skin contact was defined as contact with rubbing of the surfaces five times up and down in one direction, followed by 15 minutes of close contact of the skin surfaces, then rubbing five times up and down in other direction. The contacted areas of groups C and D were placed in a sleeve. The sleeves were removed after 24 hours and the dosed skin area was washed with soap and water five times. All samples were counted for radioactivity [46]. The majority of the topical doses resided on the skin surface during the 24-hour period and the percentage of dosages recovered are shown in Table 2.8.

This study does not assess the duration of residual topical drug availability for transfer relative to the skin contact time, differences in formulation, or routine skin washing effects. The topical bioavailability determined by the urinary recovery of estradiol was 8.2 ± 6.3% of the doses in Group B, meaning a large portion of active substance is still available for transfer or absorption.

Franklin and Geffner [12] documented the transfer of estradiol and testosterone. "The cream," or topical testosterone, is frequently illegally used in sport. Additionally, fentanyl transfer has been reported [47]. Transfer is possible for any bioactive topical chemical, and hazardous environmental chemicals including pesticides, herbicides, and pollutants can settle topically and be transferred to another person. Yerasi only investigated one rub/contact sequence. However, the potential of topical transfer of bioactive chemicals has been shown in humans in vivo [46]. In reality, skin contact occurs under many conditions with a multitude of variables contributing to overall chemical skin transfer. Further investigation is thus warranted.

Penetration Enhancement and Retardation

Penetration Pathway

Human SC has a unique hierarchical structure. Dead, flattened, keratin-rich corneocytes are "bricks" embedded in an intercellular lipid-rich matrix [10]. Viable epidermis and dermis are relatively impermeable, and the SC constitutes the rate limiting barrier for percutaneous absorption of many different permeants.

Chemicals penetrate the SC by passive diffusion. To successfully deliver a drug to the skin from a vehicle requires [18] dissolution and diffusion from the vehicle to the vehicle-skin interface and the SC, diffusion through the SC and viable epidermis, and diffusion through the dermis and into the microcirculation. Three major skin diffusion pathways [2] are the transcellular route, the intercellular route, and the appendage route. The intercellular pathway is the most prominent, and the degree of transdermal delivery is largely dependent upon the interaction of SC lipid bilayers.

Drug transport in SC lipid bilayers is highly anisotropic and size-dependent. The lipid bilayers exhibit strong structural heterogeneity resulting in a wide spectrum of drug partition and diffusion coefficients. As a result, hydrophobic molecules are believed to diffuse by a tortuous pathway through the tail-group region and hydrophilic molecules by the head-group region. Transport between bilayers can occur at bilayer interfaces or sites of structural discontinuity. The SC barrier restricts molecule diffusion, allowing only molecules with certain physicochemical properties including low molecular weight (<500 Daltons), good aqueous solubility (1 mg/ml), moderate liposolubility (10 < Ko/w < 1000), and a low melting point (<200 °C) to pass. Consequently, a very limited number of chemicals can permeate the skin [24, 25].

Penetration Enhancement

To ensure therapeutically effective doses are achieved via drug penetration, considerable investigation into strategies to enhance penetration has been done. Methods to improve delivery rely on chemical penetration enhancers (CPE) to overcome the skin barrier. CPEs such as menthol and fatty acids can be obtained naturally, while others including Azone® and DMSO can be synthesized artificially. Chemical enhancement to promote transdermal drug absorption can be classified by their mechanism of action [3]:

1. Alteration of SC hydration: Water, chemical, or physical occlusion can increase the SC hydration, changing the solubilities of permeants by opening the SC structure and modifying the partitioning from the vehicle into the membrane.

2. Lipid disruption or fluidization: Azone, DMSO, alcohols, fatty acids, terpenes, and compounds with a polar head and long alkyl chain can increase permeability by disrupting or fluidizing the lipid structure of the SC. They are more effective for hydrophilic permeants, although their use with lipophilic permeants has been reported to increase delivery.
3. Extraction of SC lipids: Solvents including DMSO and various alcohols can extract lipids from the SC by forming aqueous channels to increase permeability.
4. Interaction with keratin: DMSO, decyl methyl sulfoxide, urea, and surfactants can interact with keratin in the corneocytes, changing the diffusion coefficient and increasing permeability. However, chemical interaction with the peptide/protein material of the lipid bilayer domain may also increase permeability.
5. Increased partitioning and solubility in the SC: Solvents including ethanol, propylene glycol, and *n*-methyl pyrrolidones increase permeant penetration by enhancing the solubility and its level of partitioning.

Numerous compounds have been reported to enhance drug permeability. Several enhancer classification systems have been developed based on the chemical structure, functional group, area of action, or solubility. Commonly, classifications are based on the chemical structure [9] or the basis of their activity [1]. Recently, Songkro [34] combined information on CPE chemical structure and their functional groups resulting in 17 classes: water, sulfoxides and similar compounds, pyrrolidones, alcohols, glycols, urea and derivatives, azone and derivatives, enzymes, iminosulfuranes, cyclodextrins, fatty acids, fatty acid esters, surfactants, terpenes, polyers, monoolein, and oxazolidinones. Common chemical penetration enhancers with their corresponding mechanisms of action, safety, and adverse effect profiles can be referenced [24, 25].

Penetration Retardation

An improvement in chemical delivery, transdermal penetration, and dermal absorption can be problematic when cosmetics, pesticides, or chemical warfare agents are exposed to the skin. The effectiveness of the SC barrier can be altered by variations in SC thickness, hair follicle anatomy and location, moisture, temperature, and the presence of chemical enhancers. Various strategies may reduce the ability of undesirable materials to cross the SC barrier. They can be classified by their mechanism of action [4]:

1. Active ingredient design manipulation to facilitate physicochemical properties that decrease permeation
2. Permeant chemical modification such as bonding it to a polymer to prevent dermal uptake

3. Formulation modification to:
   (a) Reduce its thermodynamic activity
   (b) Reduce its solubility in the skin lipids
   (c) Increase the microviscosity of the skin lipids

Penetration retardation has been used in cosmetic products, sunscreen agents, and topical antifungal treatments. This method is also imperative to the US military for reducing the threat of chemical warfare agents and potential biochemical threats.

Barrier Creams

The application of topical barrier cream prior to that of a chemical compound has demonstrated a protective effect against percutaneous absorption and chemical toxicity. However, the heterogeneous character of the SC, the lipophilicities of the three skin layers, and the physicochemical properties alter chemical penetration. Zhai and Maibach [48] performed an in vivo study evaluating three barrier creams' ability to protect against hydrophilic and lipophilic dyes. The importance of using the appropriate protective formulation was shown as the surface biopsies detecting dye in the skin post barrier cream and dye application proved that one cream was capable of decreasing both dyes from penetrating. Another formulation protected against the lipophilic dye, but not against the hydrophilic dye. The third cream increased the levels of both dyes within the tissue. In a similar in vivo model, Zhai and Maibach [49] also showed the effectiveness of various barrier creams for contact irritant and allergen exposure protection in humans. Therefore, careful selection of an appropriate barrier cream to protect against and not enhance penetration of undesirable chemicals is extremely important.

Chemical Retarders

Penetration retarders promote the SC lipid bilayer to chemically bind more closely and rigidly to increase its barrier potential [23].

Azone is a percutaneous penetration enhancer; however, some of its analogues act as chemical retardants. Hadgraft et al. [14] found that azone and its analogue N-0915 have opposite actions: enhancing and reducing transdermal delivery of dipalmitoylphosphatidylcholine and diethyl *m*-toluamide, respectively. Azone has a larger area per molecule necessitating a "soup spoon" conformation, shifting the charge over its head group. This structure differs from that of typical, more linear permeation retarders. Meanwhile, N-9015 pulls ceramides together by electrostatic interaction [14].

Comparison of In Vitro Stratum Corneum Binding/Partitioning, In Vitro Skin Absorption, and In Vivo Percutaneous Absorption

Comparison of Stratum Corneum/Water Partition Coefficients Between Powdered and Sheet Samples

Powdered SC is prepared with membrane SC containing little lipid. Correlation of the log P SC P/W and log P SC S/W of seven chemicals with different solubilities was performed in one study [35, 36]. The results by chemicals are theophylline (log $P_{SC\ P/W}$–0.91, log $P_{SC\ S/W}$0.66), hydrocortisone (−0.16, 0.98), salicylic acid (0.02, 1.83), atrazine (0.77, 1.57), estradiol (1.23, 2.1), PCB (2.8, 2.3), and acitretin (2.69, 2.4). Figures 2.2, 2.3, and 2.4 show that log P o/w and log P powdered SC/w have the best linear relationship fit (correlation coefficient = 0.99, $p = 0.00001$).

Comparison of p-Nitroaniline Binding to Powdered Stratum Corneum and In Vitro and In Vivo Percutaneous Absorption

Isolated SC is a tool to examine the skin binding and absorption of environmental chemicals that contaminate water. To determine whether it penetrates transdermally, results from in vitro and in vivo percutaneous absorption studies were evaluated for correlation.

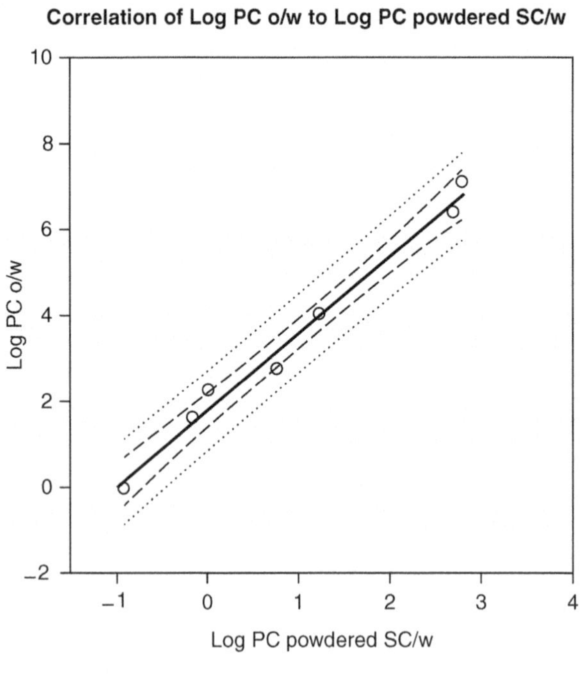

Fig. 2.2 Correlations of log P o/w and log P powdered SC/w in seven model chemicals. Correlation coefficient of log Po/w and log P powdered SC is 0.993, *p*-value 0.00001. (Data were cited with permission from Surbe et al. [35, 36])

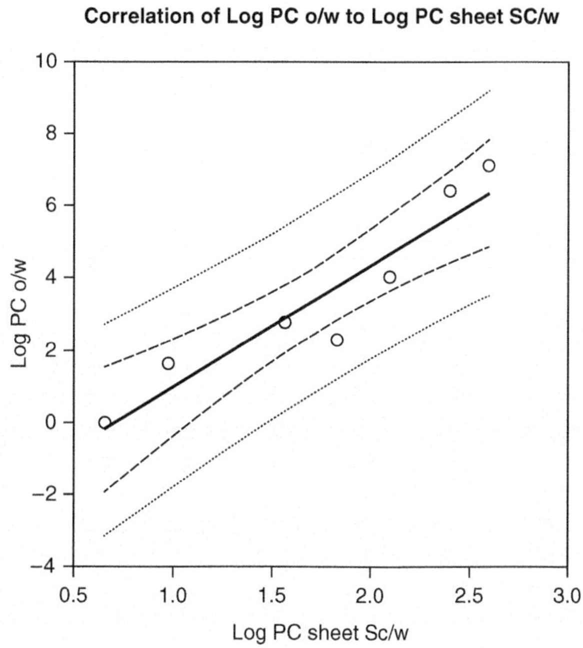

Fig. 2.3 Correlations of log P o/w and log P sheet SC/w in seven model chemicals. Correlation coefficient of log Po/w and log P sheet SC is 0.944, *p*-value 0.00138. (Data were cited with permission from Surber et al. [35, 36])

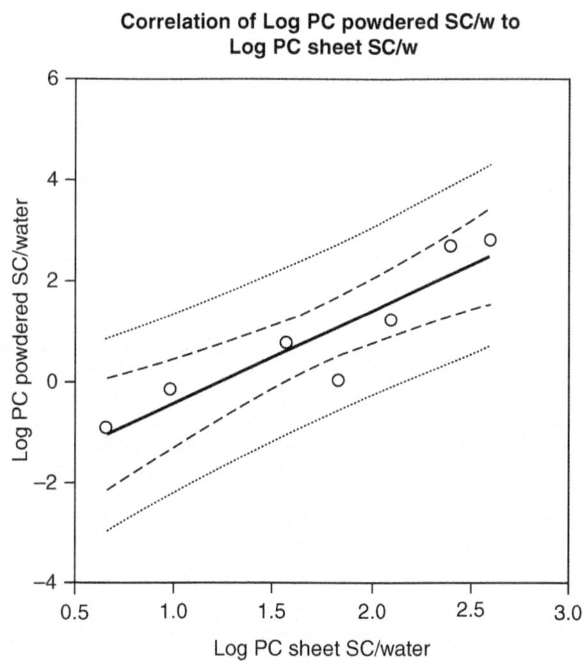

Fig. 2.4 Correlations of log P powdered SC/w and log P sheet SC/w in seven model chemicals. Correlation coefficient of log Po/w and log P sheet SC is 0.922, *p*-value 0.0031. (Data were cited with permission from Surber et al. [35, 36])

The in vivo percutaneous absorption of nitroaniline post 30-minute exposure is 4.1 ± 2.3% of applied dose versus 5.2 ± 1.6% absorbed in vitro through human cadaver skin and 2.5 ± 1.1% bound to human SC P. The values obtained for in vivo absorption, in vitro absorption, and in vitro binding to human SC P of *p*-nitroaniline agree with prior reports [39].

Powdered Stratum Corneum and QSAR Predictive Modeling

To predict chemical partitioning into SC in vitro, most data uses structurally related chemicals or quantitative structure-activity relationships (QSARs) with little focus on structurally unrelated chemicals. Because the range of molecular structure and physico-chemical properties of chemicals is extremely wide, a predictive model must address a broad scope of partitioning behavior [15]. To accomplish this, the partitioning mechanism between SC powder and water was examined. To determine how PC powdered SC/W is affected by chemical concentration, incubation time, and chemical lipophilicity, an in vitro model for predicting dermal exposure to hazardous chemicals was created.

Figure 2.5 shows the relationship between the log P powdered SC/*w* and the log P o/w for a number of chemicals. The lipophilicities and hydrophilicities of

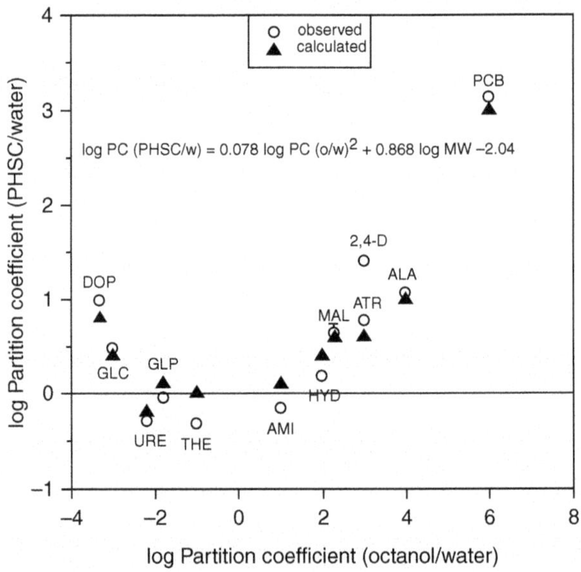

Fig. 2.5 The graph is modified with permission from Hui et al. [29]. Correlation of the logarithm of stratum corneum/water partition coefficients (log PC SC P/w) and logarithm of octanol/water partition coefficients of the 12 test chemicals. The prediction formulation seems nicely to fit the observed values ($r^2 = 0.90$). Open symbols are expressed as observed values and each represented the mean of a test chemical +/− S.D. ($n = 5$). Close symbols expressed as calculated values by Eq. 2.3. DOP dopamine, GLC glycine, URE urea, GLP glyphosate, THE theophylline, AMI aminopyrine, HYD hydrocortisone, MAL malathion, ATR atrazine, 2,4-D 2,4-dichlorophenoxyacetic acid, ALA alachlor, PCB polychlorinated biphenyls

compounds were defined as log PC o/w, larger or smaller than 0, respectively. The logarithms of SC P/water partition coefficients for the lipophilic chemicals were proportional to the logarithms of the octanol and water partition coefficients.

$$\log \text{PC powdered SC} / \text{W} = 0.59 \log \text{PCo} / \text{w} - 0.72 \tag{2.1}$$

$$\text{Student } t \text{ values}: 9.93$$

$$n = 7 \quad r^2 = 0.95 \quad S = 0.26 \quad F = 98.61$$

For the hydrophilic chemicals, the log PC powdered SC/w values are approximately and inversely proportional to log PC o/w.

$$\log \text{PC powdered SC} / \text{w} = -0.60 \log \text{PCo} / \text{w} - 0.27 \tag{2.2}$$

$$\text{Student } T \text{ value}: \quad -4.86$$

$$n = 5 \quad r^2 = 0.88 \quad s = 0.26 \quad F = 23.61$$

However, the overall relationship of the PC powdered SC/w of these chemicals and their PC o/w is nonlinear, as described by the following equation:

$$\log \text{PC powdered SC} / \text{w} = 0.078 \log \text{PCo} / \text{w}^2 + 0.868 \log \text{MW} - 2.04 \tag{2.3}$$

$$\text{Student } T \text{ values}: \quad 8.29 \quad 2.04$$

$$n = 12 \quad r^2 = 0.90 \quad s = 0.33 \quad F = 42.59$$

The logarithm of molecular weight (MW) gave a stronger correlation than MW ($T = 1.55$) alone. The calculated log PC powdered SC/w values are compared to the observed values for these chemicals with the calculated values acceptably close. This implies that this equation could be useful in predicting the in vitro partitioning of important environmental chemicals in P SC [15].

Percutaneous penetration is a complex process with multiple steps related to absorption and excretion kinetics, vehicle characteristics, wash effects, and other steps that each offers insights to better understand penetration, how we can design newer assays, and how we can optimize decontaminants to improve our prognostic estimates and outcomes in those dermally exposed to hazardous chemical agents.

Acknowledgments This publication was supported by the Skin Disease Research Foundation—The San Francisco Foundation.

References

1. Asbill CS, Michniak BB. Percutaneous penetration enhancers: Local versus transdermal activity. Pharm Sci Technol Today. 2000;3:36–41.
2. Barry BW. Structure, function, diseases, and topical treatment of human skin. In: Barry BW, editor. Dermatological formulations: percutaneous absorption. New York: Marcel Dekker; 1983. p. 1–48.
3. Benson HAE. Transdermal drug delivery: penetration enhancement techniques. Curr Drug Deliv. 2005;2:23–33.
4. Braue EH, Doxzon BF, Lumpkin HL, Hanssen KA, Stevenson RS, Deckert RR, Graham JS. Military perspectives in chemical penetration retardation. In: Smith EW, Maibach H, editors. Percutaneous penetration enhancers. 2nd ed: Taylor & Francis Group, LLC; 2006. p. 385–97.
5. Bronaugh RL, Congdon ER. Percutaneous absorption of hair dyes: correlation with partition coefficients. J Invest Dermatol. 1984;83:124–7.
6. Bucks DW, Wester RC, Mobayen MM, Yang D, Maibach HI, Coleman D. In vitro percutaneous absorption and stratum corneum binding of alachlor: effect of formulation dilution with water. Toxicol Appl Pharmacol. 1989;100:417–23.
7. Chadrasekaran SK, Campbell PS, Watanabe T. Application of the 'dual sorption' model to drug transport through skin. Polym Eng Sci. 1980;20(1):36–9.
8. Chan HP, Zhai H, Hui X, Maibach H. Skin decontamination: principles and practices. Toxicol Ind Health. Published online Jul 30, 2012. https://doi.org/10.1177/0748233712448112.
9. Chattaraj SC, Walker RB. Penetration enhancer classification. In: Smith EW, Maibach HI, editors. Percutaneous penetration enhancers. Florida: CRC Press; 1995. p. 5–20.
10. Elias PM. Epidermal lipids, barrier function, and desquamation. J Invest Dermatol. 1983;80:44S–9S.
11. Federal Working Group on Pest Management. Occupational exposure to Pesticides – Report to the Federal Working Group on Pest Management from the Task Group on Occupational Exposure to Pesticides. Washington, D.C.; 1974
12. Franklin SF, Geffner ME. Precocious puberty secondary to topical testosterone exposure. J Pediatr Endocr Metab. 2003;16:107–10.
13. Gogoleva TE, Ademola JI, Wester RC, Magee PS, Maibach HI. Relative contributions of human skin layers to partitioning of chemicals with varying lipophilicity. In: Bronaugh R, Maibach HI, editors. Percutaneous absorption- drugs- cosmetics- mechanism- methodology. 3rd ed. New York; Chapter 26,: Marcel Dekker; 1999. p. 451–62.
14. Hadgraft J, Peck J, Williams DG, Pugh WJ, Allan G. Mechanisms of action of skin penetration enhancers/retarders: azone and analogues. Int J Pharm. 1996;141:17–25.
15. Hui X, Wester RC, Magee P, Maibach HI. Partitioning of chemicals from water into powdered human stratum corneum (callus): a model study. Vitro Toxicol. 1995;8(2):159–67.
16. Hui X, Wester RC, Zhai H, Cashmore AK, Barbadillo S, Maibach HI. Chemical partitioning into powdered human stratum corneum: a useful in vitro model for studying interactions of chemicals and human skin. In: Zhai H, Wilhelm KP, Maibach HI, editors. Marzulli and Maibach's dermatotoxicology. 7th ed. Boca Raton: CRC Press, Taylor and Francis Group; 2008. p. 87–94.
17. Idson B. Vehicle effects in percutaneous absorption. Drug Metab Rev. 1983;14(2):207–22.
18. Kalia YN, Guy RH. Modeling transdermal drug release. Adv Drug Deliv Rev. 2001;48:159–72.
19. Kintz P, Tracqui A, Morgin P. Accidental death caused by the absorption of 2, 4-dichlorophenol through the skin. Arch Toxicol. 1992;66:298–9.
20. McMaster J, Maibach HI, Wester RC, Bucks DAW. Dose rubbing enhance in vivo dermal absorption? In: Bronaugh RL, Maibach HI, editors. Percutaneous absorption, mechanisms – methodology – drug delivery. New York/Basel: Marcel Dekker, Inc; 1985. p. 359–61.

21. Moody RP, Maibach HI. Skin decontamination: importance of the wash-in effect. Food Chem Toxicol. 2006;44(11):1783–8.
22. Noonan PK, Wester RC. Cutaneous metabolism of xenobiotics. In: Bronaugh RL, Maibach HI, editors. Percutaneous Absorption. New York: Marcel Dekker; 1989. p. 53–75.
23. Purdon CH, Smith EW, Surber C, Pellanda C. Assessment of vehicle effects by skin stripping. In: Smith EW, Maibach HI, editors. Percutaneous penetration enhancers. 2nd ed. Florida: CRC Press; 2005. p. 299–309.
24. Quan D, Hui X, Maibach HI. Chemical enhancements of transdermal drug delivery systems: advantages and challenges—Part 1. TransDermal. 2010a;(March):5–10.
25. Quan D, Hui X, Maibach HI. Chemical enhancements of transdermal drug delivery systems: advantages and challenges—Part 2. TransDermal. 2010b;(May):15–20.
26. Raykar PV, Fung MC, Anderson BD. The role of protein and lipid domains in the uptake of solutes of human stratum corneum. Pharm Res. 1988;5(3):140–50.
27. Ross JH, Driver JH, Harris SA, Maibach HI. Dermal absorption of 2,4-D: a review of species differences. Regul Toxicol Pharmacol. 2005;41:82–91.
28. Rougier A, Dupuis D, Lotte C, Roguet R, Wester RC, Maibach HI. Regional variation in percutaneous absorption in man: measurement by the stripping method. Arch Dermatol Res. 1986;278:465–9.
29. Rougier A, Lotte C, Maibach HI. The hairless rat: a relevant animal model to predict in vivo percutaneous absorption in human? J Invest Dermatol. 1987a;88:577–81.
30. Rougier A, Lotte C, Maibach HI. In vivo percutaneous penetration of some organic compounds related to anatomic site in humans: predictive assessment by the stripping method. J Pharm Sci. 1987b;76(6):451–545.
31. Rougier A, Rallis M, Krien P, Lotte C. In vivo percutaneous absorption: a key role for stratum corneum/vehicle partitioning. Arch Dermatol Res. 1990;282:498–505.
32. Schalla W, Jamoulle J, Schaefer H. Localization of compounds in different skin layers and its use as an indicator of percutaneous absorption. In: Bronaugh RL, Maibach HI, editors. Percutaneous absorption. New York: Marcel Dekker; 1989. p. 283–312.
33. Scheuplein RJ, Blank IH. Mechanisms in percutaneous absorption. IV. Penetration of nonelectrolytes (alcohols) from aqueous solutions and from pure liquids. J InvestDermatol. 1973;60(5):286–96.
34. Songkro S. An overview of skin penetration enhancers: penetration enhancing activity, skin irritation potential and mechanism of action. Songklanakarin J Sci Technol. 2009;31(3):299–321.
35. Surber C, Wilhelm KP, Hori M, Maibach HI, Guy RH. Optimization of topical therapy: partitioning of drug into stratum corneum. Pharm Res. 1990a;7(12):1320–4.
36. Surber C, Wilhelm KP, Hori M, Maibach HI, Guy RH. Partitioning of chemicals into human stratum corneum: implications for risk assessment following dermal exposure. Fundam Appl Toxicol. 1990b;15:99–107.
37. Wester RC, Maibach HI. Cutaneous pharmacokinetics: 10 steps to percutaneous absorption. Drug Metab Rev. 1983;14(2):169–205.
38. Wester RC, Bucks DW, Maibach HI, Anderson J. Polychlorinated biphenyls (PCBs): dermal absorption, systemic elimination, and dermal wash efficiency. J Toxicol Environ Health. 1983;12:511–9.
39. Wester RC, Mobayen M, Maibach HI. In vivo and in vitro absorption and binding to powdered stratum corneum as methods to evaluate skin absorption of environmental chemical contaminants from ground and surface water. J Toxicol Environ Health. 1987;21:367–74.
40. Wester RC, Maibach HI, Bucks D, McMaster J, Mobayen M, Sarason R, Moore RP. Percutaneous absorption and skin decontamination of PCBs: in vitro studies with human skin and in vivo studies in the rhesus monkey. J Toxicol Environ Health. 1990;31:235–46.
41. Wester RC, Melendres J, Sarason R, McMaster J, Maibach HI. Glyphosate skin binding, absorption, residual tissue distribution, and skin decontamination. Fundam Appl Toxicol. 1991;16(4):725–32.

42. Wester RC, Maibach HI, Sedik L, Melendres J. Percutaneous absorption of PCBs from soil: In vivo rhesus monkey, in vitro human skin, and binding to powdered human stratum corneum. J Toxicol Environ Health. 1993;39(3):375–82.
43. Wester RC, Melendres J, Logan F, Hui X, Maibach HI. Percutaneous absorption of 2,4-dichlorophenoxyacetic acid from soil with respect to soil load and skin contact time: In vivo absorption in rhesus monkey and in vitro absorption in human skin. J Toxicol Environ Health. 1996;47:335–44.
44. Wester RC, Melendres J, Sedik L, Maibach HI, Riviere J. Percutaneous absorption of salicylic acid, theophylline, 2,4-dimethylamine, diethyl hexyl phthalic acid and p-Aminobenzoic acid in the isolated perfused porcine skin flap compared to man in vivo. Toxicol Appl Pharmacol. 1998;151:19–165.
45. Wester RC, Maibach HI, Hui X, Tanojo H. Progress Report of Environmental Management Science Program (DOE grant #DE-FG07-97ER62509): Bioavailability of organic solvents in soils: input into biologically-based dose-response models for human risk assessment; 1999.
46. Wester RC, Hui X, Maibach HI. In vivo human transfer of topical bioactive drug between individuals: estradiol. J Investig Dermatol. 2006;126:2190–3.
47. Yerasi AB, Butts JD, Butts JD. Disposal of used fentanyl patches. Am J Health Syst Pharm. 1997;54:85–6.
48. Zhai H, Maibach HI. Effect of barrier creams: human skin in vivo. Contact Dermatitis. 1996;35(2):92–6.
49. Zhai H, Maibach HI. Barrier creams – skin protectants: can you protect skin? J Cosmet Dermatol. 2002;1(1):20–3.
50. Zhai H, Chan HP, Hui X, Maibach HI. Skin decontamination of glyphosate from human skin in vitro. Food Chem Toxicol. 2008;46:2258–60.

Chapter 3
Recent Knowledge: Human/Animal Skin Decontamination

Christina Phuong and Howard I. Maibach

Introduction

Humans are constantly exposed to substances of varying toxicities, ranging from chemical warfare agents and pesticides to topical creams and cosmetics of everyday use. Thus, the ability to prevent or slow absorption of these toxicants is vital.

Human skin (HS) provides the first line of defense, functioning as a physical barrier against external agents. Barrier function is primarily due to SC, a multicellular membrane at the uppermost layer of the epidermis [28]. This layer plays an important role in the homeostatic regulation of water in the body as well as controlling skin permeability to external substances [7].

Percutaneous absorption through the SC is a highly complex process composed of at least 15 steps [13, 14]. Skin decontamination is a critical step to mitigate absorption of deleterious toxicants. The scientific and practical knowledge of skin decontamination has been examined previously [6]. Here, more recent highly varied literature (post [6]) is placed into a biological and clinical perspective to elucidate the mechanism and challenges of skin decontamination.

C. Phuong (✉)
Department of Dermatology, University of California, San Francisco, San Francisco, CA, USA

H. I. Maibach
Department of Dermatology, University of California San Francisco, San Francisco, CA, USA
e-mail: howard.maibach@ucsf.edu

H. Zhu, H. I. Maibach (eds.), *Skin Decontamination*,
https://doi.org/10.1007/978-3-030-24009-7_3

Discussion

Diffusion and Partitioning in SC Membrane

SC membrane's complex structure creates an effective, wide-ranging defense system (Table 3.1). Layers of cross-linked corneocytes are embedded within a continuous lipid matrix, composed mainly of free fatty acids, cholesterol, and ceramides, to create a tightly bound cornified envelope [5, 31]. Fluidity of this cornified epithelium results from its water content [3]. Raman spectroscopy revealed water molecules primarily bound to biomolecules of the membrane [8]. The differing properties of these phases regulate the skin's permeability.

Absorption and desorption rates have previously been measured according to diffusion models from a simple two-dimensional homogeneous SC to a brick-and-mortar model considering the lipoidal pathway [15, 18]. However, knowledge of the anatomical heterogeneity complexities of skin demands a more sophisticated model that further breaks down the diffusion and partitioning steps. With the addition of a homogenous epidermal/dermal compartment, the model membrane is represented as three phases, corneocytes, surrounding lipids, and the deep skin layer (DSL). Partition coefficients among these phases, thereby considering $K_{lip/don}$, $K_{DSL/lip}$, and $K_{SC/DSL}$ in addition to simply $K_{SC/don}$, provide more accurate insight into the rate of transport of compounds through skin [11].

Water content has a significant effect on partitioning of substances. For example, flufenamic acid enters the DSL by both binding to proteins and by water of hydration, while caffeine only enters through solvation in water [11]. Thus, partitioning between phases is majorly dependent on the molecule's lipophilicity and hydrophilicity.

In addition, partition and diffusion coefficients heterogeneity exist, as molecules penetrate deeper in the SC [33]. It is suggested that the diffusion gradient results from three distinct layers of the SC with distinct barrier properties. The upper layer allows passive movement of exogenous ions, the middle layer functions in skin hydration and as a selective barrier to specific ions such as K and Cr (VI), while the lower layer defends against different ions such as Cr (III) [16]. Nonetheless, constant coefficients may be used as good predictors of penetrant concentration – depth-profiles, indicating that diffusion and partitioning are coupled such that one may compensate for the other [24].

Attention has increasingly been put on slow desorption kinetics from keratin binding, believed a major drive for the SC reservoir, which results in prolonged existence in the body even after removal of the substance from the skin [29]. Slow

Table 3.1 Abbreviations list

Don	Donor
DSL	Deep skin layer
Lip	Lipid
SC	Stratum corneum

desorption kinetics appear largely related to lipophilicity. Nonlipophilic molecules also accumulate in a reservoir, indicating additional factors involved in this retention [29].

In sum, much progress has been made to determine more accurate parameters that affect rates of diffusion and partitioning of molecules through the SC as well as properties driving formation of an SC reservoir, partly explaining difficulties in decontamination methods and predicting toxicant penetration behavior through SC.

Decontamination in Alternative In Vitro Models

An in vivo HS experiment is an ideal method to study chemical permeation through the skin for accurate risk assessment and decontamination analysis. However, this sometimes proves difficult due to financial, ethical, and safety considerations, as some chemicals are too toxic to be tested in vivo.

Alternative models using excised skins from humans and animals result in generally accepted good correlation with in vivo experiments and can help elucidate factors influencing dermal absorption, but an ideal model to confidently use vitro data as a predictive tool for in vivo behavior does not currently exist [17, 32]. Thus, there is continued exploration of different models that may give further insight into transfer of toxicants across the skin. The potential of using synthetic or natural membranes provides a novel approach toward decontamination studies. In addition, less expensive and more readily accessible models would be advantageous.

In vitro experiments regarding organophosphorus compounds (OPCs) provide insight into important considerations that affect dermal transfer. Frozen HS samples showed that chemical interactions between OPCs and the vehicle of application also affect absorption profiles; thus, the physicochemical properties, such as lipophilicity and vapor pressure, of the vehicle of application must be considered [23].

Recent use of synthetic membranes shed additional light on decontamination and diffusion kinetics of OPCs. Hydrophilic and lipophilic adsorptive powders are able to reduce toxicant transfers across the membrane [19]. Transfer of OPCs also exhibited first order processes, which agrees with in vitro HS experiments; however, synthetic membranes had a significantly less evident initial accumulation period of toxicant [19]. This accumulation period is an important phase of percutaneous absorption, as it reflects the reservoir effect.

Natural membranes such as peach skin, tomato, onion, egg, and cellophane have also been considered as possible alternatives to HS for in vitro studies. They have hydrophilic properties that allow small to middle size hydrophilic drugs to permeate and diffuse in a manner similar to human skin [2]. Extent of similarity for each membrane to HS depends on the specific drug tested, which ranged in lipophilicity and MW [2, 25]. Thus, the physicochemical nature of the drug and membrane are important considerations in understanding diffusion mechanism. These studies promote exploration of possible novel models to be used in chemical penetration experiments and to test decontamination methods.

Challenges to Mass Decontamination Methods

Optimal decontamination procedures are a necessary precaution to any toxic exposure. Use of water and/or detergents are generally considered safe and historically used for mass decontamination for their ease of use and low cost, although risk assessment remains ongoing as progressive insights are made [21].

Passive diffusion is involved in the transfer of toxicants across skin. Compounds prefer to remain in their own physicochemical environment unless there is an external driving force to push compounds into a new environment. Analyzing the solubility within the layers of the skin helps explain diffusion behavior of different substances through the donor fluid to the skin compartment to the receptor fluid. Since the skin compartment is more lipophilic than the donor fluid, diffusion is slower for hydrophilic compounds, so wash off after 6 hours more effectively reduces skin deposition of hydrophilic compounds compared to lipophilic compounds [26]. Moreover, receptor fluid is more hydrophilic than the skin compartment; thus, there is preference for the formation of a skin reservoir for lipophilic compounds [26]. With this understanding, immediate action to reduce the concentration of any substance in the donor fluid will subsequently reduce the amount available in the reservoir and the risk of later entry into the systemic circulation.

Use of water and/or detergents pose risk for a wash in effect, in which percutaneous absorption is enhanced after decontamination attempts with skin washing [22]. Increased skin hydration and the surfactant effect are two of a variety of explanations for the wash in effect [22]. Wet swine skin resulted in an increased amount of permeated paraoxon (pox) compared to dry skin, warm, or cold skin [20]. Moreover, decontamination through showering with the detergent Argos (solution containing, e.g., sodium alkylethersulphate, sodium alkylbenzensulphonate, and cocamide DEA) or FloraFree (mainly consisting of surfactants, e.g., potassium tallate and potassium cocoate) added to the water, regardless the use of physical removals, increased pox permeation [20].

Risks of detergents themselves remain under investigation. Detergents can remove skin lipids, disrupt epidermal barrier function, and are considered permeation enhancers [27, 30]. Furthermore, detergents can include anionic, cationic, nonionic, or zwitterionic surfactants, but a majority are anionic surfactants such as sodium lauryl sulfate (SLS) [4]. Repeated exposure to alkaline agents, including SLS, impairs skin barrier function and reduces natural moisturizing factors (NMF), which are necessary to regulate water balance in the SC [1]. Thus, anionic detergents threaten SC membrane integrity and may enhance risk of irritant contact dermatitis [1].

However, detergents Argos (containing, e.g., sodium alkylethersulphate, sodium alkylbenzesulphonate, and cocamide DEA) and triton X (polyethylene glycol p-(1,1,3,3-etramethylbuyl)-phenyl ether), themselves, did not permeate the skin either as a 5% water solution or as a concentrate [21]. Permeation rate of the detergent althosan MB 50% (50% benzalkonium chloride) as a concentrate, not a 5% water solution, was detectable, although not at an acutely toxic level [21]. Thus, more data are needed to elucidate the toxicity of detergent based mass decontamination.

Disinfectant Wipes to Measure Dermal Absorption

Skin wipes are a useful tool to measure toxicant levels on the skin surface, which provide insight into the potential harm humans are exposed to. For example, lead is a ubiquitous toxic element known to cause development health problems. Surface wipes of floor dust showed lead contamination levels that significantly correlated with blood lead levels in children [10]. Thus, improved measures to decontaminate households from lead-filled dust are necessary.

In addition, concerns of phthalates in indoor dust in China also led to investigation. Phthalates commonly used in many commercial products can cause adverse health effects such as asthma and neurodevelopment problems [12, 34]. Skin wipe samples showed detectable levels of di(isobutyl) phthalate (DiBP), di(n-butyl) phthalate (DnBP), and di(20ethylhexl phthalate (DEHP) in multiple regions of the body [9]. Dermal absorption estimations of these phthalates from the measured skin surface levels represented a significant percent of total phthalate uptake, thereby indicating a need to limit dermal exposure to phthalates [9]. However, due to the complexities of HS, accurate predictions of dermal absorption rates from skin surface concentrations remain difficult. Thus, skin wipes have helped to shed light on the need to limit dermal exposure to phthalates, but a quantified contribution assessment of dermal absorption to total phthalate uptake requires further investigation.

Conclusion

Effective methods of skin decontamination are critical to mitigate the percutaneous absorption of deleterious toxicants into the body. More data show the complexities of diffusion across the SC and the importance of the water component. Furthermore, increased investigation shows the potential harm of decontamination methods used today. While in vivo HS experiments are preferred, alternative models are still being designed for efficiency, cost effectiveness, and ethical concerns. These recent data findings update the available knowledge pertaining to decontamination and its challenges.

References

1. Angelova-Fischer I, Dapic I, Hoek AK, Jakasa I, Fischer TW, Zillikens D, Kezic S. Skin barrier integrity and natural moisturising factor levels after cumulative dermal exposure to alkaline agents in atopic dermatitis. Acta Derm Venereol. 2014;64:640–4.
2. Ansari M, Kazemipour M, Aklamli M. The study of drug permeation through natural membranes. Int J Pharm. 2006;327:6–11.
3. Blank IH. Factors which influence the water content of the stratum corneum. J Invest Dermatol. 1952;18:433–40.
4. Skin decontamination of chemical exposures. Cincinnati: National Institute for Occupational Health and Safety; 2005.

5. Bouwstra JA, Dubbelaar FER, Gooris GS, Weerheim AM, Ponec M. The role of ceramide composition in the lipid organisation of the skin barrier. Biochim Biophys Acta. 1999;1419:127–36.
6. Chan HP, Zhai H, Hui X, Maibach HI. Skin decontamination: principles and perspectives. Toxicol Ind Health. 2012;29:955–68.
7. Elias PM, Cooper ER, Korc A, Brown BE. Percutaneous transport in relation to stratum corneum structure and lipid composition. J Invest Dermatol. 1981;76:297–301.
8. Gniadecka M, Faurskov Nielsen O, Christensen DH, Wulf HC. Structure of water, proteins, and lipids in intact human skin, hair, and nail. J Invest Dermatol. 1998;110:393–8.
9. Gong M, Zhang Y, Weschler CJ. Measurement of phthalates in skin wipes: estimating exposure from dermal absorption. Environ Sci Technol. 2014;48:7428–35.
10. Gulson B, Anderson P, Taylor A. Surface dust wipes are the best predictors of blood leads in young children with elevated blood lead levels. Environ Res. 2013;126:171–8.
11. Hansen S, Henning A, Naegel A, Heisig M, Witum G, Neumann D, Kostka KH, Zbytovska J, Lehr CM, Schaefer UF. In-silico model of skin penetration based on experimentally determined input parameters. Part I: experimental determination of partition and diffusion coefficients. Eur J Pharm Biopharm. 2008;68:352–67.
12. Hsu NY, Lee CC, Wang JY, Li YC, Chang HW, Chen CY, Bornehag CG, Wu PC, Sundell J, Su HJ. Predicted risk of childhood allergy, asthma, and reported symptoms using measured phthalate exposure in dust and urine. Indoor Air. 2012;22:186–99.
13. Hui X, Lamel S, Qiao P, Maibach HI. Isolated human/animal stratum corneum as a partial model for 15 steps in percutaneous absorption: emphasizing decontamination, part I. J Appl Toxicol. 2013a;33:157–72.
14. Hui X, Lamel S, Qiao P, Maibach HI. Isolated human and animal stratum corneum as a partial model for the 15 steps of percutaneous absorption: emphasizing decontamination, part II. J Appl Toxicol. 2013b;33:173–82.
15. Johnson ME, Blankschtein D, Langer R. Evaluation of solute permeation through the stratum corneum: lateral bilayer diffusion as the primary transport mechanism. J Pharm Sci. 1997;86:1162–72.
16. Kubo A, Ishizaki I, Kubo A, Kawasaki H, Nagao K, Ohashi Y, Amagai M. The stratum corneum comprises three layers with distinct metal-ion barrier properties. Sci Rep. 2013;3:1731.
17. Leo MS, MS HIM. Percutaneous absorption. In: Vinod SP, Maibach HI, Jenner J, editors. Topical drug bioavailability, bioequivalence, and penetration. New York: Springer; 1993. p. 3–19.
18. Manitz R, Lucht W, Strehmel K, Weiner R, Neubert R. On mathematical modeling of dermal and transdermal drug delivery. J Pharm Sci. 1998;87:873–9.
19. Mircioiu C, Voicu VA, Ionescu M, Miron DS, Radulescu FS, Nicolescu AC. Evaluation of in vitro absorption, decontamination and desorption of organophosphorous compounds from skin and synthetic membranes. Toxicol Lett. 2013;219:99–106.
20. Misik J, Pavlikova R, Josse D, Cabal J, Kuca K. In vitro skin permeation and decontamination of the organophosphorus pesticide paraoxon under various physical conditions-evidence for a wash-in effect. Toxicol Mech Methods. 2012a;22:520–5.
21. Misik J, Pavlikova R, Cabal J, Josse D, Kuca K. In vitro skin permeation of detergents and detergent-based decontamination mixture. Mil Med Sci Lett. 2012b;81:96–9.
22. Moody RP, Maibach HI. Skin decontamination: importance of the wash-in effect. Food Chem Toxicol. 2016;44:1783–8.
23. Moore CA, Wilkinson SC, Blain PG, Dunn M, Aust GA, Williams FM. Percutaneous absorption and distribution of organophosphates (chlorpyrifos and dichlorvos) following dermal exposure and decontamination scenarios using in vitro human skin model. Toxicol Lett. 2014;229:66–72.
24. Naegel A, Hansen S, Neumann D, Lehr CM, Schaefer UF, Wittum G, Heisig M. In-silico model of skin penetration based on experimentally determined input parameters. Part II: mathematical modelling of in-vitro diffusion experiments. Identification of critical input parameters. Eur J Pharm Biopharm. 2008;68:368–79.

25. Nawale R, Mayee R. Behavior of natural membrane on drug permeation. Int J Pharm Innov. 2013;3:45–54.
26. Nielsen JB. Efficacy of skin wash on dermal absorption: an in vitro study on four model compounds of varying solubility. Int Arch Occup Environ Health. 2010;83:683–90.
27. Okuda M, Yoshiike T, Ogawa H. Detergent-induced epidermal barrier dysfunction and its prevention. J Dermatol Sci. 2012;30:173–9.
28. Scheuplein RJ. Permeability of the skin. Handbook of physiology, reactions to environmental agents. Baltimore: Waverly Press Inc; 1975. p. 299–322.
29. Seif S, Hansen S. Measuring the stratum corneum reservoir: desorption kinetics from keratin. J Pharm Sci. 2012;101:3718–28.
30. Shokri J, Nokhodchi A, Dashbolaghi A, Hassan-Zadeh D, Ghafourian R, Barzegar-Jalali M. The effect of surfactants on the skin penetration of diazepam. Int J Pharm. 2001;228:99–107.
31. Swartzendruber DC, Wertz PW, Madison KC, Downing DT. Evidence that the corneocyte has a chemically bound lipid envelope. J Invest Dermatol. 1987;88:709–13.
32. Vallet V, Cruz C, Josse D, Bazire A, Lallement G, Boudry I. In vitro percutaneous penetration of organophosphorus compounds using full-thickness and split-thickness pig and human skin. Toxicol in vitro. 2007;21:1182–90.
33. Watkinson AC, Bunge AL, Hadgraft J, Naik A. Computer simulation of penetrant concentration-depth profiles in the stratum corneum. Int J Pharm. 1992;87:175–82.
34. Whyatt RM, Liu X, Rauh VA, Calafat AM, Just AC, Hoepner L, Diaz D, Quinn J, Adibi J, Perera FP, Factor-Litvak P. Maternal prenatal urinary phthalate metabolite concentrations and child mental, psychomotor, and behavioral development at 3 years of age. Environ Health Perspect. 2012;120:290–5.

Chapter 4
Decontamination of Chemically Contaminated Remains

Jill A. Harvilchuck, Dan Noort, Glenn Lawson, Kelly Kyburz, Miranda Verschraagen, and Alison Director-Myska

Introduction

"Our government has a solemn promise, and it's a sacred trust…We will not forget our fallen heroes. We will recover them. We will bring them home…A mother never forgets her son. The tears are as real today as they were 50 years ago. That was her son, and he was lost in combat, and she wants him home." These words were spoken by a senior US Department of Defense (DoD) official [1] in 2004 to the families of unaccounted-for service members from America's past conflicts. Twelve years later, this somber reality continues to inspire experts within the US DoD to keep our solemn vow and underwrite for all warfighters the ethos that they "will never leave a fallen comrade." However, the challenges of keeping that promise are significantly more complex if the fallen hero perished after being contaminated with a chemical, biological, or radiological agent. Despite the myriad of obstacles, dedicated US DoD stakeholders continue to collaborate on developing a strategy, informed by scientific studies, to repatriate contaminated human remains while managing the safety of handlers and transporters and mitigating the risk to public health.

J. A. Harvilchuck (✉)
Battelle Memorial Institute, Columbus, OH, USA
e-mail: harvilchuckj@battelle.org

D. Noort
TNO Defence, Security and Safety, Rijswijk, The Netherlands

G. Lawson · A. Director-Myska
Defense Threat Reduction Agency, Ft. Belvoir, VA, USA

K. Kyburz
Office of the Assistant Secretary of the Army for Manpower and Reserve Affairs, Pentagon, Washington, DC, USA

M. Verschraagen
Netherlands Forensic Institute, The Hague, The Netherlands

H. Zhu, H. I. Maibach (eds.), *Skin Decontamination*,
https://doi.org/10.1007/978-3-030-24009-7_4

This chapter will provide a brief history of the US DoD's efforts to establish a capability to repatriate chemically contaminated human remains. It will address current doctrine and gaps and explain current research studies conducted by the US DoD to determine the residual toxic hazards and postmortem risks of chemically contaminated remains. Implications of the study results on operational concepts and procedures will be addressed, and recommendations for future studies will be suggested.

History of Chemically Contaminated Remains

The US military, as well as the international community, has not yet effectuated the daunting task of repatriating chemically contaminated remains from an overseas theater to the continental United States or home country. The historical usage of chemical weapons against US service members in previous wars overwhelmed mortuary affairs capacity and eventuated in the institution of American cemeteries overseas. However, that is no longer considered an acceptable option for bringing closure to the families of America's fallen warfighters. The expectation within the United States is a commitment to ensuring that our fallen heroes return to American soil with honor and dignity, and this has become firmly ingrained in our national psyche. Since September 11, 2001, "a 'new normal' has changed expectations and approaches to caring for the deceased and their families"[2]. As a result, the intent to safely return the remains of service members who have been chemically contaminated to their families is of paramount importance for the US DoD.

The complexities of such an undertaking are immense.To safely conduct the repatriation process, significant regulatory and policy constraints must be adhered to across many jurisdictions. In 2003, the Deputy Secretary of Defense published a policy [3] that required the US DoD to intercontaminate human remains in the theater of operations until a safe means of transporting them back to the continental United States was established. The updated US DoD policy [4], which was published in 2015, now allows for temporary storage or interment of US DoD-affiliated contaminated human remains until the remains can be returned safely through routine mortuary channels.

Current Doctrine and Gaps

While mortuary affairs is a logistics function, safe repatriation of contaminated remains requires integrated activities in the theater of operations between medical, mortuary affairs, chemical, biological, radiological, and nuclear (CBRN) defense, transportation specialists, and the medical examiner. Current logistics doctrine provides for a theater-level mortuary affairs contaminated remains mitigation site (MACRMS) where personnel from various disciplines coalesce to reduce the contamination hazard from exposure to the remains, collect information to provide a scientific identification for the decedent, and place the remains into a package that allows for safe handling during evacuation and transportation to the United States [5]. The integrated MACRMS mission is focused on avoiding second-order contamination effects throughout the repatriation process. Primary functions within the MACRMS include maintaining a chain of custody of the remains, preserving forensic evidence, mitigating the contamination hazard, collecting specimens for positive identification, preparing remains for evaluation, and packaging the remains in a containment system for eventual evacuation to and throughout the United States for final disposition. The medical examiner conducts only a limited postmortem examination at the MACRMS, and there is no embalming on chemically contaminated human remains (C-CHR) at any point. The safety of the MACRMS staff and other personnel who may come in contact with the remains takes priority over the rapid repatriation of the C-CHR.

An enduring capability to repatriate C-CHR requires materiel and nonmateriel solutions. While interim equipment systems have been developed since 2002, the need for approved and fielded equipment systems for the end-to-end capability persists. The MACRMs mission is untested, and procedures have only been developed and validated for a limited number of contaminants. Additionally, service members handling contaminated remains must have appropriate protection during every phase of the repatriation process. Past efforts at identifying equipment requirements determined the need for a contaminated remains recovery pouch, a remains decontamination system to be used at the MACRMS, and a contaminated remains transportation package. Recent efforts have suggested that the requirement for other possible materiel solutions to provide protection during intratheater evacuation to the MACRMS may also exist. Additionally, there is a need for more research on alternatives for low-level chemical contamination detectors, indicators, and decontaminants.

Nonmateriel gaps include shortfalls in current doctrine, which does not adequately address CHR decontamination guidelines when there are multiple contaminants. Moreover, guidelines for decontaminating remains prior to emplacing them into the recovery pouch for hasty burial, temporary storage, or temporary interment need to be further developed. Similarly, doctrinal guidelines to address how to transport CHR from the incident site and/or contaminated casualty collection site to the MACRMS must be developed. Due to the dynamic nature of the CBRN effects on the battlefield and the resultant time lag for standing up an incident-specific MACRMS capability, the US DoD should determine how the decomposition effects due to hasty burial, temporary storage, or temporary interment affect the efficacy of MACRMS operations. Processes for collection and disposition of decontamination waste products at the MACRMS require further development as well.

Other nonmateriel gaps include necessary policies, processes, and procedures to support the return of contaminated remains which have been rendered safe through mitigation and/or containment. Effective protocols are dependent upon the engineering standards of the transportation package that will be developed. In the absence of a CHR transportation package that meets stringent international and federal HAZMAT packaging requirements, the US DoD has been unable to provide specific recommendations to ensure safe and satisfactory final disposition of CHR within the United States. Currently, the US DoD is testing a transportation package which may be an acceptable solution to use for certain C-CHR. Based on the progress made to date in the development of this containment system, the US DoD is able to move forward with coordination between joint, interagency, intergovernmental, and industry stakeholder organizations to develop business practices that can be used as benchmarks during specific instances to transport C-CHR across jurisdictions within the United States and to meet safe and effective standards for final disposition consistent with the laws, policies, and regulations.

The US DoD's commitment to treating the deceased and their families with the "utmost compassion, respect, professionalism, and dignity throughout the casualty and mortuary, and medical examiner processes" [2] requires that these issues be addressed as expeditiously as possible. Unresolved issues include the need to develop a strategic messaging plan that addresses requirements for nonviewability and direct burial, the need to develop training packets for C-CHR casualty notification and assistance officers and military escorts, and the need to determine if special information briefings for families would be beneficial. The US DoD must determine the requirements for transportation markings and labeling for the C-CHR containment package, develop technical escort protocols for airlift, establish contracts for transportation of the C-CHR within the United States, and determine communication processes to facilitate information exchange throughout the repatriation process. The US DoD should identify potential federal cemeteries that would enter C-CHR and address the possibility of exceptions to eligibility criteria. Other disposition options for families also need to be explored (e.g., interment in private or state cemeteries and cremation). Procedures for burial in a cemetery must be identified. For example, cemeteries may require cement vaults, special markings, and/or periodic monitoring. Finally, the US DoD should determine cremation standards for the C-CHR and the containment package, identify approved cremation facilities, and coordinate contracts to ensure compliance with the existing US DoD standards for cremation.

To develop effective protocols, the US DoD needs to also explore opportunities to resolve gaps in science and technology. The lack of clearance levels specifically for contaminated human remains necessitates the containment of the hazard in a safe package. Until a determination can be made that exposed remains can be considered decontaminated to a safe level, commanders will need to know when and how to categorize chemically exposed remains as C-CHR. In addition to further studies to determine the distribution and persistency of the hazards associated with different agents, there is a need for investigating the effects of certain decontaminants on the distribution and persistence of hazards from different agents on and within the remains to determine both the short-term risks to handlers and transporters and the long-term risks to public health. Development of additional decontaminants that reduce water requirements and waste would be beneficial. Research efforts to determine if there is a point at which decontamination operations should not be done or if large volumes of decontaminants (spray or submersion) can be used to reduce processing time for CHR should be done in the future. Processes for dealing with contaminated personal effects disposition and regulated medical waste must also be informed by scientific studies.

Current Research

Background

To date, little research has been done to support the decontamination or safe handling of C-CHR. Instead, research efforts have mainly focused on the protection against exposure to chemical warfare agents (CWAs) and therapy to increase the survivability of victims after a CWA exposure. However, after a severe intoxication, chances are profound that victims will not survive, despite aggressive treatment. During the handling of CHR and personal effects, the agent may still be present on the skin, in bodily fluids or tissues, or on/in personal effects and may pose a contact and inhalation hazard to unprotected personnel. Agents may be present for a longer period of time in human remains compared to living human beings due to the postmortem changes of physiological processes that influence the biological and chemical fate of the agents.

The presence of toxic agents on or inside the body of deceased victims, as well as on their clothes, poses a threat to (unprotected) personnel handling the remains. Several (civil) cases are known from history, in which handling contaminated victims leads to intoxication of rescuers. For example, in 1943, German bombers attacked ships in the harbor of Bari, including one which was carrying sulfur mustard. Rescuers were unaware that they were dealing with sulfur mustard casualties, and many additional victims were caused among the rescuers by contact with the contaminated skin and clothing of victims.

Additionally, secondary exposure of ambulance personnel and medical personnel also took place after the terrorist attack in the Tokyo subway with sarin gas in 1995. Secondary exposure took place because victims were not decontaminated and their outer clothing was not removed before transportation to hospitals, personnel did not wear adequate protection, and ambulances were not ventilated. Thus, 135 ambulance workers [6] and 110 members of the medical staff [7] became intoxicated. It has been assumed that the secondary exposure resulted from off-gassing of sarin from the clothing of victims [6, 8]. No information was found on the off-gassing from the bodies of (deceased) victims.

The 1994 sarin attack in Matsumoto also led to the contamination of rescuers, but this was probably due to direct contamination on-site, rather than secondary effects. The severity of intoxication was directly related to the time after the incident at which the rescuers arrived [9].

It has been estimated that 80% of the contamination will be present on the clothing of victims after a chemical incident. Contaminated clothing and/or outer gear should be removed from the body as soon as possible to reduce the risk of secondary contamination. These contaminated items will present both a contact and inhalation hazard. Especially porous materials, such as rubber, are known to absorb CWAs, leading to a prolonged hazard. Obviously, the hazard of contaminated clothing is also relevant in the case of surviving victims.

The secondary hazard from decontaminated human remains may seem less important than the hazard from contaminated clothing. However, after removal of clothing and decontamination of skin and hair, the hazard may not be completely removed as deceased victims may continue to emit fluids or gases after decontamination. A vapor concentration may build up when a body has been temporarily stored in a refrigerated body bag or coffin at a morgue or temporary site. After opening the coffin at room temperature, e.g., for autopsy examination, the vapor may be released and pose an unexpected hazard.

An essential tool for the determination of the actual hazard of CHR and personal effects is the use of effective chemical agent monitors. This handheld detection equipment responds to the presence of vaporized agents and is required for ongoing detection, identification, and monitoring of human remains to detect the presence of hazards [10]. It is vital that the current detection equipment be able to detect low-level concentrations of vapor from all CWAs.

The expected hazard will depend on the type of CWA. For sulfur mustard, the contact and evaporation hazards are equally important. VX is known to be a slowly evaporating CWA. It was recently confirmed that the agent poses a greater contact hazard than an evaporation hazard [11]. On the other hand, sarin is known to evaporate rapidly. The agent poses an inhalation hazard, but only for a short period of time since the agent is rapidly fully evaporated. It is anticipated that the hazard of sarin will be more significant on contaminated clothing materials than on human remains.

Biological Fate of CWAs in Healthy Humans

The distribution and metabolism of CWAs in living organisms have been studied extensively. After exposure, agents will be absorbed, distributed, metabolized, and excreted, depending on the route of administration. Some useful data were obtained from experiments on human volunteers in the 1940s and 1950s [12–14], as well as from extensive toxicokinetic studies on laboratory animals [15–17].

The biological fate of nerve agents is relatively simple [18–21]. The predominant process consists of hydrolysis (either spontaneous or enzymatic) to relatively non-toxic phosphonic acids that are readily excreted in urine. In addition to binding to its physiological target acetylcholinesterase, scavenging by butyrylcholinesterase (BuChE), carboxylesterase (CaE), and even albumin has been well documented [22]. The metabolism of sulfur mustard is complex, among other things, because of the agent's bifunctional alkylating character, resulting in a wide range of mixed hydrolysis/oxidation products and glutathione-derived conjugates in various oxidation stages, DNA adducts, and cancer. Also, an extensive binding to proteins occurs [18–20, 23].

Enzymatic activities and hydrolysis rates of CWAs in plasma and tissue homogenates have been well documented. These data were used to develop a physiologically based pharmacokinetic (PBPK) model to predict the toxicokinetics of nerve agents in intoxicated (living) human beings [17, 24].

Postmortem Biological Fate of CWAs

After death, physiological processes start to change rapidly, many of which will have an effect on the biological and chemical fate of CWAs. When a victim dies slowly, some changes may start even before death (such as a reduced blood circulation and a change in percutaneous uptake). It is anticipated that CWAs will remain present in their parent form for a longer period of time in human remains compared to healthy human beings, because of the slowed or terminated processes of natural detoxification. On the other hand, certain biochemical mechanisms may be activated following death which may enhance the destruction of CWAs.

It is important to understand the postmortem physiological changes that are likely to occur when investigating the hazard remaining on chemically contaminated human remains. The following changes are likely to affect the potential hazard postmortem:

- The transportation of agent through the body by the blood circulation stops immediately after death. As a result, metabolism of the agent by the liver ceases.
- The body temperature gradually cools from 37 °C to ambient temperature (*algor mortis*).
- Gradual muscular stiffening (*rigor mortis*) will occur approximately 6 hours after death and is caused by a physicochemical change in muscle protein.
- Postmortem decomposition of the soft tissues (putrefaction) by enzymes and bacteria starts between 36 and 72 hours after death, depending on external factors such as outside temperature, location of body (e.g., in the water), etc. Putrefaction starts in the anterior abdominal wall and results in the gradual dissolution of all tissues into gases, liquids, and salts.
- Saponification is the hydrolysis of fatty tissues with the release of free fatty acids. This process starts within weeks after death at room temperature.
- Postmortem redistribution of the agent may occur throughout the body. Immediately after death, blood circulation is terminated. Still, agent concentrations in body fluids and organs may change, similar to drugs, due to postmortem redistribution [25]. Agents may be redistributed from "reservoir" organs such as the gastrointestinal tract, liver, and lungs to surrounding tissues. This may occur immediately after death by diffusion through blood vessels and transparietal diffusion toward the surrounding organs.
- Postmortem scavenging by enzymes and proteins may still continue to occur, although to a limited extent. Natural detoxification of nerve agents occurs by

binding to scavenging enzymes. The total amount of available enzyme (BuChE and CaE) is normally limited to about 60 nM in human blood. Victims that succumbed to a lethal dose of nerve agent will have enzyme activity levels that approach zero and detoxification by scavenging to these enzymes is no longer possible. Some enzyme activity may still be present, if there has been an alternate cause of death (e.g., the blast of an explosion) in addition to a nerve agent intoxication. Although enzyme activity will decrease in time due to the decrease in temperature, it has been shown that cholinesterase activity levels in the postmortem blood of nonintoxicated patients were almost identical to those in serum samples from healthy controls [26]. However, in the case of nerve agent exposure, it is estimated that postmortem scavenging will play a limited role in detoxification when it is assumed that the received dosage will be far higher than the amount of available binding sites. Nonetheless, binding to sites with less affinity (e.g., the tyrosine-411 residue in albumin) might occur under these conditions. In the case of sulfur mustard, alkylation of proteins (e.g., hemoglobin and albumin) and DNA will contribute to the postmortem detoxification of this agent.

- Postmortem metabolism of CWA is expected to occur, but at a much slower rate, due to the decrease in body temperature and the cessation of liver metabolism. It has been shown that the decomposition of organophosphate pesticides continues postmortem [27]. Nerve agents will be detoxified by spontaneous and enzymatic hydrolysis, whereas sulfur mustard will undergo hydrolysis and oxidation. In addition, alternative, yet unknown degradation pathways may arise, e.g., by bacteria during putrefaction. In general, metabolism leads to agent detoxification, but it cannot be excluded that under postmortem conditions, metabolism may be incomplete or slightly altered and consequently might give rise to the formation of toxic reaction products, such as desethyl-VX (EA2192) in the case of VX and mustard sulfone in the case of sulfur mustard. Many factors play a role during postmortem agent degradation. The process is complex and is expected to be slow, especially for the more persistent agents. This was shown, for example, by the reported presence of unmetabolized sulfur mustard in postmortem tissue samples from Iranian victims [28, 29].

Current Research

There have only been two major studies performed in recent years, both funded by the Defense Threat Reduction Agency (DTRA), which investigated the hazard remaining on chemically contaminated remains. Both studies were designed as first steps to fill the knowledge gap surrounding this topic and provide information into the hazard to personnel handling chemically contaminated remains.

Guinea Pig Contaminated Remains Hazard (VX, Sulfur Mustard)

In the first study, performed by TNO in the Netherlands, the biological and chemical fate of a number of CWAs [VX and sulfur mustard (HD)] was determined in euthanized and CWA-contaminated hairless guinea pigs. Both the residual contact and inhalation hazards were determined through 96 hours following contamination and euthanasia (30 min after contamination). Animals were contaminated with eight 1-μL drops of liquid VX (>100 percutaneous LD_{50}) or HD (<1 percutaneous LD_{50}). Additionally, animals were exposed to a whole-body vapor exposure of HD, and the residual vapor and contact hazard were evaluated.

In VX-contaminated hairless guinea pigs, it was determined that the amount of VX on the skin decreased gradually but was still present after 96 hours at levels between 20 and 90 μg/cm^2. VX levels in the blood were also determined through 22 hours, with levels remaining fairly constant (low ng/ml range) over time. VX was determined to be present at much higher levels in the liver (up to 7 μg/g liver) than in the blood, especially after 5 hours, which might be an indication of agent redistribution. The metabolism of VX into its hydrolysis product, EMPA, could only be analyzed in liver samples at variable levels (2–200 ng/mL), which was in agreement with the high and variable VX concentrations found in the liver. The toxic metabolite of VX (desethyl VX; EA2192; V27A) was only found in one of the blood and liver samples, and it was at extremely low levels (0.2 ng/mL).

In HD-contaminated hairless guinea pigs, HD on the skin was found to not be very persistent after death, when at ambient room temperature. Approximately 3 hours after application (2.5 hours after death), HD could no longer be detected on the skin using tape stripping. In the blood, intact HD could be detected through the last blood sampling time point (23 hours post death), with levels gradually decreasing from 20 to 3 ng/ml. In the liver, HD was detected for up to 48 hours post-death (up to 25 ng/g liver) following contamination, with gradually decreasing levels. Sulfur mustard in the liver was detected at much lower levels than VX in the liver, probably reflecting the much higher intrinsic reactivity of sulfur mustard compared to VX. The vapor hazard from these remains was most pronounced in the first 24 hours after death, with amounts of off-gassed HD up to 500 μg/h. However, when liquid HD was applied to hairless guinea pigs at low temperatures (5–7 °C), agent levels in the blood and liver were significantly higher than those found at ambient temperatures. This might be caused by a lower reactivity of the agent at lower temperatures, and/or because more agent had penetrated the skin. The latter explanation is in agreement with the decreased off-gassing observed during the initial (0.5–1 hours) postexposure time period, immediately following contamination. Also, it seems that cooling of the remains prolongs the process of off-gassing.

The relatively nontoxic sulfur mustard metabolite, sulfur mustard sulfoxide, was found in the blood of the remains of hairless guinea pigs, after percutaneous contamination with sulfur mustard. In addition, protein adduct formation was determined by mass spectrometric analysis of a cysteine sulfur mustard adduct, after pronase digestion of whole blood. Similar adduct formation has been observed under normal in vivo conditions. From a practical point of view, it is worthwhile to note that the detection equipment appears to respond at later time points (> 72 hours post death), probably because of natural putrefaction products which are formed after death.

Hairless guinea pigs that were exposed to whole-body HD vapor (applied dose 10,000 mg.min.m^{-3}, 250 mg.m^{-3} during 40 min) had, as expected, much lower levels (up to 0.04 μg/cm^2) of HD on the skin compared to those found following a liquid exposure. The vapor hazard levels were also found to be lower (up to 7 μg/h off-gassed HD) than that compared to a liquid exposure. However, the internal levels of free HD (as measured in blood and liver) were of the same order of magnitude as found following a percutaneous liquid exposure.

Swine Contaminated Remains Hazard (VX)

In a study performed by Battelle (Columbus, OH, USA), the contact and inhalation hazard remaining on VX-contaminated Yorkshire swine was determined through 1 week post-death (unpublished data). To mimic a more realistic situation, the remains were stored at room temperature following death for approximately 24 hours prior to decontamination. Cold storage conditions (1.1° to 4.4 °C) were used after 24 hours post-death to mimic the procedures and storage conditions likely to be followed by the US Mortuary Affairs in the event C-CHR would need to be processed. Half of the animals were nondecontaminated controls, and half of the animals were decontaminated in accordance with the US MACRMS Protocol, to determine the effectiveness of the current US MACRMS Protocol against a gross VX contamination.

The contact and inhalation hazard remaining on female weanling Yorkshire swine due to a gross VX contamination was determined through 1 week post-death. In addition, the rinsate used as part of the decontamination process was collected and sampled for parent compound and EA2192, a toxic metabolite of VX, to determine the hazard that would be present in the run-off fluids during the decontamination process.

Deeply anesthetized animals were exposed to approximately 9.5 mL neat VX (purity of 96.3%, provided by Edgewood Chemical Biological Center) percutaneously on the ventral abdomen. Although the application of 9.5 mL of VX (approximately 9.5 grams) on a swine for the purposes of determining the contamination hazard of remains may seem extreme, the purpose of this study was to mimic a worst-case scenario that would be found on a battlefield as closely as possible in order to provide relevant information that would inform the tactics, techniques, and procedures (TTPs) on safe handling and decontamination of chemically contaminated remains. In 2004, 155-mm artillery shells were found in Iraq that contained 3–4 L of sarin. A service member that was near "ground zero" during an explosion of one of these shells would easily be expected to be exposed to the quantities used on this study (9.5 mL), and possibly more. Additionally, in a technical report produced by the US Army, it was estimated that a worst-case scenario for contamination of remains would be 200 grams per man following exposure to a "puddle" of agent, and contamination due to a tactical ballistic missile attack with VX would be approximately 2–6 grams per man (Papirmeisteret al., 1993). As a result, the 9.5 grams of VX used in this study provided a reasonable potential exposure for a service member near the site of the attack and potentially a worst-case scenario for decontamination.

Due to the large volume of neat agent that was used, the surface area of the swine abdomen was not large enough to prevent run-off of excess agent. As a result, an unknown amount of agent rolled off the side of the animals, resulting in an overall contamination of less than 9.5 mL of neat VX. Animals remained anesthetized through death. Following death, the remains were kept at room temperature for 24 hours and were either transferred to containment boxes without decontamination or were decontaminated and then transferred to containment boxes for storage at 1.1° to 4.4 °C.

The following procedure was performed for remains that were decontaminated in accordance with the US MACRMS Protocol:

- The remains were washed with warm, soapy water using a soft sponge.
- Remains were then rinsed with 750 mL of room temperature tap water. A sample of this rinsate was collected and analyzed for the contact hazard of VX and EA2192 that would remain.
- Following the soapy water scrub and rinse, the remains were placed in a 5% sodium hypochlorite solution (pH >11; temperature between 20 and 25 °C) for 60 minutes. (Note: It is important for VX to be decontaminated with a pH less than 7 or greater than 10. Between pH 7-10, toxic metabolites of VX are likely to form.)
- After a 60-minute soak in the hypochlorite solution, the remains were transferred to a room temperature rinse water bath for 5 minutes.
- Following decontamination, remains were then placed in cold storage as detailed above.

The contact and inhalation hazards were determined immediately following transfer to containment boxes at 24 hours, while the remains were at room temperature (and after decontamination, as appropriate). Additionally, the contact and inhalation hazards were determined at 72, 120, and 168 hours post-death, during which time the remains were still cool from having been removed stored in the CSU.

Following death, the remains remained at room temperature for approximately 24 hours prior to decontamination and/or cold storage. As expected, significant bloating was noted along with the expelling of liquid from the mouth and nose of the remains during this time. The bloating of the remains proved problematic for those that were decontaminated. The thinness of the skin due to the bloating resulted in tears following the 60-minute 5% sodium hypochlorite decontamination, leading to exposed muscle and organs.

Inhalation Hazard of Remains

On average, the VX inhalation hazard remaining following a gross contamination decreased over time and was lower in remains that had been decontaminated. The US Army has provided guidance regarding the short-term exposure limit (STEL; 15-minute exposure limit that should never be exceeded) and the immediately dangerous to life and health (IDLH) limits for human exposure to nerve agents [30]. Although the greatest hazard was immediately following death when the remains were at room temperature prior to decontamination (169 times greater than IDLH), nondecontaminated remains 1 week post-death (following immediate removal from the cold storage unit) still presented a significant hazard (62 times greater than IDLH) (Table 4.1). When these numbers are put in terms of the risk to those handling or decontaminating the contaminated remains, the results are that Level A, or equivalent, personal protective equipment (PPE) would be required when handling contaminated remains that have not yet been decontaminated.

It is important to note that although the inhalation hazard was significantly deceased in remains that were decontaminated, a hazard still existed to the point where PPE would be required when handling the decontaminated remains. Immediately following decontamination and while at room temperature, the inhalation hazard of the remains was found to average over 1600 times the STEL for VX (or over five times the IDLH), dropping to an average of 56 times STEL by 168 hours post-death, when the remains were still cool from removal from the cold storage unit. Immediately following decontamination, a CBRN compliant self-contained breathing apparatus (SCBA) would still be required because IDLH conditions still existed [31]. One week (168 hours) following death, the inhalation hazard decreased; however, it is likely that if the remains had been allowed to warm to room temperature prior to the hazard determination, the hazard would have been significantly higher. Additional studies would be needed to confirm the hazard.

Contact Hazard of Remains

The contact hazard on the skin of contaminated remains both before and after decontamination was determined through a wipe of the application site on the remains at various time points post-death. This wipe sample represented a touch

Table 4.1 VX Inhalation hazard: STEL and IDLH

	Nondecontaminated		Decontaminated	
Hours post-death	IDLH	STEL	IDLH	STEL
24	169 ± 66	50,656 ± 19,835	5.4 ± 3.90	1605 ± 1167
72	41 ± 8	12,320 ± 2496	0.4 ± 0.05	134 ± 52
120	55 ± 22	16,594 ± 6455	0.3 ± 0.20	98 ± 66
168	62 ± 24	18,598 ± 7283	0.2 ± 0.05	56 ± 15

contact hazard of the chemically contaminated remains, as it was only wiped on one spot of the challenge site to determine the VX levels.

On average, a decrease in the contact hazard over time from the dose site was observed in the control and decontaminated remains for both VX and EA2192 (Table 4.2). As expected, the largest hazard was found 24 hours post-death, while the remains were at room temperature. Remains that were not decontaminated had an average of 311 mg VX, or 104 times the median lethal dose (LD_{50}) for a 70 kg man (Table 4.4) present as a touch contact hazard on the skin. (Note: This is only the amount of VX contained in a single spot, not the total VX contamination on the entire animal.) Additionally, 17 mg EA2192, the toxic metabolite of VX, was found as a touch contact hazard on nondecontaminated remains.

In decontaminated remains, the hazard was significantly reduced, but still present, with 1.6 mg VX, or 0.6 times the LD_{50} for a 70 kg man and 166 times the no-observable adverse effect level (NOAEL) for a single acute exposure in humans, found as a touch contact hazard on the skin at room temperature (Table 4.3). Additionally, 14 μg EA2192 was found as a touch contact hazard immediately following decontamination.

The rinsate of remains that were decontaminated was collected and sampled for VX and EA2192 to determine any potential contact hazard that would be present during the decontamination process. VX levels in the rinsate ranged from approximately 120 mg up to over 21,000 mg VX, and EA2192 levels ranged from approximately 6 mg to over 1500 mg, indicating that the rinsate used during the decontamination process is likely to present an extremely significant hazard to those that may come in contact with it. Additionally, the high levels of VX present in the rinsate indicate that decontamination of the rinsate would need to be performed prior to removal of the water.

Table 4.2 VX contact hazard on skin

	Nondecontaminated		Decontaminated	
Hours post-death	VX (mg)	EA2192 (mg)	VX (mg)	EA2192 (mg)
24	311 ± 69	16.6 ± 3.7	1.6 ± 0.9	0.014 ± 0.007
72	132 ± 64	4.0 ± 2.1	0.8 ± 0.7	0.006 ± 0.005
120	9 ± 2	0.2 ± 0.1	0.2 ± 0.1	0.002 ± 0.001
168	24 ± 12	1.0 ± 0.5	0.4 ± 0.2	0.002 ± 0.001

Table 4.3 VX contact hazard on skin: MLD or NOAEL

	Nondecontaminated		Decontaminated	
Hours post- death	MLD	NOAEL	MLD	NOAEL
24	104 ± 23	31,705 ± 6900	0.6 ± 0.3	166 ± 92
72	44 ± 21	13,225 ± 6364	0.3 ± 0.2	81 ± 66
120	3.0 ± 0.7	875 ± 225	0.1 ± 0.0	18 ± 10
168	8.0 ± 3.8	2425 ± 1153	0.1 ± 0.1	42 ± 19

Color Change in Skin

An interesting observation was discovered when the contaminated remains were removed from the CSU at 72 hours post-death. Both decontaminated and control remains were found to have a greenish hue to the skin where the VX had been applied or where it had run down the sides of the animal. An initial hypothesis was that there was an interaction with the bleach [32] and the VX on the remains' skin; however, the greenish hue was observed on both control and decontaminated remains. The greenish hue color was only observed where VX had contacted the skin of the remains. The greenish hue was not observed on the back of the remains, which had no access to agent. Since investigative studies were not conducted, the cause of the greenish hue in the skin is presently unknown, although it is hypothesized that the cause may be the binding of the thiol-leaving group of VX to heme in the blood and tissues, creating a sulfhemoglobin. Sulfhemoglobin consists of a heme that has been irreversibly bound to a thiol, resulting in a greenish hue in the blood [33, 34]. This has been reported previously in the literature with overdoses of drugs containing sulfur compounds [35].

Representative pictures are presented of the greenish hue observed in the remains in Figs. 4.1 and 4.2 for control and decontaminated remains, respectively. Although remains that were decontaminated were generally observed to have a lighter shade of green, a greenish hue was still observed.

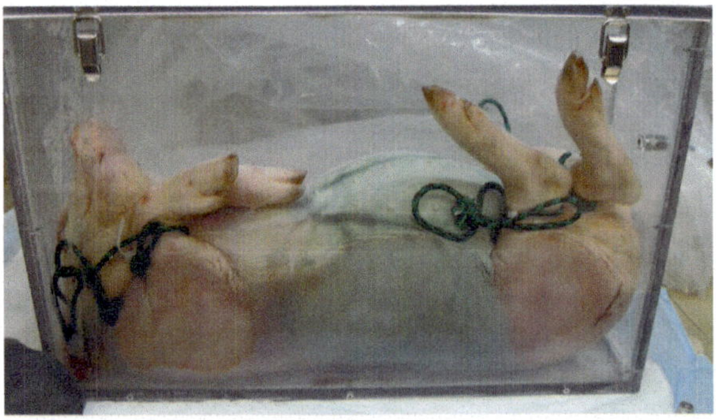

Fig. 4.1 Representative color change on nondecontaminated remains

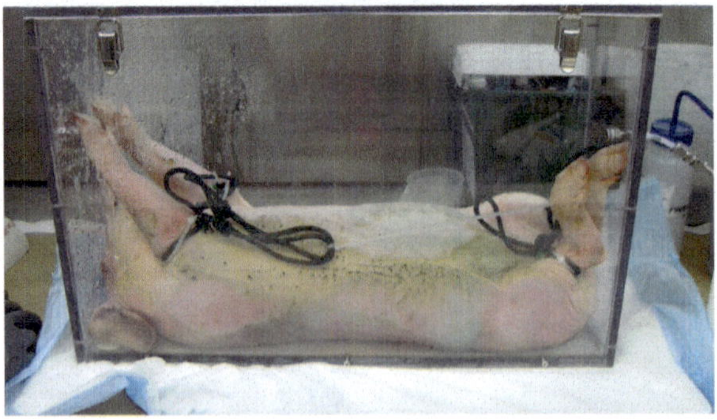

Fig. 4.2 Representative color change on decontaminated remains

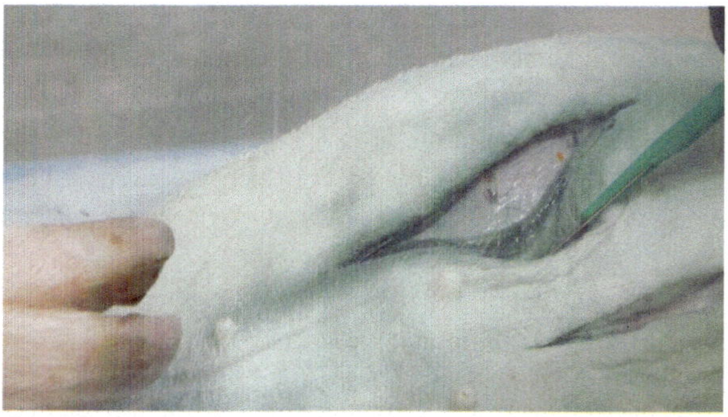

Fig. 4.3 Representative color change depth through skin

Table 4.4 Representative color change quantification (hue)

Area quantified	Group	Hue
Unexposed leg	Nondecontaminated	2
	Decontaminated	8
Exposed abdomen (dark)	Nondecontaminated	98
	Decontaminated	102
Exposed abdomen (light)	Nondecontaminated	105
	Decontaminated	45

In addition, following completion of the last sample collection, an incision was made into the skin to determine the depth of the greenish hue. As illustrated in Fig. 4.3, the greenish color extended through all layers of skin, down to the muscle layer of the remains, and remained through the end of the study at 1 week post-death.

The color difference between the representative remains from each group was quantified (Table 4.4). In areas that were not exposed to VX (e.g., the leg of both decontaminated and nondecontaminated remains), no differences were found. However, in areas where the agent had been applied to the skin, the nondecontaminated remains had a color hue approximately twice that of the decontaminated remains.

Overall, this study has demonstrated that the MACRMS protocol does not result in effective decontamination of VX through 1 week post-death. While decontaminated remains presented significantly less of a hazard than those that were not decontaminated, a contact hazard of 40× NOAEL and an inhalation hazard of 56× STEL at 1 week post-death would not allow the removal of PPE when handling these remains. Also, it is likely that storage in the CSU may have decreased the vapor hazard that would normally be present if the remains were stored in conditions warmer than 1.1 to 4.4 °C or if the remains were allowed to warm to room temperature prior to handling or manipulation.

Remains that were decontaminated post-death were found to have a touch contact hazard of approximately 40× (the NOAEL) and an inhalation hazard of approximately 56× STEL at 168 hours post-death, when stored in a CSU. Immediately following decontamination (24 hours post-death and at room temperature), the hazard was even greater. A contact hazard of 160× the NOAEL and an inhalation hazard of over 1600× STEL or over 5× IDLH conditions were observed. The inhalation hazard represents a closed environment, allowing the concentration of VX to build. An open-air environment would likely lessen the inhalation hazard immediately following decontamination. However, even at 168 hours post-death when the remains were stored within a CSU, which would decrease the inhalation hazard due to the cold environment, the headspace above the remains was found to be 56× STEL. This result would indicate that appropriate PPE would be required along with an appropriately ventilated environment prior to opening a body bag that contained VX-contaminated human remains. If the remains were stored at a temperature greater than 1.1 to 4.4 °C, it is possible that the inhalation hazard would increase.

Remains that were not decontaminated, representing conditions that would be present transporting the contaminated remains from the battlefield to the site for decontamination, presented a much greater hazard. After remaining untouched for 24 hours, remains that were not decontaminated had an initial contact hazard of 31,100× NOAEL (or 104× LD_{50}) and an initial inhalation hazard of approximately 51,000× STEL (or 169× IDLH). However, VX-contaminated human remains that were in an open environment for an extended period of time would not likely present as great of an inhalation hazard as described, although, if the contaminated remains were placed within a body bag and that bag was opened for any reason, the hazard would likely be much greater than an IDLH environment.

Discussion and Implications

The recent studies performed by TNO and Battelle indicate the most significant hazard of chemically contaminated human remains will be, as expected, the handling prior to decontamination. The lethal dose to 50% of the population (LD_{50}) for VX is approximately 3.0 mg per 70 kg man by the percutaneous route. Because lethality can result from an extremely small exposure (Fig. 4.4), safe handling and processing of even moderately or minimally contaminated human remains is critical. When a worst-case scenario is postulated, safely being able to process and decontaminate chemically contaminated human remains becomes even more problematic.

The potential for exposure to those recovering nondecontaminated remains is likely to be significant, especially in a warm and/or enclosed environment. Cooler temperatures are more likely to decrease the immediate inhalation hazard but are likely to increase the length of the inhalation and contact hazard (as was observed in HD contaminated guinea pig remains). Remains that have been exposed to a liquid exposure of CWA are likely to present a significant contact and inhalation hazard, even when only parts of the body are contaminated. For victims of a vapor-only hazard, the remaining agent is likely to decrease significantly in a much shorter period of time, thereby decreasing the overall hazard to those recovering the remains.

The results of the Battelle study indicated that the current MACRMs decontamination protocol is not sufficient to reduce the hazard to a safe handling level for

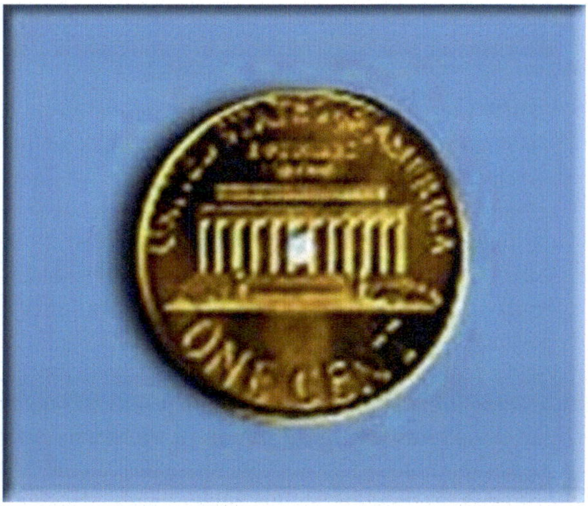

Fig. 4.4 VX LD50 in a 70 kg person

VX-contaminated remains, below which workers would not have to wear PPE. However, it is important to note that bleach, which was used in the MACRMS protocol for decontamination, is not the preferred decontaminant to use for VX. High-test hypochlorite (HTH) is the preferred decontaminant for VX, not bleach, especially for larger levels of contamination. RSDL has been shown to work extremely well against VX and the other CWAs as a decontaminant for personal decontamination [36–38]. It is possible that the use of RSDL would provide better decontamination than the bleach used in the MACRMS protocol, especially for VX. However, it is important to remember that even with adequate external decontamination, there is still the potential for exposure due to internal contamination of the remains. As decomposition occurs, bodily fluids are expelled, which may present a potential contamination risk. Additionally, the contamination in the blood and tissues may present a contact hazard. It is possible that the use of embalming fluids containing a proper decontaminant may help to decrease or eliminate the contamination risk inside the remains. However, a previous study investigated the Polar Cavity Firmindex® 53, Rex 36, and Hexaphene MA64 embalming fluids and found they had limited ability to decontaminate VX or HD [39].

As discussed above, one of the most obvious and important conclusions from these studies in terms of doctrine, policy, and training is that C-CHR and contaminated personal effects pose significant residual contact and vapor hazards if they are not decontaminated. Implications of the studies affirmed C-CHR hazard mitigation options that can be used to further develop doctrine, policy, and training (including the combination of clothing removal, time, decontamination, and containment):

- Prior to these studies, the US DoD had an approved program to develop a Contaminated Human Remains Pouch (CHRP), which was intended to safely contain the contamination hazard during recovery of remains from the incident site and while transporting the remains to the MACRMS. When the CHRP did not meet certain standards during operational testing, results of these studies informed an alternate course of action using the existing human remains pouch in conjunction with special handling procedures. In 2014, efforts to develop the CHRP were canceled, and the alternative recovery procedures were recommended for use until an approved CHR recovery pouch is fielded. Study results indicated that the development of adsorptive carbon liners inside the human remains pouch for vapor reduction may provide significant hazard mitigation in the future.

- Subject matter experts from US DoD stakeholder organizations agreed after reviewing the study results that removing most of the decedent's clothing and personal equipment as early as practicable in the recovery process would significantly reduce external contamination. Consequently, the C-CHR recovery process requires additional analysis that will inform the development of doctrine and procedures both during recovery operations and at the MACRMS to mitigate the residual hazard throughout the entire chain of custody during repatriation. US DoD discussions on this subject since the studies were completed indicate that recovery procedures may also be dependent upon the nature of the exposure incident and will be influenced by evidentiary requirements for a forensic investigation by the Armed Forces Medical Examiner.

The studies assured the need to employ the MACRMS concept to integrate decontamination tasks prior to packaging contaminated remains and transporting to the United States for final disposition. While further testing to determine the effects from a broader spectrum of CBRN hazards on human remains is needed, we have been able to leverage results of these research studies to achieve momentum and make progress in the development of equipment and related procedures to mitigate the secondary hazards while handling C-CHR. Based on the conclusions from these studies, US Army functional proponents for Mortuary Affairs acknowledged the need to change the proposed MACRMS protocols for decontaminating human remains to decrease the hazards posed to personnel operating at the MACRMS.

- Results of the study did not change the expectation of refrigeration requirements for C-CHR during the time it takes to establish the MACRMS, which could take as long as 4 weeks. Although cooling the remains will not reduce the contact risk of HD, the benefits derived from the retardation of the decomposition process may outweigh the associated risks if remains are able to undergo the necessary tasks within MACRMS. Also, data show that holding the remains for a longer time period, may allow for additional agent degradation.
- Prior to these studies, the original MACRMS protocols included the sorting of contaminated decedents upon arrival by type of exposure (liquid and VX and Lewisite vapor versus nonliquid contamination) based on previous literature reviews. However, this sorting procedure was changed based on the determination that we can expect that compounds will not become completely detoxified during the biological and chemical processes that contribute to agent degradation after death. Thus, unit personnel should transport all contaminated remains to the MACRMS to undergo the decontamination mitigation process regardless of the exposure type.

- Initial draft MACRMS decontamination procedures using bleach and water were changed to include the use of RSDL to decrease the hazards associated with the decontamination process, in part due to the conclusion that rinsates from the decontamination process potentially pose a significant contact and inhalation hazard. Additionally, results from testing of bleach submersion indicated that draft procedures using a bleach solution on remains should be changed due to the likelihood that the advanced stage of decomposition of the C-CHR when the MACRMS is established can be expected to impact the efficacy of the decontamination process. For this reason, the subject matter experts within US DoD agreed that the use of refrigeration to slow the decomposition process should be sustained as part of the process. When the bleach soak procedures were eliminated and RSDL application procedures were incorporated into the MACRMS protocols, the need for point detection was also eliminated, thereby reducing the number of steps and equipment requirements for the MACRMS. Using RSDL reduces the need for water and lowers the splash and removal hazards associated with contaminated water. Moreover, using RSDL may provide the ability to neutralize the contamination as opposed to removing it.
- Low-level detection at the MACRMS will be done using MINICAMS®. The inner receptacle of the transportation package will be cleaned with a sponge and warm soapy water. By using RSDL instead of a sodium hypochlorite solution, MACRMS personnel are able to avoid potential scenarios where the bleach solution interferes with the MINICAMS®. However, it is important to note that potential interferences with the MINICAMS® and RSDL are still possible if the RSDL is not completely removed from the skin. An internal study performed by Battelle in 2011 indicated that RSDL resulted in a false positive for sarin (GB) and a false negative for GB and VX (unpublished data).
- MACRMS Personnel Protective Equipment requirements must be re-evaluated and Just-In-Time training must be developed based upon these and other contamination studies as part of incident specific planning each time the MACRMS is deployed.

The studies confirmed that a potential hazard exists from CWA that may still be present in and on the C-CHR even after the decontamination process. In addition, the studies revealed that agent may persist for a longer time period in decedents than in living persons.

- These findings confirmed the need to continue doctrine development and analysis of the complete C-CHR repatriation process from the point of exposure through final disposition, and they validated the need for a performance oriented package that complies with 49 CFR Class 6.1 Inhalation Hazard *not other specified (n.o.s.)* (name of CWA) Hazard Zone A to contain the residual hazard while transporting C-CHR from the MACRMS to the place of final interment.
- The progress made to date with the development of the MACRMS protocols and materiel solutions has laid the foundation for US DoD to start the coordination with Whole of US Government and industry stakeholders to establish effective processes and procedures that can be used on a case by case basis for transportation to the continental United States and for final disposition of C-CHR within

the United States. However, results of the studies underscore the importance of communicating to jurisdictional authorities the need to restrict access to the remains once inside the containment package.

Finally, the US Army will need to update doctrine, procedures, and training requirements related to the processing of contaminated personal effects such as uniforms and boots, which the study determined, pose a significant hazard due to the high persistence of CWA on and in these materials. Personal effects will not be decontaminated at the MACRMS. Instead, they will be placed into storage and/or destroyed until effective protocols can be developed to ensure they are safe for disposition to the family. Storage of grossly contaminated personal effects will need to be investigated as they will continue to pose an off-gassing and contact hazard until effectively decontaminated.

Future Studies/Path Forward

Future studies should include investigations into the performance of RSDL on remains to confirm its effectiveness as a decontaminant on C-CHR and to determine its effectiveness in neutralizing contamination and reducing the residual hazard on decedents and other surfaces. Studies should also include the evaluation of the agent coming back to the surface of the remains during decomposition, and again posing an inhalation and contact hazard. Compatibility testing, in the presence of RSDL, should be conducted with low-level detectors used at the MACRMS to verify effective decontamination and detection within the MACRMS and to investigate the potential interferences with the decontaminants used. Additional studies would be required to determine the effectiveness of the MACRMS protocol (current or modified) with more volatile agents using a field-relevant exposure.

Depending on the outcome of the RSDL studies, determining the effects of other decontaminants on both the residual hazards to handlers and transporters and the long-term risks to public health is another area that may warrant additional investigation. These studies could also be aimed at determining if alternative decontaminants can be used to expedite the decontamination process at the MACRMS. Similarly, research is needed to validate the process for dealing with CHR decontamination waste products at the MACRMS.

Although not investigated in the most current studies, the role of wounds in combination with a CWA exposure should be evaluated, with regard to the effectiveness of a decontaminant and the processes and procedures being used to decontaminate C-CHR with wounds. Additionally, consideration during the MACRMs process should be given to shrapnel, clothing, or other objects that may be embedded in the wounds. It is possible that contaminated wounds on C-CHR will present a significant agent hazard, as the agent will locally accumulate in the wounds due to a lack of circulation. Effective decontamination and detection of any potential residual hazard in the wound is critical on C-CHR. It is important to remember that protocols for effective decontamination of wounds on C-CHR may not be compatible with wound healing therapies on a living casualty.

The US DoD should continue low-level, long-term contamination exposure studies and conduct additional experiments to determine the level at which decomposition pursuant to temporary interment and/or hasty burial affects the procedures at the MACRMS. Additionally, the same potential gaps exist with biologically contaminated remains as well. Preliminary studies with *Bacillus anthracis* have been funded by the Defense Threat Reduction Agency and conducted by TNO, the Netherlands, to investigate effective decontamination of these remains.

Eventual studies to determine if and how development of protocols for separating decedents contaminated by a combination of agents should be done. In addition to investigating potential indicators to determine if personal effects are contaminated, confirmation studies on the effectiveness of decontamination protocols for personal effects made of different types of material must be conducted before the US DoD can release them to the family.

Overall, additional efforts in this area will help to determine the appropriate procedures and hazard mitigation for effectively decontaminating and safely returning Service member remains for burial.

References

1. Jennings JD. Deputy Assistant Secretary of defense for prisoner of war/missing personnel affairs, January 5, 2004.
2. Department of Defense, Final Report of the Executive Steering Committee, Mortuary Affairs, Medical Examiner System, and Casualty Assistance Support Study, 27 November 2012, p. 8.
3. Wolfowitz P. Deputy Secretary of Defense, 2003.
4. Department of Defense Directive (DoDD) 1300.22 Mortuary Affairs Policy, October 30, 2015.
5. Joint Publication (JP) 4-06 Mortuary Affairs and Army Techniques Publication (ATP) 4-46.2, Mortuary Affairs Contaminated Remains Mitigation Site, [draft].
6. Okumura T, Kouichiro S, Fukuda A, Kohama A, Takasu N, Ishimatsu S, Hinohara S. The Tokyo Subway sarin attack: disaster management, Part 1: community emergency response. Acad Emer Med. 1998;5:613–7.
7. Okumura T, Suzuki K, Fukuda A, Kohama A, Takasu N, Ishimatsu S, Hinohara S. The Tokyo Subway sarin attack: disaster management, Part 2: hospital response. Acad Emer Med. 1998;5:618–24.
8. Tucker JB. War of nerves: chemical warfare from World War I to Al-Qaeda. New York: Pantheon Books; 2006.
9. Nakajima T, Sato S, Morita H, Yanagisawa N. Sarin poisoning of a rescue team in the Matsumoto sarin incident in Japan. Occup Environ Med. 1997;54:697–701.
10. Joint Publication 4-06. Mortuary Affairs. 12 October2011.
11. Boone CM, Chau LF, Gaasbeek RC. Evaporation of residual chemical warfare agents and the relation to the response of chemical agent monitors. TNO-DV 2008 A106. 2008.
12. Heinen JH, Carhart HW, Taylor WH, Stolp BN, Conner JC Jr, Clausen NM. Chamber tests with human subjects IX. In: Basic tests with H vapor. 1945. Final report AD-396 275. Washington, DC: Naval Research Laboratory.
13. Cullumbine H. Chemical warfare experiments using human subjects. Brit Med J. 1946;19:576–8.

14. Sinclair DC. Disability produced by exposure of skin to mustard-gas vapour. Brit Med J. 1950;11:346–9.
15. Van der Schans MJ, Lander BJ, van der Wiel H, Langenberg JP, Benschop HP. Toxicokinetics of the nerve agent (±) VX in anesthetized and atropinized hairless Guinea pigs and marmosets after intravenous and percutaneous administration. Toxicol App Pharm. 191:48–62.
16. Van der Schans MJ, Benscop HP, Whalley CE. Toxicokinetics of nerve agents. In: Romano Jr JA, et al., editors. Chemical warfare agents. Chemistry, pharmacology, toxicology, and therapeutics. 2nd ed. Boca Raton: CRC Press; 2008.
17. Sweeney RE, Langenberg JP, Maxwell DM. A physiologically based pharmacokinetic (PB/PK) model for multiple exposure routes of soman in multiple species. Arch Toxicol. 2006;80:719–31.
18. Noort D, Benschop HP, Black RM. Biomonitoring of exposure to chemical warfare agents: a review. Toxicol Appl Pharmacol. 2002;184:116–26.
19. Noort D, Black RM. Methods for the retrospective detection of exposure to toxic scheduled chemicals. Part B: mass spectrometric and immunochemical analysis of covalent adducts to proteins and DNA. In: Mesilaakso M, editor. Chemical weapons convention related analysis. Chichester, UK: Wiley; 2005.
20. Black RM, Noort D. Methods for the retrospective detection of exposure to toxic scheduled chemicals. Part B: analysis of covalent adducts to proteins and DNA. In: Mesilaakso M, editor. Chemical weapons convention related analysis. Chichester, UK: Wiley; 2005.
21. Black RM, Noort D. Chapter 5: Biological markers of exposure to chemical warfare agents. In: Marrs TT, Maynard RL, Sidell F, editors. Chemical warfare agents: toxicology and treatment. West Sussex: John Wiley and Sons, Ltd; 2007.
22. Williams NH, Harrison JM, Read RW, Black RM. Phosphylated tyrosine in albumin as a biomarker of exposure to organophosphorus nerve agents. Arch Toxicol. 2007;81:627–40.
23. Noort D, Fidder A, Degenhardt-Langelaan CEAM, Hulst AG. Retrospective detection of sulfur mustard exposure by mass spectrometric analysis of adducts to albumin and hemoglobin: an in vivo study. J Anal Toxicol. 2008;32:25–30.
24. Langenberg JP, Van Dijk C, Sweeney RE, Maxwell DM, De Jong LPA, Benschop HP. Development of a physiologically-based model for the toxicokinetics of C(±)P(±)-soman in the atropinized Guinea pig. Arch Toxicol. 1997;71:320–31.
25. Pélissier-Alicot AL, Gaulier JM, Champsaur P, Marquet P. Mechanisms underlying postmortem redistribution of drugs: a review. J Anal Toxicol. 2003;27:533–44.
26. Klette KL, Levine B, Dreka C, Smith ML, Goldberger BA. Cholinesterase activity in postmortem blood as a screening test for organophosphate/chemical warfare agents. J Forensic Sci. 1993;38:950–5.
27. Kupfermann N, Schmoldt A, Steinhart H. Rapid and sensitive quantitative analysis of alkyl phosphates in urine after organophosphate poisoning. J Anal Toxicol. 2004;28:242–8.
28. Vycudilic W. Detection of sulfur mustard gas Bis (2-Chloroethyl sulfid in urin). Forensic SciInt. 1985;28:131–6.
29. Drasch G, Kretschmer E, Kaverr G. Concentration of sulfur mustard in the tissue of a victim of vesicant exposure. J Forensic Sci. 1987;32:1788–9.
30. Department of the Army. Toxic Chemical Agent Safety Standards. DA Pamphlet 385-61. 13 November 2012.
31. DHHS (NIOSH) Publication Number 2008-132. Guidance on Emergency Responder Personal Protective Equipment (PPE) for Response to CBRN Terrorism Incidents. June 2008.
32. Adair TW, Dobersen MJ, Lear-Kaul K. Appearance of chemical burns resulting from the washing of a deceased body with bleach. J Forensic Sci. 2007;52:709–11.
33. Bandenburg RO, Smith HL. Sulfhemoglobinemia: a study of 62 clinical cases. Am Heart J. 1951;42:582–8.
34. Haggard HW. The fate of sulfides in the blood. J Bio Chem. 1921;49:519–29.
35. Flexman AM, Del VG, Schwarz SK. Dark green blood in the operating theatre. Lancet. 2007;369:1972.

36. Hayes TL, Snider TH, Sabourin CL, Olson CT, Estep JE. Phases I and II: Canadian Reactive Skin Decontamination Lotion (RSDL). Final report. Contract no. DAMD17–99-D-0010, Task Order 0008. 2004.
37. Braue EH Jr, Hanssen KA, Doxzon BK, Lumpkin HL, Clarkson ED. Evaluation of RSDL, M291 SDK, 0.5% bleach, 1% soapy water and SERPACWA. Part 1: Challenge with VX. U.S. Army Medical Research Institute of Chemical Defense.USAMRICD-TR-09-01. 2009.
38. Schwartz MD, Hurst CG, Kirk MA, Reedy SJD, Braue EH. Reactive Skin Decontamination Lotion (RSDL) for the Decontamination of Chemical Warfare Agent (CWA) dermal exposure. Current Pharm Biotech. 2012;13:1971–9.
39. Snider TH, Babin MC, Hayes TL. Evaluation of decontamination solutions for use on remains. Final report. Contract no. DAMD17–99-D-0010, Task Order 0020. 2004.

Chapter 5
Effectiveness of Chemical, Biological, Radiological, and Nuclear (CBRN) Skin Decontaminants: Toward Tests Standardization

Denis Josse

Introduction

Decontamination is a crucial step in the care to victims exposed to CBRN agents [1]. To be beneficial to victims, it must be performed as quickly as possible following exposure, and as thoroughly as possible on the body surface which not only includes skin but also wounds, hair, eyes, and other mucous membranes.

Decontamination is defined by NATO as the process of making any person, object, or area safe by absorbing, destroying, neutralizing, making harmless, or removing chemical or biological agents, or by removing radioactive material clinging to or around it [2]. Human decontamination has two main objectives [3]: firstly, to improve the prognosis, functional and vital, of contaminated victims, and secondly, to reduce the transfer of contamination from the body surface to media, including noncontaminated skin, with which it interacts.

From a practical point of view, decontamination is usually performed in two consecutive steps: the first one, "emergency decontamination" (ED) consists in partial disrobing and use of emergency decontamination kit on the unprotected body surfaces, and the second one, "thorough decontamination" (TD) consists in total disrobing followed with showering.

Emergency decontamination kits include absorbents, for example, handkerchief, paper, towel, clean fabric, and adsorbent powders such as Fuller's earth, talcum, flour, clean sand, and cat litter [3]. Adsorbent powders are poured on the contaminated area, then either left until a shower can be performed or, after a short contact time, removed with a towel or more effectively with water.

For instance, Fuller's earth has a relatively high affinity for lipophilic chemicals and has been shown to be highly effective as a skin decontaminant against SM and

D. Josse (✉)
Colonel in the French Fire and Rescue Services, Alpes-Maritimes, Villeneuve-Loubet, France
e-mail: denis.josse@sdis06.fr

H. Zhu, H. I. Maibach (eds.), *Skin Decontamination*,
https://doi.org/10.1007/978-3-030-24009-7_5

VX [4, 5]. However, if the decontamination is delayed after exposure, it is slightly less effective than the RSDL® kit, which consists of a polylethylene glycol (PEG) and oximate-based lotion, applied with a sponge [4, 6, 7].

Showering can be performed with different systems, for example, fixed shower, mobile decontamination unit, ladder pipes from the Fire Services, and by implementing different protocols varying according to the duration, water temperature, additive to water, water flow rate, and pressure [8].

When choosing a decontamination kit, one has to consider not only effectiveness but also skin, wound and eye biocompatibility, ease and restrictions of use, cost, stability and storage conditions, and elimination after usage.

Evaluation of human skin decontamination effectiveness against CBRN agents is limited by at least two factors: firstly, for obvious ethical reasons, highly toxic or infectious CBRN agents cannot be used on human volunteers, and secondly, their disposal is restricted to a few laboratories, usually from the Army.

To cope with this issue, laboratories refer to human skin models and, if they cannot dispose of CBRN agents, they use simulants, that is, agents with physicochemical properties very close to that of the real agents and, usually, much less toxic or pathogenic [9].

Human skin models currently consist of in vitro human or animal skin, or in vivo pig or rodent skin [10].

Without standardized tests available at the international level, evaluation of skin decontamination effectiveness relies on highly variable models and procedures [11–16]. Tests heterogeneity is mainly related to agents (liquid or vapor, amount, diluted or not in a solvent), skin models (in vitro or in vivo; animal species: human, pig, rat, guinea pig, etc.; anatomic site: ear, flank, back, abdomen, etc.), skin preparation (e.g., hair cut or not, in vitro full-thickness skin or split-thickness skin), environmental conditions (temperature, relative humidity, and air flow rate), exposure duration before decontamination (1 min, 5 min, 15 min, 30 min, etc.), and decontaminant operating procedures.

In such heterogeneous conditions, results are not comparable from one test laboratory to another. Furthermore, it is quite complex for the users to evaluate the efficacy claims and determine whether the products correspond to their operational needs, particularly since the results have to be extrapolated to human beings who would be exposed to real agents in the same test conditions.

In this context, a French working group comprising scientists from tests and research laboratories, end users and industrials, supported by the national standardization institute (AFNOR), has recently validated a French standard test method (FSTM) (NF X 52-122) to evaluate the effectiveness of skin decontaminants against CBRN agents [17]. The main objectives of this STM are to provide relevant information to the customers and to facilitate comparison between tests through the evaluation of normalized parameters.

The main elements of this STM are addressed in this chapter.

Effectiveness of a Skin Decontamination Kit or System: What Does It Mean?

In this STM, decontamination effectiveness is defined as the ability to remove CBRN agents from the skin surface or neutralize them on the skin surface, without enhancing deleterious effects of CBRN agents already absorbed in the skin before the use of decontaminant. The skin surface is the interface between the first layer of cells from the *stratum corneum* and the environment. It includes the hair and skin appendages such as the hair follicles and sweat glands.

Emergency Versus Thorough Decontamination

ED aims at improving the vital and functional prognosis of contaminated victims and at reducing the irreversible cellular lesions due to CBRN agents. The main goal of ED is therefore to reduce the exposure duration to CBRN agents and skin absorption of these agents.

The main objective of TD is to limit the transfer of contamination from the skin to other surfaces.

Evaluation of Skin Decontamination Effectiveness (DE) Relatively to Nondecontaminated Skin

According to the FSTM, effectiveness of skin decontamination must be evaluated relative to nondecontaminated skin, exposed to CBRN agents in the same conditions as decontaminated skin.

Agents

Decontamination effectiveness must be evaluated against the same CBRN agents as those claimed by the provider. Storage and use of CBRN agents must be in accordance with the regulations. When CBRN agents cannot be used, they will be substituted with simulants. The choice of simulants must be justified and scientifically validated with references.

Skin Models

There are numerous examples in the literature of reliable correlations between in vitro and in vivo skin permeation studies [18–20].

In vitro skin models must be animal or human skin samples, the latter being more relevant. Pig skin can be an alternative to human skin since their structure and permeability is similar [21, 22]. Rat or guinea pig skin, from the abdomen or back, can also be used. Skin samples are placed into diffusion cells which must be used in nonocclusive conditions and as recommended by the OECD guidelines n°428 [23]. For practical reasons, the donor compartment can be shortly removed to better implement the decontamination protocol.

Freshly excised human skin must be used if CBRN agents are significantly metabolized in the skin (i.e., at least 10% of the applied dose is enzymatically degraded). If the skin metabolism of CBRN agents is relatively low, then samples frozen at –20 °C can be used. Skin integrity of each sample must be checked as recommended [23].The skin thickness must be measured and be lower than 1 mm. Skin surface must be at least 0.6 cm^2.

Use of animal models in vivo must follow the regulations. The best choice is pig but rat or guinea pig can also be used.

Tests can be performed on human volunteers if the regulations are respected and only with nontoxic or nonpathogenic contaminants. The choice of the anatomic site to be contaminated must be in accordance with real exposure scenarios and must consider health risks assessment.

Skin Contamination

The agent purity must be higher than 95% unless it can be justified. The exposed skin area must be totally covered by the contaminant. As a result, the contaminant can be diluted but the vehicle, preferentially volatile, must not modify the skin permeability or the agent physicochemical properties.

The amount of agent loaded on the skin (Q_0) must be as realistic as possible, that is, for chemicals from a few μg to a few $mg.cm^{-2}$. For radioactive agents, it could be between 1 and 10,000 $Bq.cm^{-2}$. For biological agents, it must be expressed in colony-forming units $(cfu).cm^{-2}$ for bacteria or fungi, or in plaque-forming units $(pfu).cm^{-2}$ for virus.

Exposure Durations

Exposure durations, that is, time between contamination (T_0) and decontamination (T_1) will be representative of the context of use. When ED kits are evaluated, they must be of 5 and 30 min, whereas for TD systems, they will be of 30 and 60 min.

Operating Instructions

They must scrupulously respect the instructions of use as given by the provider. In particular, they should indicate how the decontaminant is applied on the skin surface, for example, apply the absorbent on the skin without wiping or wipe back-and-force twice, each time with a new absorbent, or rub the skin in a circular motion. The contact duration with the skin surface and the amount of decontaminant applied per area of contaminated skin must be mentioned. Operating instructions can include several successive steps (e.g., washing, rinsing, and drying).

Skin decontamination with a liquid must include a final drying step, which will be performed with an absorbent applied softly on the skin surface, that is, without scrubbing. This drying process can be repeated several times, each time with a new absorbent sample, until the skin surface becomes dry.

Mass Balance

Mass balance must be evaluated since it is an important parameter to validate the operating procedure. The average mass balance must be of 100 ± 10% for nonvolatile and stable agents, that is, that are not degraded on and in the skin, as recommended by the OECD guidelines number 428 [23].

Indicators of Decontamination Effectiveness

It has been clearly established that chemical agents, more particularly the most lipophilic of them, constitute a reservoir in the skin *stratum corneum*, from which they are more or less rapidly resorbed in blood [24]. Toxic effects can target the skin itself and/or be systemic. Local skin effects are directly related to the amount of agents present on and in the skin. Systemic effects mainly depend on the amount of agents resorbed and on their skin permeation rate. Skin decontamination must not increase the local and systemic deleterious effects of CBRN agents. Amount of agents and their effects must be evaluated according to scientifically validated or referenced analytical methods.

For in vitro skin models, the amount of agents on the skin surface, in the skin and penetrating through the skin, and the rate of skin permeation must be evaluated. For decontaminated (Q) and nondecontaminated (Q_t) skin samples, the following amounts of agent have to be determined:

- Q_0 and Q_{0t}, loaded on the skin
- Q_1, eliminated from the skin surface
- Q_2 and Q_{2t}, present on the skin surface immediately after decontamination
- Q_3 and Q_{3t}, present in the skin at the end of the experimentation

- Q_4 and Q_{4t}, absorbed through the skin (in the receptor fluid) at the end of the experimentation
- Absorbed through the skin every 30 min and for at least 1h 30 min

as well as the lag time τ and the maximum resorption rate J_{max} (expressed as amount of agent.cm^{-2}.h^{-1} or min^{-1}). Agents present on the skin surface will be absorbed using cotton balls then by tape-stripping the skin with two adhesives. Agents will be extracted from cotton balls and strips then quantified.

Extraction recoveries (average and standard deviation) from each matrix (skin, cotton ball, tape-strip, and decontaminant) have to be determined. In vitro tests alone will be sufficient for evaluating the skin decontamination effectiveness if it has been shown that correlation between in vitro and in vivo results is reliable.

For in vitro tests, the total number of skin samples have been evaluated to be at least 18 for nondecontaminated skin (12 to evaluate Q_{2t} at two different exposure times and six to measure the resorption kinetic data), and 12 for decontaminated skin (six for each exposure duration) to evaluate Q_1, Q_2, Q_3, Q_4, and the resorption kinetic data.

For in vivo animal models, the following parameters will be evaluated: Q_0, Q_{0t}, Q_1, Q_2, Q_{2t}, Q_3, and Q_{3t} and, whenever possible, τ and J_{max} for the decontaminated and nondecontaminated animals. For lethal agents, the survival rate after a minimal duration (equal to the experimental time) over which the death cannot result from contamination, and the average life duration after exposure will be estimated. For nonlethal agents, toxic effects will be evaluated directly or indirectly by using biomarkers.

For studies on human volunteers, Q_2 and Q_{2t} will be determined.

Expression of Results in the Test Report

Mass Balance (MB)

For decontaminated samples, MB (%) = $(Q_1 + Q_2 + Q_3 + Q_4) \times 100 / (Q_0)$.

When Q_1 cannot be evaluated then it is estimated by the difference between Q_{2t} and Q_2.

For nondecontaminated samples, MB (%) = $(Q_{2t} + Q_{3t} + Q_{4t}) \times 100 / (Q_{0t})$.

Effectiveness of Emergency Decontamination

It is determined by the DE (Q_1) (in vitro or in vivo), DE (τ) and DE (J_{max}) (in vitro), FP (in vitro or in vivo) or DE(S), and FP_δ (in vitro or in vivo) values as following:

- Ability to eliminate and/or neutralize CBRN agents that are present on the skin surface, DE(Q_1) (%) = $Q_1 \times 100/Q_{2t}$.

- Ability to modulate the lag time τ, DE (τ) = ($\tau-\tau_t$) × 100/τ_t, where τ_t is the lag time for the nondecontaminated samples.

DE (τ) is either negative or positive depending on whether the decontamination enhances or delays the agent resorption, respectively.

- Ability to modulate J_{max}, DE (J_{max}) = (J_{max} – J_{maxt}) × 100/J_{maxt}, where J_{maxt} is the maximum resorption rate for the nondecontaminated samples.

If decontamination enhances the skin resorption of agents, then DE (J_{max}) is positive, and if decontamination slows it down, then DE (J_{max}) is negative.

If the in vitro results can be reliably extrapolated to in vivo models, then the ability to improve the functional prognosis is evaluated according to the ratio FP = (Q_{2t} + Q_{3t} + Q_{4t}) / (Q_2 + Q_3 + Q_4). The higher the FP, the better the DE.

If not, then in vivo studies will be performed and effect of decontamination on the survival rate will be evaluated according to the DE(S) and FP_δ values calculated as following:

DE(S) = (N_{ds} – N_{cs}) × 100/N, where N_{ds} and N_{cs} are the number of animals that survived among the decontaminated and nondecontaminated ones, respectively, and N is the number of animals in each set.

FP_δ = D_d/D_c, where D_d and D_c are the average survival duration for the decontaminated and nondecontaminated animals, respectively.

From the toxicity biomarker, the functional prognosis could be evaluated from FP and FP_δ values as given in the following: FP = Q_c/Q, where Q_c and Q are the amounts of toxicity biomarkers for the nondecontaminated and decontaminated animals. Effect of decontamination on the time for initial detection of toxicity biomarkers: FP_δ = D_{id} / D_{ic}, where D_{id} and D_{ic} are the corresponding values for the decontaminated and nondecontaminated animals.

Effectiveness of Thorough Decontamination

It is determined from the DE (Q_1) (in vitro or in vivo), DE (τ), and DE(J_{max}) (in vitro) values.

Test Report

The test report is divided into five parts: (1) identification of the test laboratory, (2) of the customer, (3) of the decontaminant, (4) experimental conditions, and (5) results.

Identification of the decontaminant must indicate whether it is used as an ED and/or a TD product.

Experimental conditions must specify the skin models, the environmental conditions (temperature and relative humidity), the agent physicochemical characteristics, including the Log $K_{o/w}$, the water solubility limit and the vapor pressure, and give information on the analytical methods in relationship with the agent quantification and extraction.

The conclusion must indicate the effectiveness of decontamination product according to its ability to neutralize specific CBRN agents on the skin surface or to eliminate them from the skin surface (ED and TD), to modulate the toxic or pathogenic effects (ED and TD), and to improve the functional or vital prognosis (for ED only).

Conclusion

Tests standardization for evaluating the effectiveness of skin decontaminants against CBRN agents is quite important not only to help the users to get reliable information, thereby allowing them to make an informed choice when buying a decontamination product, but also for companies to promote their products on the basis of standardized, scientifically validated criteria. In this respect, the FSTM [17] constitutes a framework on the way toward international standardization.

References

1. Lukey BJ, Slife HF, Clarkson ED, Hurst CG, Braue EH. Chemical warfare agent decontamination from skin. In: Romano JA, Lukey BJ, editors. Chemical warfare agents: chemistry, pharmacology, toxicology, and therapeutics. Boca Raton: CRC Press/Taylor/Francis Group; 2008. p. 611–25.
2. NATO Standard, AEP-66, NATO handbook for sampling and identification of biological, chemical and radiological agents (SIBCRA), Edition 1 Version 1, final draft, February 2012 , Published by the NATO standardization agency (NSA).
3. Josse D, Barrier G. Emergency decontamination in low-resource settings. In Arora R, Arora P, editors. Disaster management: medical preparedness, response and homeland security. CAB International; 2013, chapter 18, p 325.
4. Taysse L, Daulon S, Delamanche S, Bellier B, Breton P. Skin decontamination of mustards and organophosphates: comparative efficiency of RSDL and Fuller's earth in domestic swine. Hum Exp Toxicol. 2007;26(2):135–41.
5. Taysse L, Dorandeu F, Daulon S, Foquin A, Perrier N, Lallement G, Breton P. Cutaneous challenge with chemical warfare agents in the SKH-1 hairless mouse(II): effects of some currently used skin decontaminants (RSDL and Fuller's earth) against liquid Sulphur mustard and VX exposure. Hum Exp Toxicol. 2011;30(6):491–8.
6. Bjarnason S, Mikler J, Hill I, Tenn C, Garrett M, Caddy N, Sawyer TW. Comparison of selected skin decontaminant products and regimens against VX in domestic swine. Hum Exp Toxicol. 2008;27(3):253–61.
7. Schwartz MD, Hurst CG, Kirk MA, Reedy SJ, Braue EH Jr. Reactive skin decontamination lotion (RSDL) for the decontamination of chemical warfare agent (CWA) dermal exposure. Curr Pharm Biotechnol. 2012;13(10):1971–9.

8. Amlot R, Larner J, Matar H, Jones DR, Carter H, Turner EA, Price SC, Chilcott RP. Comparative analysis of showering protocols for mass-casualty decontamination. Prehosp Disaster Med. 2010;25(5):435–9.
9. Bartelt-Hunt SL, Knappe DR, Barlaz MA. A review of chemical warfare agent simulants for the study of environmental behavior. Crit Rev Env Sci Tech (CRC Press LLC, Boca Raton, FL). 2008;38(2):112–36.
10. Abd E, Yousef SA, Pastore MN, Telaprolu K, Mohammed YH, Namjoshi S, Grice JE, Roberts MS. Skin models for the testing of transdermal drugs. Clin Pharmacol. 2016;8:163–76.
11. Matar H, Guerreiro A, Piletsky SA, Price SC, Chilcott RP. Preliminary evaluation of military, commercial and novel skin decontamination products against a chemical warfare agent simulant (methyl salicylate). Cutan Ocul Toxicol. 2016;35(2):137–44.
12. Dennerlein K, Jäger T, Göen T, Kilo S, Schaller KH, Drexler H, Korinth G. Evaluation of the effect of skin cleaning procedures on the dermal absorption of chemicals. Toxicol In Vitro. 2015;29(5):828–33.
13. Rana S, Dutta M, Sharma N, Goel R, Khan AW, Kotta S, Ali J, Ansari SH, Sultana S, Sharma RK. Scintigraphic evaluation of decontamination lotion for removal of radioactive contamination from skin. Disaster Med Public Health Prep. 2014;31:1–6.
14. Misik J, Pavlikova R, Josse D, Cabal J, Kuca K. In vitro skin permeation and decontamination of the organophosphorus pesticide paraoxon under various physical conditions–evidence for a wash-in effect. Toxicol Mech Methods. 2012;22(7):520–5.
15. Petitot F, Moreels AM, Paquet F. In vitro evaluation of percutaneous diffusion of uranyl nitrate through intact or excoriated skin of rat and pig. Can J Physiol Pharmacol. 2004;82(2):133–9.
16. Stratilo CW, Crichton MKF, Sawyer TW. Decontamination efficacy and skin toxicity of two decontaminants against Bacillus anthracis. PLoS One. 2015;10(9):e0138491. https://doi.org/10.1371/journal.pone.0138491.
17. Norme NF. X52-122, janvier 2016, sécurité de protection du citoyen – NRBC-E – protocole d'évaluation des performances de technologies de décontamination de la peau saine.
18. Mohammed D, Matts PJ, Hadgraft J, Lane ME. In vitro–in vivo correlation in skin permeation. Pharm Res. 2014;31(2):394–400.
19. Waters LJ. Recent developments in skin mimic systems to predict transdermal permeation. Curr Pharm Des. 2015;21(20):2725–32.
20. Godin B, Touitou E. Transdermal skin delivery: predictions for humans from in vivo, ex vivo and animal models. Adv Drug Deliv Rev. 2007;59(11):1152–61.
21. Simon GA, Maibach HI. The pig as an experimental animal model of percutaneous permeation in man: qualitative and quantitative observations – an overview. Skin Pharmacol Appl Ski Physiol. 2000;13(5):229–34.
22. Jacobi U, Kaiser M, Toll R, Mangelsdorf S, Audring H, Otberg N, Sterry W, Lademann J. Porcine ear skin: an in vitro model for human skin. Skin Res Technol. 2007;13(1):19–24.
23. OECD Environment, Health and Safety Publications, Series on Testing and Assessment. Test guideline 428: skin absorption: in vitro method. Paris: OECD; 2004.
24. Hafeez F, Chiang A, Hui X, Zhu H, Kamili F, Maibach HI. Stratum corneum reservoir as a predictive method for in vitro percutaneous absorption. J Appl Toxicol. 2016;36(8):1003–10.

Chapter 6
Effects of Soap-Water Wash on Human Epidermal Penetration

Hanjiang Zhu, Eui-Chang Jung, Christina Phuong, Xiaoying Hui, and Howard I. Maibach

Introduction

The superficial layer of skin, stratum corneum (SC), represents the first barrier against external toxicants [6]. Chemicals contaminants on skin surface can be absorbed into SC within minutes and remain there to form a "chemical reservoir", which plays a critical role in percutaneous delivery and skin decontamination. Earlier studies [5, 7, 8] demonstrated the positive correlation between chemical content in the SC reservoir determined by tape stripping at 30 min postdermal exposure and systemic absorption for up to 4 days in human and/or animals in vivo. This suggests the importance of removing hazardous chemical from SC reservoir. Wash-in effect, referring to enhancement of chemical percutaneous absorption caused by water-based skin decontamination strategies, was summarized by Moody and Maibach [12]. Overhydration of SC, effects of surfactant on skin barrier integrity, and friction occurring in the washing process were believed to be factors responsible for the accelerated release of chemical from SC reservoir to deeper layer of skin [4].

Moody et al. reported significant wash-in effects in several in vitro percutaneous penetration studies of pesticides, including 2,4-dichlorophenoxyacetic acid [14], 2,4-dichlorophenoxyacetic acid dimethylamine [13], dichlorodiphenyltrichloroeth-

H. Zhu (✉) · C. Phuong · X. Hui · H. I. Maibach
Department of Dermatology, University of California San Francisco, San Francisco, CA, USA
e-mail: Hanjiang.Zhu@ucsf.edu; Xiaoying.Hui@UCSF.edu; Howard.Maibach@ucsf.edu

E.-C. Jung
Department of Dermatology, University of California San Francisco, San Francisco, CA, USA

Department of Dermatology, Gyeongsang National University Changwon Hospital, Changwon, South Korea

H. Zhu, H. I. Maibach (eds.), *Skin Decontamination*,
https://doi.org/10.1007/978-3-030-24009-7_6

ane [15] and N,N-diethyl-meta-toluamide [16] using rat, guinea pig, and human skin models. However, penetration enhancement was not observed for caffeine, benzoic acid, and malathion after a soap-water wash (5% soap solution) at 6 h post-chemical exposure time [19]. Soap-water wash can reduce the chemical residue in SC reservoir, decrease skin penetration [19], and subsequently provide modest protection in model animals against toxic chemicals [2, 3, 11].

Here, to evaluate decontamination efficacy of soap-water wash, better understand the mechanisms of wash-in effect, and provide insights into improvements for skin decontamination, in vitro human epidermal penetration studies of four model chemicals, hydroquinone, benzoic acid, paraoxon, and clonidine, were conducted with flow-through diffusion cells. We selected these compounds as they have similar Log P values and molecular weights as common chemical warfare agents and pesticides, which are the key interests of this decontamination study. Also hydrophobic compounds with relatively low molecular weight have high penetration ability and low decontamination efficiency [20]; therefore, better understanding of wash-in effect of these compounds may help improve skin decontamination. Epidermis, instead of the commonly used dermatomed skin, was chosen to monitor the real-time penetration rate of chemicals through skin barrier. SC absorption rates of these chemicals at various SC hydration levels (0–295% of the dry sample weights) were determined and compared with the results of epidermal penetration studies to verify the correlation between SC hydration and wash-in effect.

Materials and Methods

Chemicals

[^{14}C(U)]-hydroquinone (50 mCi mmol^{-1}), [7-^{14}C]-benzoic acid (55 mCi mmol^{-1}), and [^{14}C(U)]-paraoxon (77 mCi mmol^{-1}) were synthesized by American Radiolabeled Chemicals, Inc. (St. Louis, MO), and [imidazoline ring ^{14}C]-clonidine (55.77 mCi mmol^{-1}) was from Perkin-Elmer Life Sciences, Inc. (Boston, MA). Reagent-grade ethanol was from Fisher Scientific (Pittsburg, PA). Soluene-350® tissue solubilizer and ULTIMA GOLDTM scintillation cocktails were manufactured by PerkinElmer Life and Analytical Sciences (Boston, MA). Nonradiolabeled hydroquinone, benzoic acid, paraoxon and clonidine as well as trypsin 1:250 for epidermis digestion were obtained from Sigma-Aldrich (St Louis, MO).

Dosing solutions of hydroquinone, benzoic acid, paraoxon, and clonidine were prepared in ethanol with 0.05 mCi ml^{-1} specific radioactivity and 20 mg ml^{-1} corresponding nonradiolabeled chemicals. Receptor fluid was 0.01 mole L^{-1} PBS aqueous solution containing 5% (v/v) polyethylene glycol and was prepared with phosphate-buffered saline (PBS) tablets obtained from Diagnostic BioSystems (Pleasanton, CA) and polyethylene glycol form Sigma-Aldrich (St Louis, MO).

Epidermal Absorption/Penetration Experiment

Adult human cadaver skin was obtained from the Pathology Department of the University of California, San Francisco. Skin was taken from the abdominal region of eight donors and dermatomed using a Padgett Electro-dermatome (Padgett Instruments, Inc., Kansas City, MO) with a target thickness of 400 μm, immediately sealed in aluminum foil, and stored at 4 °C until use. Prior to experiments, epidermis was separated from dermis by heating for 30 seconds in a 60 °C water bath and cut into circular sections to fit diffusion cells. Physical condition of skin samples was assayed visually to exclude any surface damage.

Circular epidermis samples were clamped onto a glass diffusion cell (Laboratory Glass Apparatus, Inc. Berkeley, CA) in a continuous flow-through diffusion cell system, with 1 cm^2 surface area open to air. Circular metal nets were placed underneath skin samples to prevent epidermis from collapsing into diffusion cells. Receiving chambers (below the skin, 3 ml volume) were filled to capacity with receptor fluid stirred magnetically at ~600 rpm. Temperature of diffusion cells was maintained using a Lauda E100 Heating Circulator (Lauda Dr. R. Wobser Gmbh & Co. Kg, Germany) to achieve a skin surface temperature of 32 °C. Receptor fluid was pumped to the diffusion cell at a rate of 30 mL/h using a Pump Pro® MPL (Watson-Marlow, Inc., Wilmington, MA), and collected every 10 minutes using a Retriever Fraction Collector (Teledyne ISCO, Inc., Lincoln, NE) for 90 minutes. Surface of epidermis was dried with cotton pad and allowed to air dry for another 30 min before topical dosing.

A volume of 5 μl dosing solution was applied on skin surface. After 30 minutes, the dosed set was washed once with a small cotton ball soaked with 2% hand soap solution (Softsoap, New York, NY), twice with cotton balls soaked with distilled deionized water, and then dried with two dry cotton balls. Each wet cotton ball was placed on the dosed set for 3 minutes. No wiping was applied during the washing process. Sixty minutes after dosing, epidermis was removed from the diffusion cell and digested for 2 hours with 2 mL Soluene® 350. A volume of 15 mL scintillation cocktail was added to each collected sample and stabilized overnight before assayed.

Stratum Corneum Absorption Experiment

Human cadaver skin was prepared into SC membranes with modified method of Kuriharabergstrom, T et al. [9]. After immersing skin in 60 °C water for 1 min, epidermis was carefully peeled off from the dermis and placed on a cotton pad soaked with 0.5% (wt/wt) trypsin solution with SC side up for at least 15 hours at 36 °C. The pH of trypsin solution was adjusted between 8.0 and 8.6 with 5%

(wt/wt) sodium bicarbonate. After digestion, SC was thoroughly rinsed with water three times and then dried under vacuum overnight at room temperature.

To control SC hydration levels, prepared SC membranes were equilibrated in humidity chambers containing saturated magnesium chloride and potassium nitrate solutions at room temperature for at least a week before use. The percentage relative humidity of humidity chambers was measured to be 28% and 90%, respectively. Dried SC sample were conditioned with Drierite desiccant (anhydrous calcium sulfate, mesh size: 8, Xenia, OH) in a vacuum oven at 50 °C under 18 mmHg of vacuum for a week. Over-hydrated samples were prepared by soaking in deionized water for an hour before use.

Water content of samples was measured by determining the difference between before and after drying weights; prepared SC membranes were accurately weighed and then dried with Drierite desiccant at 50 °C under 18 mmHg vacuum for a week. Weights of vacuum-dried samples were immediately measured after removal from the vacuum oven.

SC absorption was measured as per the modified procedure described previously [21]. Briefly, SC membranes were cut into 17-mm long squares for each dosing. After spreading 5 μL of dosing solution on the SC, scintillation glass vials containing SC samples were immediately capped to avoid change in the SC water content. After exposure (15 s, 5, 15, 30 and 60 min), SC membranes were washed by swirling for 10 s in 1 mL water thrice in different vials (additional wash was applied to certain samples to make certain the radioactivity of last wash was less than 1/10 of the radioactivity in SC sample). A 15 mL of scintillation cocktail was added to each collected fraction and left overnight before being measured for radioactivity in the liquid scintillation counter.

Radioactivity Measurement

Radioactivity measurements were performed in a Model 1500 Liquid Scintillation Counter (Packard Instrument Company, Downer Grove, IL, USA). ^{14}C counting accuracy was audited by quenched and unquenched standards. Counting efficiency was ≥95%. Background control and test samples were each counted for 3 min for radioactivity.

Results

Epidermal Absorption/Penetration

Mass balance of ^{14}C-labeled hydroquinone, benzoic acid, paraoxon, and clonidine in collected fractions of soap-water wash, epidermis, and receptor fluid is provided in Table 6.1. Total mass balance radioactivity recoveries of all four chemicals ranged from 92.3% to 97.5%.

Table 6.1 Epidermal absorption/penetration levels of model chemicals in ethanol as percentage applied dose

	MW[a] (g mol^{-1})	Log P[b]	Nonwash		Soap-water wash		P-value[e]
Hydroquinone	110.11	0.59	$n = 4$[c]		$n = 8$		
			–	–	Decontamination	83.0 ± 4.8	
			Epidermis	92.6 ± 0.8	Epidermis[d]	11.9 ± 0.8	
			Receptor fluid	1.4 ± 0.5	Receptor fluid	0.5 ± 0.2	0.006
			Mass balance	93.6 ± 0.9	Mass balance	95.5 ± 1.9	
Benzoic acid	122.12	1.63	$n = 4$		$n = 4$		
			–	–	Decontamination	82.3 ± 7.1	
			Epidermis	92.9 ± 1.3	Epidermis	8.0 ± 5.1	
			Receptor fluid	3.9 ± 0.3	Receptor fluid	4.2 ± 2.0	>0.05
			Mass balance	96.8 ± 1.2	Mass balance	94.5 ± 1.9	
Paraoxon	275.2	1.98	$n = 5$		$n = 5$		
			–	–	Decontamination	82.4 ± 10.8	
			Epidermis	96.5 ± 2.0	Epidermis	9.8 ± 8.7	
			Receptor fluid	1.2 ± 0.2	Receptor fluid	3.1 ± 1.2	0.001
			Mass balance	97.5 ± 2.1	Mass balance	95.8 ± 1.0	
Clonidine	230.09	2.49	$n = 8$		$n = 8$		
			–	–	Decontamination	89.0 ± 3.1	
			Epidermis	91.9 ± 3.8	Epidermis	9.2 ± 2.5	
			Receptor fluid	0.2 ± 0.1	Receptor fluid	0.2 ± 0.2	>0.05
			Mass balance	92.3 ± 3.7	Mass balance	95.8 ± 1.3	

[a]MW, molecular weight

[b]Log P, logarithm octanol/water partition coefficients was searched from the PubChem BioAssay database. (National Center for Biotechnology Information) [17]

[c]Data represent mean ± standard deviation of each group, n is number of trials

[d]Note that the considerable amounts of chemicals remained in epidermis after soap-water wash

[e]*Statistical analysis performed by one-way ANOVA* showed no significant difference between nonwash and soap-water wash groups for benzoic acid and clonidine. Soap-water wash decreased total penetration of hydroquinone (% dose in receptor fluid), and increased that of paraoxon at 90 min

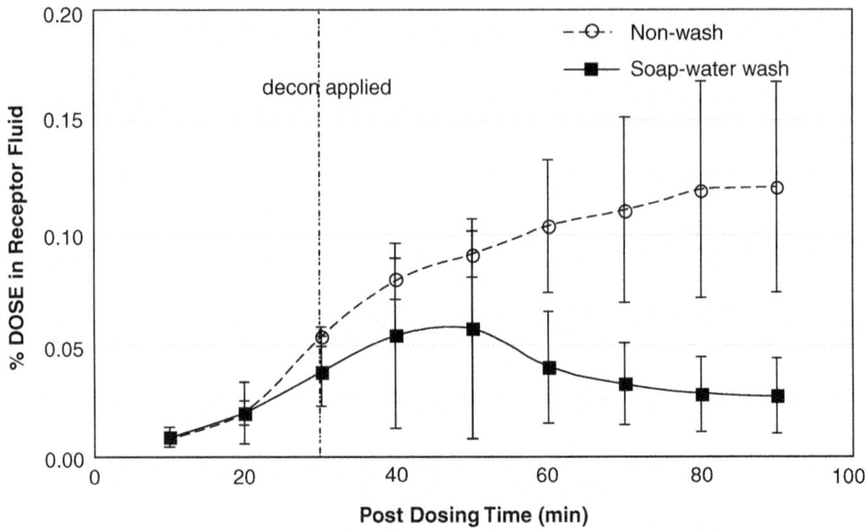

Fig. 6.1 Epidermal penetration curves of hydroquinone compared for soap-water wash at 30 min postexposure ($n = 8$) and nonwash ($n = 4$). Note that the penetration rate of nonwash group continuously increased during 90 min experiment, soap-water wash group showed decreased penetration rate after washing at 30 min postdosing

Soap-water wash applied at 30 min postexposure failed to remove completely the chemicals in epidermis; 8.0–11.9% remained in epidermis after 90 min exposure. Statistical analysis was performed with one-way ANOVA to compare the total penetration amounts (percentage dose in receptor fluid) in the soap-water wash groups and nonwash groups. Total penetration of hydroquinone decreased significantly from 1.4% to 0.5% ($P = 0.006$) by surface washing, yet soap-water wash caused no significant differences in the total penetration of benzoic acid and clonidine compared to the corresponding nonwash groups. Significantly higher concentration of paraoxon was determined in receptor fluid with the soap-water wash ($P = 0.001$).

Figures 6.1, 6.2, and 6.3 shows penetration fluxes of hydroquinone, benzoic acid, and paraoxon, respectively. Nonwash groups of benzoic acid and paraoxon reached constant penetration rates after 30 min exposure. Without surface wash, penetration rate of hydroquinone continuously increased until the end of the experiment. Before decontamination, soap-water wash group and nonwash group of the same chemical show similar penetration curves. As soap-water wash was applied 30 min postexposure, penetration rate of hydroquinone gradually decreased and reached a significant lower level compared to its nonwash group 50 min postdosing (20 min postdecontamination, Fig. 6.1). Increased % dose of benzoic acid in receptor fluid was determined 30 min to 60 min postdosing (0 min to 30 min postdecontamination); 30 min after decontamination (60 min postdosing), less penetration was observed in the soap-water wash group compared to that in the nonwash group (Fig. 6.2). The "wash in" peak for benzoic acid resulted in no significant difference in the total penetration amount of benzoic acid at the end of the experiment (Table 6.1). Penetration curve of paraoxon was accelerated by soap-water wash during the 90-min experimental period (Fig. 6.3)

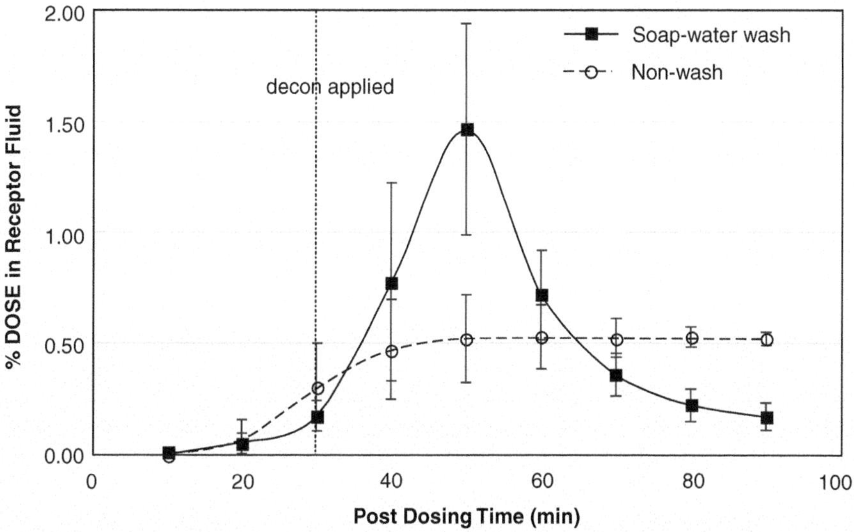

Fig. 6.2 Epidermal penetration curves of benzoic acid compared for soap-water wash at 30 min postexposure ($n = 4$) and nonwash ($n = 4$). Note that nonwash group reached constant penetration rate after 30 min penetration; a penetration enhancement peak of soap-water wash group showed after decontamination. The amount of penetration enhancement suggests extractable chemical portion that can be removed by appropriate decontamination systems

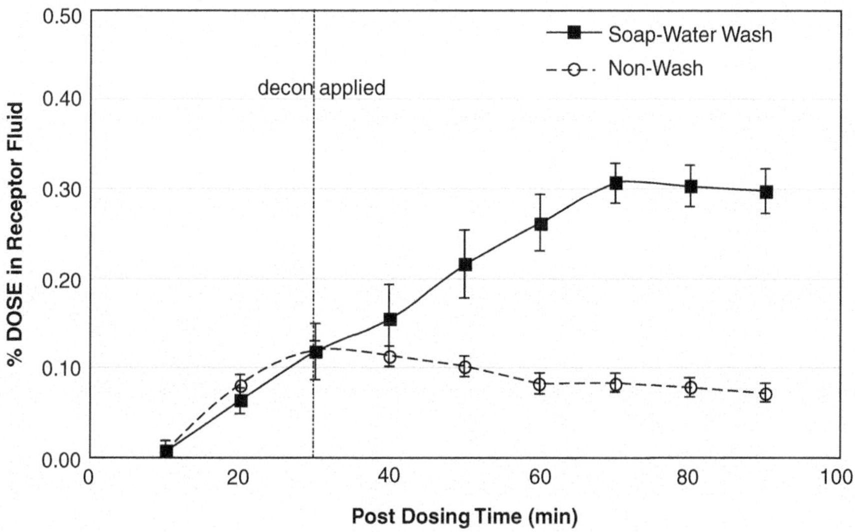

Fig. 6.3 Epidermal penetration curves of paraoxon compared for soap-water wash at 30 min postexposure ($n = 5$) and nonwash ($n = 5$). Note that soap-water wash group showed an accelerated penetration curve after washing at 30 min postdosing; nonwash group reached constant penetration rate after 20 min penetration. The amount of penetration enhancement suggests extractable chemical portion that can be removed by appropriate decontamination systems

resulting in a significant higher total amount penetrated in receptor fluid compared to nonwash samples (Table 6.1). Limited level of clonidine (0.2%) penetrated through human epidermis in 90 min, and the skin wash at 30 min showed no effect on penetration flux (figure not shown).

Stratum Corneum Absorption Rate

Chemical absorption rate into SC was conducted with isolated human SC membranes. Vacuum-dried isolated SC membrane was considered to have 0% of water. Hydration levels of SC conditioned in three humidity chambers were measured to be 35%, 174%, and 295% of the dry sample weights.

Figure 6.4a, b shows the dose absorption curves of benzoic acid and clonidine into SC with different water contents. Each point represents the average of five trials. A linear regression was performed to the linear range of each absorption curve in Fig. 6.4 to permit the equation, D = aT+b, where D is percent dose of chemical absorbed in SC; T is time of chemical exposure, a is the slope of the line, representing chemical absorption rate in percentage per min; and b is the intercept in percentage units. The unit of chemical absorption rates (a) was then converted into nmol min^{-1} and plotted against SC water content for each chemical (Fig. 6.5a–d). Slopes of chemical absorption rates decreased as water content increased for hydroquinone (Fig. 6.5a) and clonidine (Fig. 6.5d), while those of benzoic acid (Fig. 6.5b) and paraoxon (Fig. 6.5c) increased as SC water content increases, suggesting that overhydration of SC has greater effects on chemical absorption of benzoic acid and paraoxon than the other two model chemicals

Discussion

Skin decontamination of toxicants in humans is still difficult after a half century of extensive study. The chemicals of main interest include chemical warfare agents and pesticides, such as sulfur mustard (MW = 159.07, Log P = 2.41), tabun (MW =162.13, Log P = 0.38), soman (MW = 182.17, Log P = 1.78) and VX (MW = 159.07, Log P = 2.41). All of these chemicals are hydrophobic compounds with medium molecular weights, which are the key descriptors for chemicals with high penetration ability [20]. Therefore, we selected the four model chemicals with log P values ranging from 0.59 to 2.49 and molecular weights from 110.11 to 203.09 to study their transportation behavior under soap-water wash conditions (Table 6.1). Moreover, the model chemical, paraoxon is the most potent acetylcholinesterase-inhibiting pesticide, as well a close simulant to G and V series nerve agents.

To track real-time changes of chemical diffusion rates through skin barrier (SC), epidermis was separated from the dermis and employed as skin sample. Significant increases in diffusion rates following soap-water wash were observed for benzoic

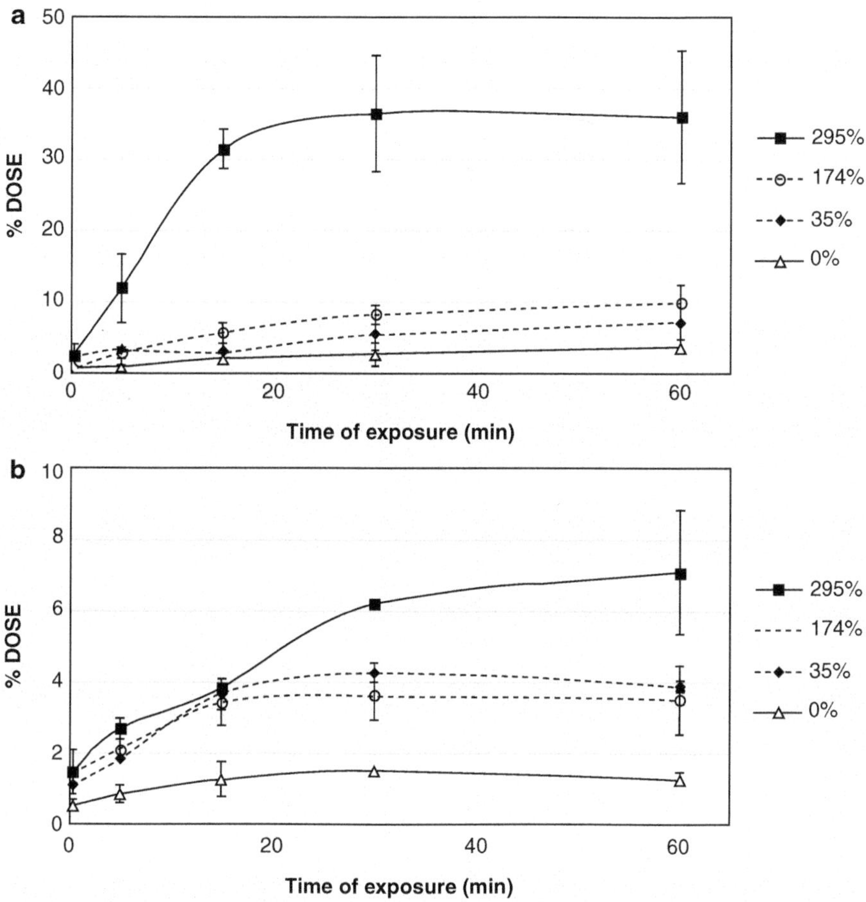

Fig. 6.4 Absorption curves of (**a**) benzoic acid and (**b**) clonidine into SC membranes with four hydration levels, 0%, 35%, 174% and 295% of water/SC dry weight. Each point was mean of five trials. Note that the enhancement effect of SC overhydration on chemical absorption rate is more significant to benzoic acid than clonidine. SC absorption rates in nmol min^{-1} (y-axis vales of Fig. 6.5) were calculated from the slopes of the linear ranges of absorption curves. SC, stratum corneum

acid and paraoxon compared to that of nonwash groups (Figs. 6.2 and 6.3). This penetration enhancement phenomenon agrees with Moody et al.'s (2006) observation in the in vitro percutaneous absorption studies of pesticides, where skin wash was conducted at 24 h postdosing. As diffusion rate of benzoic acid decreased from 30 min postdecontamination (60 min postdosing), the penetration enhancement occurred rapidly after soap-water wash was counteracted and caused no significant difference in total penetration amount at 90 min. This may explain why a wash-in effect was not observed in the previous in vitro percutaneous penetration study of benzoic acid [19], where the existence of dermis and the longer collection period of receptor fluid (2 h)

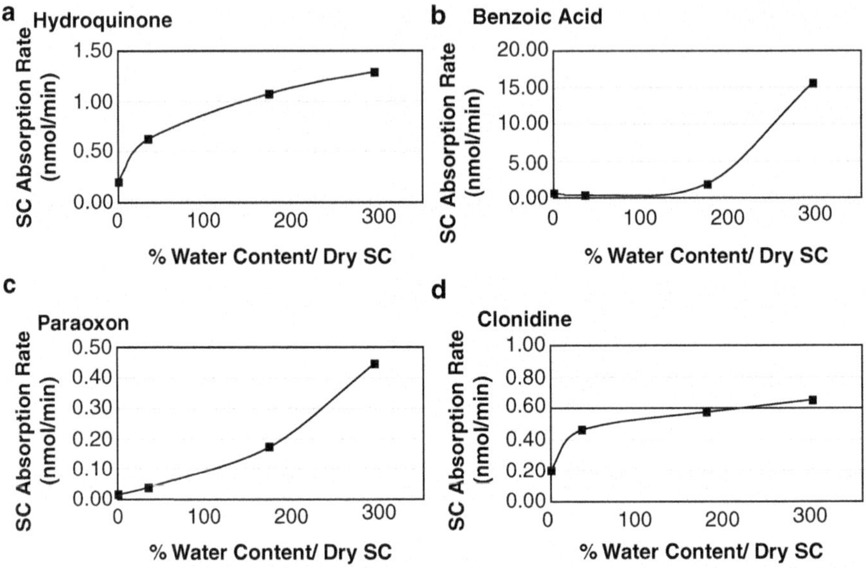

Fig. 6.5 SC absorption rates (nmol min^{-1}) of (**a**) hydroquinone, (**b**) benzoic acid (**c**) paraoxon, and (**d**) clonidine versus SC water content. Note that the slopes of hydroquinone and clonidine, which show no wash-in effect in epidermal penetration experiment, decreased as water content increased; the slopes of benzoic acid and paraoxon, observed significant wash-in effect, which increased as the water content increased. These results suggest that wash-in effect is chemical dependent, which correlates with SC hydration during skin wash

may neglect and override the relative brief diffusion rate increase by the penetration reduction derived from reduced amount of chemical in SC reservoir.

Our pervious 24 h in vitro percutaneous penetration study of paraoxon using human dermatomed skin and diffusion cells indicated that a soap-water wash conducted at 30 min postexposure resulted in no significant difference in total penetration amount at 24 h (unpublished data). Although the soap-water wash group of paraoxon showed an accelerated penetration curve (Fig. 6.3) and significant higher absorption amount than those of nonwash group (Table. 6.1) in this 90 min experiment, skin wash may still be able to reduce the paraoxon penetration rate in the longer term, so that the total penetration amount at 24 h would be comparable with its nonwash group. It has to be noted that the accelerated intake of toxins into dermis and subsequently circulatory system caused by skin wash may enhance toxicity and reduce the time window and chance for successful medical interventions.

Different from benzoic acid and paraoxon, wash-in effect was not observed for hydroquinone and clonidine. Figure 6.1 shows a consistent rising penetration curve of hydroquinone nonwash group, suggesting a longer lag time for hydroquinone to cross epidermis than benzoic acid and paraoxon. Therefore, hydroquinone could be still in its relative early stage of penetration while soap-water wash was applied here (30 min postexposure). Even if the skin barrier integrity was affected by surfactant and overhydration of SC [4], chemical absorbed in superficial layer of SC would be more likely removed by surface wash than diffusion into deeper layer of skin and receptor fluid. In the case of clonidine, penetration amounts were limited for both wash and nonwash groups in the 90 min penetration (Table. 6.1), indicating a long retention time in SC. Although no effect of soap-water wash was observed in the experimental period, as 89.0% ± 3.1% of chemical was removed by skin decontamination, a lower penetration amount could be expected in the long term. Results of hydroquinone and clonidine indicate the significant effect of delayed application time on decontamination efficacy of soap-water wash; surface washing would perform better in removing chemicals during their early stage of skin absorption [10].

Even though soap-water wash had different effects on the epidermal penetration profiles of four model chemicals, similar levels of chemical remained in epidermis and receptor fluid after the decontamination (Table. 6.1), suggesting that chemicals absorbed into SC cannot be completely removed by this decontamination system, regardless of their physicochemical properties.

Both surfactant and overhydration of SC could be responsible for the wash-in enhancement effect [4]. The main surfactant of Softsoap hand soap is sodium olefin sulfonate (SLS), and the common amount of surfactant in hand soap is 10–20%. As we only used 2% hand soap solution in the first round of washing, SLS concentration applied on skin would be 0.2–0.4%, which was then quickly removed in the second water wash. SLS demonstrated a penetration enhancement effect on rat skin in vitro when present in dosing solution with concentration higher than 1% [18]; therefore, SC hydration may be a primary cause of wash-in effect, which opens up the compact structure of SC by increasing intercellular regions and swelling corneocytes [1]. We studied the effect of isolated SC hydration levels on the absorption rates of the four model chemicals, to verify the correlation of SC hydration and wash-in effect. Total chemical absorption in isolated SC membranes at 60 min exposure time increased as SC hydration levels increased (Fig. 6.4), suggesting that wet decontamination methods may increase the capacity of SC reservoir by hydrating SC. For benzoic acid (Fig. 6.5b) and paraoxon (Fig. 6.5c), the increased SC hydration level intensively enhanced the absorption rate at high water levels. Increase in SC absorption rates of hydroquinone and clonidine was less than the increase in proportion of SC water content (Fig. 6.5a and Fig. 6.5d, respectively). Comparing the results with epidermal absorption / penetration data, chemicals absorbing significantly faster into SC membranes at high hydration level showed a penetration enhancement after skin wash (benzoic acid and paraoxon), and chemicals that displayed no wash-in effect was less affected by the SC water content in SC absorption assays (hydroquinone and clonidine). This indicates that wash-in effect is chemical dependent. Chemicals absorbed into SC much faster under high water content conditions are more likely to show penetration enhancement following skin wash.

Conclusion

Soap-water wash applied at 30 min postexposure removed the majority of chemicals on skin surface, but considerable amounts of chemical remained in epidermis. A "Wash-in" skin penetration enhancement effect was observed for benzoic acid and paraoxon, but not for hydroquinone and clonidine. The different effects of soap-water wash on chemical penetration rate could be explained by the timing of decontamination and effect of SC hydration on chemical SC absorption. Surface washing tends to have greater decontamination efficiency on chemicals in their early stage of skin absorption and cause wash-in effect of chemicals, which could be intensely accelerated by increasing SC water content. Although soap-water wash could decrease total chemical penetration amount in the long term by reducing "chemical reservoir" in SC, it should be noted that the brief accelerated percutaneous absorption of chemical toxins, particularly chemical warfare agents, caused by skin wash may enhance intoxication and reduce the opportunity for successful medical interventions. The penetrated amounts of benzoic acid and paraoxon enhanced by soap-water wash suggest that the chemical portion reversibly bond in SC, which indicates skin decontamination methods can be improved.

We do not wish to overgeneralize the interpretation of the above data. Clearly, hydration/wash-in effect remains complex in biology and will benefit from in-depth investigation, including extension to in vivo human studies.

Acknowledgments This research is supported by Defense Threat Reduction Agency (DTRA) Grant: HDTRA1-14-0005 UCSF (BRBAA11-PerC-9-2-0054 – Base).

References

1. Bouwstra JA, de Graaff A, Gooris GS, Nijsse J, Wiechers JW, van Aelst AC. Water distribution and related morphology in human stratum corneum at different hydration levels. J Invest Dermatol. 2003;120:750–8.
2. Braue EH Jr, Smith KH, Doxzon BF, Lumpkin HL, Clarkson ED. Efficacy studies of reactive skin decontamination lotion, M291 skin decontamination kit, 0.5% bleach, 1% soapy water, and skin exposure reduction paste against chemical warfare agents, Part 1: Guinea pigs challenged with VX. Cutan Ocul Toxicol. 2011a;30:15–28.
3. Braue EH Jr, Smith KH, Doxzon BF, Lumpkin HL, Clarkson ED. Efficacy studies of reactive skin decontamination lotion, M291 skin decontamination kit, 0.5% bleach, 1% soapy water, and skin exposure reduction paste against chemical warfare agents, Part 2: Guinea pigs challenged with soman. Cutan Ocul Toxicol. 2011b;30:29–37.
4. Chan HP, Zhai H, Hui X, Maibach HI. Skin decontamination: principles and perspectives. Toxicol Ind Health. 2013;29:955–68.
5. Dupuis D, Rougier A, Roguet R, Lotte C. The measurement of the stratum-corneum reservoir – a simple method to predict the influence of vehicles on in vivo percutaneous-absorption. Brit J Dermatol. 1986;115:233–8.
6. Elias PM, Cooper ER, Korc A, Brown BE. Percutaneous transport in relation to stratum-corneum structure and lipid-composition. J Invest Dermatol. 1981;76:297–301.
7. Hui X, Lamel S, Qiao P, Maibach HI. Isolated human and animal stratum corneum as a partial model for the 15 steps of percutaneous absorption: emphasizing decontamination, part II. J Appl Toxicol. 2013a;33:173–82.
8. Hui X, Lamel S, Qiao P, Maibach HI. Isolated human/animal stratum corneum as a partial model for 15 steps in percutaneous absorption: emphasizing decontamination, Part I. J Appl Toxicol. 2013b;33:157–72.

9. Kuriharabergstrom T, Knutson K, Denoble LJ, Goates CY. Percutaneous-absorption enhancement of an ionic molecule by ethanol water-systems in human skin. Pharm Res. 1990;7:762–6.
10. Loke WK, U SH, Lau SK, Lim JS, Tay GS, Koh CH. Wet decontamination-induced stratum corneum hydration – effects on the skin barrier function to diethylmalonate. J Appl Toxicol. 1999;19:285–90.
11. Misik J, Pavlikova R, Cabal J, Kuca K. Percutaneous toxicity and decontamination of soman, VX, and paraoxon in rats using detergents. Arh Hig Rada Toksikol. 2013;64:211–7.
12. Moody RP, Maibach HI. Skin decontamination: importance of the wash-in effect. Food Chem Toxicol. 2006;44:1783–8.
13. Moody RP, Nadeau B. In vitro dermal absorption of two commercial formulations of 2,4-dichlorophenoxyacetic acid dimethylamine (2,4-D amine) in rat, Guinea pig and human skin. Toxicol In Vitro. 1997;11:251–62.
14. Moody RP, Nadeau B, Chu I. In-vitro dermal absorption of pesticides: 5. In-vivo and in-vitro comparison of the herbicide 2,4-dichlorophenoxyacetic acid in rat, Guinea-pig, pig, human and tissue-cultured skin. Toxicol In Vitro. 1994a;8:1219–24.
15. Moody RP, Nadeau B, Chu I. In-vitro dermal absorption of pesticides: 6. In-vivo and in-vitro comparison of the organochlorine insecticide DDT in rat, Guinea-pig, pig, human and tissue-cultured skin. Toxicol In Vitro. 1994b;8:1225–32.
16. Moody RP, Nadeau B, Chu I. In vitro dermal absorption of N,N-diethyl-m-toluamide (DEET) in rat, Guinea pig, and human skin. Toxicol In Vitro. 1995;8:263–75.
17. National Center for Biotechnology Information. PubChem Compound Database, http://pubchem.ncbi.nlm.nih.gov/ [10 Dec., 2014].
18. Nokhodchi A, Shokri J, Dashbolaghi A, Hassan-Zadeh D, Ghafourian T, Barzegar-Jalali M. The enhancement effect of surfactants on the penetration of lorazepam through rat skin. Int J Pharm. 2003;250:359–69.
19. Nielsen JB. Efficacy of skin wash on dermal absorption: an in vitro study on four model compounds of varying solubility. Int Arch Occ Env Hea. 2010;83:683–90.
20. Patel H, ten Berge W, Cronin MTD. Quantitative structure-activity relationships (QSARs) for the prediction of skin permeation of exogenous chemicals. Chemosphere. 2002;48:603–13.
21. Zhu H, Jung EC, Hui X, Maibach H. Proposed human stratum corneum water domain in chemical absorption. J Appl Toxicol. 2015;36:991. https://doi.org/10.1002/jat.3208.

Chapter 7
Fuller's Earth: Old and Faithful Skin Decontaminant Against Toxic Agents

Shlomit Dachir, Eliezer Fishbine, Yakov Meshulam, Hillel Buch, Nahum Allon, and Tamar Kadar

Introduction

Skin exposure to warfare agents is a major problem during nonconventional war [1] or terrorist attack. The skin, being the largest organ of the body and having the largest surface area in contact with the outside environment, is one of the principal targets for warfare agents that might either damage the skin or penetrate through it. Therefore, removal of the warfare agents by decontamination is a most important component in the individual defense doctrine against exposure to such compounds.

Liquids and solids are the only substances that can be effectively removed from the skin while it is generally not possible and not necessary to decontaminate vapor. Removal from the atmosphere containing the vapor is all that is required [2].

The purpose of the decontamination procedure performed after exposure is the removal of maximal amount of warfare agent from the skin, prevention of agent's penetration through the skin, and avoiding secondary contamination of the medical team that comes in contact with the injured individuals [3–5].

Although decontamination issues have been explored since the beginning of modern chemical warfare, currently there is no an ideal decontaminant. Many substances have been evaluated for their efficacy for skin decontamination, but only few became practical.

At present, decontamination of CWA from the skin is still considered as a difficult problem due to the necessity for both rapid action and nonaggressive performance. As yet, there is no consensus as to the optimal procedure for removing the toxic agents from the skin.

S. Dachir (✉) · E. Fishbine · Y. Meshulam · H. Buch · N. Allon · T. Kadar
Department of Pharmacology, Israel Institute for Biological Research, Ness Ziona, Israel
e-mail: shlomitd@iibr.gov.il; hillelb@iibr.gov.il; tamark@iibr.gov.il

H. Zhu, H. I. Maibach (eds.), *Skin Decontamination*,
https://doi.org/10.1007/978-3-030-24009-7_7

There are three basic methods of decontamination: physical removal, chemical deactivation, and biological deactivation of the agent. Up till now, biological decontamination has not been developed to the point of being practical.

An ideal decontaminant is required to have several essential characteristics: neutralize the agent, safety (nontoxic and noncorrosive), easy to apply, readily available, rapid action, will not produce toxic end-products, stable in long-term storage, will not enhance percutaneous agent absorption, and easy to dispose [6, 7] . Nevertheless, the most common problems with potential decontaminants are irritation of the skin, toxicity, ineffectiveness, or high cost.

The two most common chemical warfare agents (CWAs) that constitute a threat for skin exposure are sulfur mustard (HD) and VX (O-ethyl-S-(2-diisopropylaminoethyl-methylphosphothiolate).

Sulfur mustard is a potent cutaneous vesicant that penetrates rapidly through the skin, causing severe injuries. Being a blistering agent, it causes inflammation, blisters, and severe damage to the skin that might result in incapacitation of the victims. Healing time from such injuries is very long and often the healing is pathologic [8–11]. Since its first use in World War I and despite vast efforts, only limited success has been attained to find an effective treatment to prevent or reduce these lesions.

VX, on the other hand, is a very toxic nerve agent, an organophosphate and an extremely potent cholinesterase inhibitor. It is relatively stable, has a very low volatility, efficiently penetrates through the skin, and might cause death at very low doses (dermal human $LD_{50} \approx 0.04–0.14$ mg/kg) [12–14].

Removal of the CWA from the skin soon after exposure may reduce significantly the extent of damage following exposure to HD and the mortality rate and systemic clinical symptoms after exposure to VX.

The present article aimed to explore the efficacy of Fuller's earth powder as a universal decontaminant against CWA and to compare its efficacy against the two representative agents to other common decontaminants.

Fuller's earth powder is a natural substance containing silica of aluminum and magnesium which has very high adsorption properties. In addition, it contains small amounts of calcite, dolomite, and quartz.

Fuller's earth has been demonstrated to be a nontoxic and effective absorbent of classical liquid CWAs [15]. The powder is chemically inactive, is relatively cheap, and has long shelf life. Fuller's earth has been fielded by the Israeli Defense Forces and in by several North Atlantic Treaty Organization countries [6]. The decontamination doctrine for percutaneous toxic agents in Israel is based on a combination of application of Fuller's earth (×3) followed by wet decontamination (copious amount of water), which will be usually performed a few hours after Fuller's earth decontamination by the medical personnel.

A comparison between Fuller's earth and other common decontaminants is presented following exposure of pigs to HD and VX.

Experimental Models and Experimental Design

Cutaneous exposure was performed in the well-established pig model which is the preferred model for skin injury research due to its anatomical, physiological, and biochemical similarity to human skin [16–18].

Young female white pigs (supplied by the Institute of Animal Research, Kibbutz Lahav, Israel, and Topig20, the Netherlands) weighting 10–11 kg were housed in individual pans located in a temperature-controlled (21 ± 1 °C) room, with lights on from 06:00 to 18:00. Pigs were fed twice a day and had free access to tap water.

All procedures involving animals were in accordance with the Guide for the Care and Use of Laboratory Animals, National Academy Press, Washington, DC, 1996, and were approved by the Institutional Animal Care and Use Committee.

Exposure Procedure

Exposure to HD – Droplets Ten fields were marked on the female pigs' back skin (5 on each side), and three droplets of neat HD (1 μl each) were placed on the skin in each of the fields. Exposure durations varied between experiments and were 1, 2, 3, 5, 15, 30, and 60 minutes.

Exposure to VX Female pigs were exposed to 1-μl droplets of VX (0.4 mg/kg or 1.3 mg/kg) which was equivalent to $2LD_{50}$ for 24 hours (unpublished data). The shift in the LD50 dose is due to the changes in the exposure setup and newly imposed safety regulations.

VX was placed on the pigs' back skin along the midline. Exposure durations were 20 minutes and 1, 2, and 5 hours. Control pigs were exposed to VX for the duration of 12–24 hours.

The exposure procedures of both HD and VX were performed in a hood at room temperature and were terminated, after a predetermined period by decontamination with one of the tested materials.

All exposed pigs, independent of their decontamination methods, were washed with the decontamination solution IPP2 at the end of the day, before returning to their home cages (about 10–12 hours following exposure). This was a safety precaution required by our institution safety procedures. IPP2 decontamination solution was prepared by dissolving chloramine T (38 g /100 ml, (Axcentive, the Netherlands) and zinc chloride (5.5%) in water (56%) and ethanol (44%) (Sigma, Israel).

Decontamination efficacy was determined by morphometric analysis of the lesion areas (exposure to HD) or by the extent of ChE inhibition in whole-blood samples, clinical signs, and the occurrence of death (exposure to VX).

Quantitative Assessment of the Lesion Area The extent of the injury following exposure to HD droplets was measured using morphometric analysis of the damaged skin area. The exposed sites on the pigs' backs were photographed using a digital camera (Coolpix 950, Nikon, Tokyo, Japan). Pictures were analyzed for the damaged area using an image analysis system (Image-Pro Express 4.0).

Cholinesterase Inhibition in Whole Blood Blood samples (0.5–0.7 ml) were collected from the jugular vein at various time points following exposure to VX. One hundred microliters of blood was immediately transferred into a heparinized tube containing 1.2 DDW and mixed gently to cause hemolysis of red blood cells. Samples were stored at −4 °C until further analyzed.

The inhibition of the enzyme cholinesterase was determined using the radiometric method [19]. The blood samples were incubated with the substrate, H^3-acetylcholine, at a temperature of 25 °C for 30 minutes. The reaction was ended with a reaction stopper that separated between the radioactive acetate and the choline. Scintillation solution was added, and the radioactivity of the acetate in the organic phase was measured using a β counter.

Results

The Efficacy of Fuller's Earth

Fuller's earth is a clay material containing nonplastic form of kaolin with aluminum-magnesium silicate [20] that has the capability to absorb oily liquids and other liquids. Fuller's earth is used in the industry as absorbents for oil, grease, and animal waste and is widely used in cosmetics. It is also recommended for personal decontamination of warfare agents.

Decontamination of experimental animals was performed by applying a large amount of powder to the skin to cover the exposed areas and then was removed with a spatula. This was repeated three times and then was followed by thorough rinsing with copious amount of tap water before returning the animals to the pens.

Exposure to Liquid HD Percutaneous exposure of pigs to HD droplets and decontamination with Fuller's earth at various time points resulted in a distinct dose–response (Fig. 7.1). The efficacy of the decontamination procedure was higher when performed earlier after agent application. If decontamination took place within 1–5 minutes of exposure, the damage to the skin was very mild and a decrease of 60–90% in wound area was measured compared to wound area found following a 60-minute exposure. Still, there was a significant difference between 1- and 5-minute lesions ($p < 0.001$). Even decontamination at 15 minutes after the exposure resulted in a significant decrease in the size of the lesions ($p < 0.001$ vs 30 and 60 minutes; Figs. 7.1 and 7.2). No significant differences were found between exposure duration of 30 and 60 minutes though the lesion area after 30 minutes was somewhat smaller.

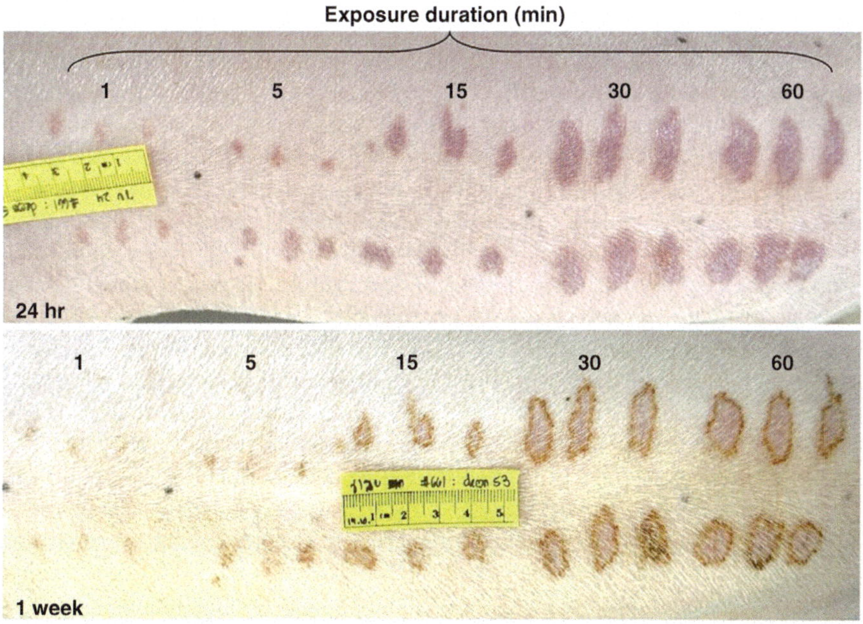

Fig. 7.1 The effect of decontamination with Fuller's earth 24 hours and 1 week following dermal exposure to HD droplets (1 μl) on the extent of the damage. Note the time-dependent effect on the skin lesions (exposure durations of: 1, 5, 15, 30, and 60 minutes)

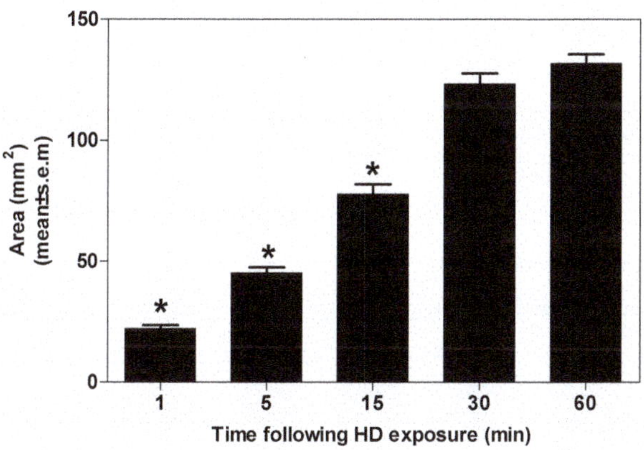

Fig. 7.2 A morphometric analysis of skin lesion area 24 hours following exposure to HD droplets (1 μl) and decontamination with Fuller's earth at various time points after exposure. Note the time-dependent response and the significant reduction in lesion area even when decontamination was performed 15 minutes post exposure ($*p < 0.001$ vs all other time points, $n = 21$ pigs)

A similar pattern of efficacy was obtained following exposure of pigs to 0.2-μl droplets up to 30 minutes [8].

Exposure to VX Exposure to 2LD50 of VX and decontamination with Fuller's earth at 20 minutes and 1, 2, 5, and 24 hours after exposure resulted in a dose–response, indicating high efficacy for early decontamination. Percutaneous exposure to VX for a duration of up to 2 hours resulted in only mild signs of intoxication that appeared starting 5 hours post exposure. Clinical signs included slight salivation, chewing, slight tremor, and restlessness that lasted up to 10 hours. None of the animals that were decontaminated up to 2 hours died and all pigs appeared healthy at 24 hours after exposure. When decontamination was performed 5 hours after exposure, all pigs developed severe signs of intoxication exhibiting salivation, tremor, and respiratory distress that deteriorated to convulsions in 50% of the animals (2/4). Similar severe clinical signs were observed in the control animals that were decontaminated 24 hours post exposure. This resulted in the death of three out of the four animals within this period, even before decontamination was performed. The inhibition of ChE activity in whole blood reached a maximal value of 50% around 4 hours after a 20-minute exposure (Fig. 7.3). When decontamination was performed 1–2 hours after exposure, inhibition increased to 60–65% within 5–8 hours. Longer exposure durations (5 and 24 hours) resulted in a maximum of 80% inhibition of ChE around 5–6 hours (Fig. 7.3).

Interestingly, the time of decontamination affected the rate of ChE inhibition development, which by itself influenced the severity of clinical symptoms. When decontamination was performed up to 2 hours post exposure, the slope was more moderate than the slope following longer periods of exposure, leading to a less severe clinical outcome (Fig. 7.3).

Another characteristic of percutaneous exposure to VX is the continuous decrease in ChE activity in blood after decontamination was performed (at least up to 2-hour exposure duration), suggesting a possible release of VX from a skin depot. When decontamination was performed after 5 hours of exposure, the inhibition was maximal most likely because all the amount of VX already reached the circulation.

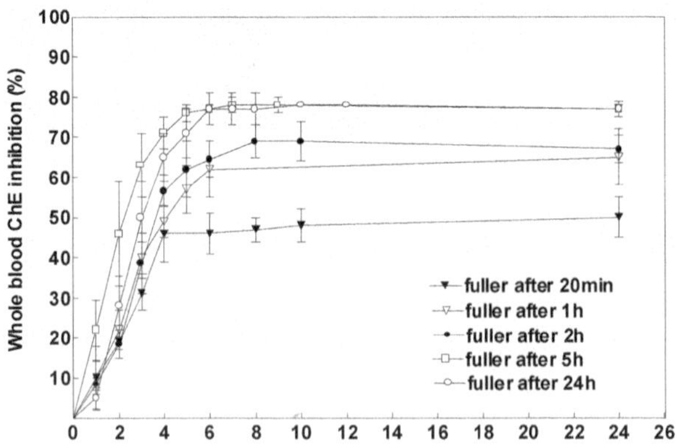

Fig. 7.3 Profile of ChE inhibition following dermal exposure to 2LD50 of VX and decontamination with Fuller's earth at various time points post exposure (20 minutes – $n = 3$, 1 hours – $n = 6$, 2 hours – $n = 2$, 5 hours – $n = 4$, 24 hours – $n = 4$)

To summarize, Fuller's earth decontamination was found beneficial, in reducing skin lesions up to 30-minute exposure durations to liquid HD and in preventing most of the VX clinical signs when performed up to 2 hours following exposure.

The Effect of Fuller's Earth Compared to Water

Rinsing the skin with water can remove or dilute substantial amounts of the agent and produce significant results. Moreover, water has the capacity to remove chemical agents not only through mechanical force but also via slow hydrolysis; however, the low solubility and slow rate of diffusion of HD and VX in water significantly limit these agents' hydrolysis rate.

Water or a solution of soap and water were suggested for decontamination if other decontaminants were not available. The solutions are well suited for mass casualty situations in which adequate water supplies are available, and they provide some protection against CWA mostly by physical removal of the agents. The following section compares the efficacy of water as a single decontaminant to the efficacy of dry decontamination with Fuller's earth.

Exposure to Liquid HD A comparison between the efficacy of water and Fuller's earth was performed following exposure to HD. The decontamination regimens that were tested were tap water (1 liter/400 cm^2), soap + water, Fuller's earth × 3, Fuller's earth × 1 + water. Analyzing all parameters that were tested it was found that Fuller's earth × 3 was the most effective decontamination method over time. The decontamination with water alone or soap + water exacerbated the effect of HD and resulted in an increase in the damaged area probably because in this experiment pigs were not rinsed with a copious amount of water but only washed with a rather small amount. Wetting the area of exposure is not efficient in removing HD from the skin.

Exposure to VX In a study that was conducted in the early 1980s, we have shown that decontamination with Fuller 20 minutes after percutaneous exposure of pigs to 10LD50 of VX (2 mg/kg) was more effective than either simple rinsing with tap water or than the combination of scrubbing with soap (WFA detergent) and rinsing with tap water. The time elapsed from agent's application to reaching 50% activity of ChE in whole blood was 39.7 ± 4.2 and 28.7 ± 3.7 minutes for water or soap + water, respectively, compared to 35.6 ± 5.3 minutes for Fuller's earth. This time interval increased up to 64.2 ± 5.9 minutes following two applications of Fuller's earth.

In addition, all pigs that were decontaminated with water or soap + water exhibited some clinical signs such as salivation. At the same time, only 50% of the pigs that were decontaminated with Fuller's earth once and none of the pigs that were decontaminated with Fuller' earth twice showed salivation.

In a later study, pigs were exposed to 2LD50 of VX and were decontaminated at either 1 or 5 hours post exposure with tap water or Fuller's earth × 3. Pigs that were decontaminated with Fuller's earth × 3 at 1 hour exhibited only mild clinical sings,

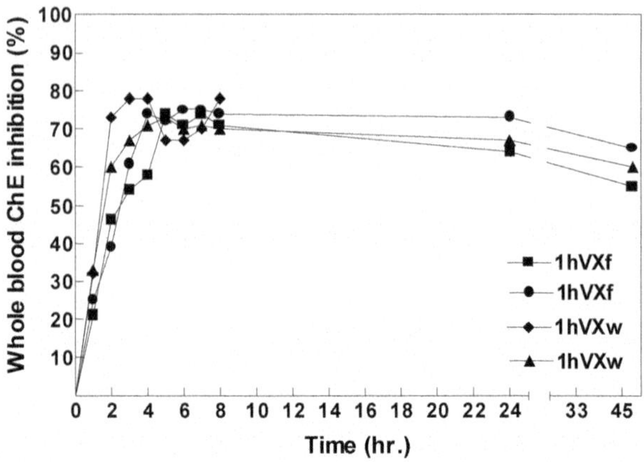

Fig. 7.4 ChE inhibition profile following dermal exposure of pigs to 2LD50 of VX and decontamination with either tap water or Fuller's earth ×3, 1 hour following exposure. Note that the slope following decontamination with water is steeper (individual pigs)

while two-thirds pigs that were decontaminated with water exhibited severe signs and one pig died within 24 hours. When decontamination with water was delayed to 5 hours post exposure, all four pigs died within 24 hours, while all the pigs that were decontaminated with Fuller's earth survived at 24 hours and only two-fourth pigs exhibited severe clinical signs.

Moreover, while following decontamination with Fuller's earth, the rate of increase in ChE inhibition was relatively moderate following decontamination with water; the increase in ChE inhibition was steep and reached a value of more than 60% at 2 hours post exposure compared to only 40–45% in pigs that were decontaminated with Fuller's earth (Fig. 7.4).

In summary, rinsing with water alone was less efficient than Fuller's earth alone when tested against both HD and VX. Furthermore, there are indications that water irrigation by itself, specifically, if used in small amounts, may exacerbate the skin lesions caused by HD and intensify the toxicity of VX, in comparison to Fuller's earth, as expressed by clinical signs and mortality rate. It appears that when using water, particularly, if using only water, it should be thorough rinsing with copious amounts of water.

In light of all the above data demonstrating the high efficacy of Fuller's earth, the procedure of decontamination with Fuller's earth application ×3 was adopted for all our future exposure scenarios.

The Efficacy of Fuller's Earth Compared to M291 Kit

The M291 SDK kit is an individual soldier decontamination kit that was first issued to US forces in 1989 as the primary countermeasure for removing CWAs from skin [4, 5]. It contains a carbonaceous adsorbent, a polystyrene polymeric, and ion exchange resins. The kit consists of a wallet-like carrying pouch containing six individual decontamination packets. Each packet contains a nonwoven, fiberfill-laminated pad impregnated with the decontamination compound, Ambergard XE-555 Resin, which is a black, free-flowing, resin-based powder. The presence of acidic and basic groups in the resin promotes the destruction of trapped chemical agents by acid and base hydrolysis. However, the neutralization process is relatively slow, and therefore, the M291 kit is considered as a nonreactive dry adsorbent decontaminant. Because the resin is black, it maps out the areas that have been decontaminated [2]. This kit was used for many years in the US Army, but a few years ago, it was replaced by RSDL [4].

Pigs were exposed to 1-μl HD droplets, and decontamination was performed 1, 2, 3, and 5 minutes following exposure. In all animals, regardless of the method of decontamination, the severity of the skin lesions increased as exposure duration increased. The efficacy of M291 and Fuller's earth were very similar after 1- and 2-minute exposure. Yet, decontamination with Fuller's earth allows an immediate coverage of large body areas, while the M291 kit provides decontamination of only smaller limited areas.

The Efficacy of Fuller's Earth Compared to M295 Decontamination Kit

The M295 decontamination kit was originally developed for the decontamination of individual equipment. It consists of a pouch containing four decontamination mitts. Each mitt is filled with an alumina-based sorbent and sealed within a waterproof protective package [21]. Similar to M291, the M295 kit decontaminates the exposed area by absorption and physical removal of the agent.

When decontamination of pig skin following exposure to HD droplets was performed with M295 kit, the extent of the lesions was substantially larger. The efficacy of decontamination with Fuller's earth was clearly superior in all time points tested. Following the short-duration exposures: 1, 5, and 15 minutes, the lesions' area that developed was about four times larger on M295 decontaminated sites than on Fuller's earth decontaminated sites (Figs. 7.5 and 7.6). In fact, the size of the

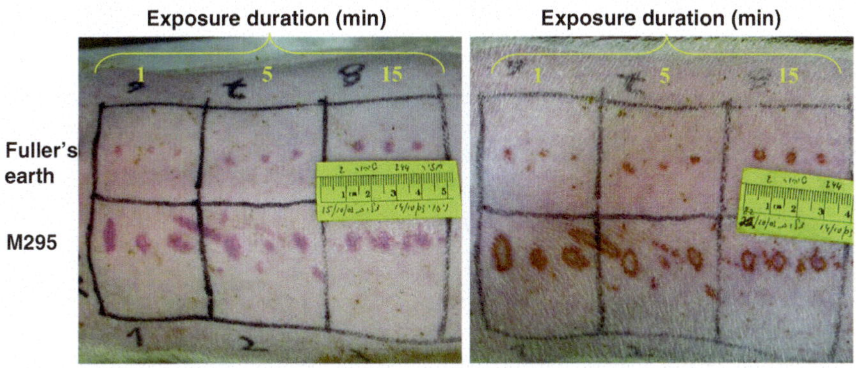

Fig. 7.5 The effect of decontamination with M295 decontamination kit compared to decontamination with Fuller's earth at various time points after dermal exposure to HD droplets (1 μl) on the extent of the damage at 24 hours and 1 week following exposure. Note the exacerbation of the lesions on the sites that were decontaminated with M295

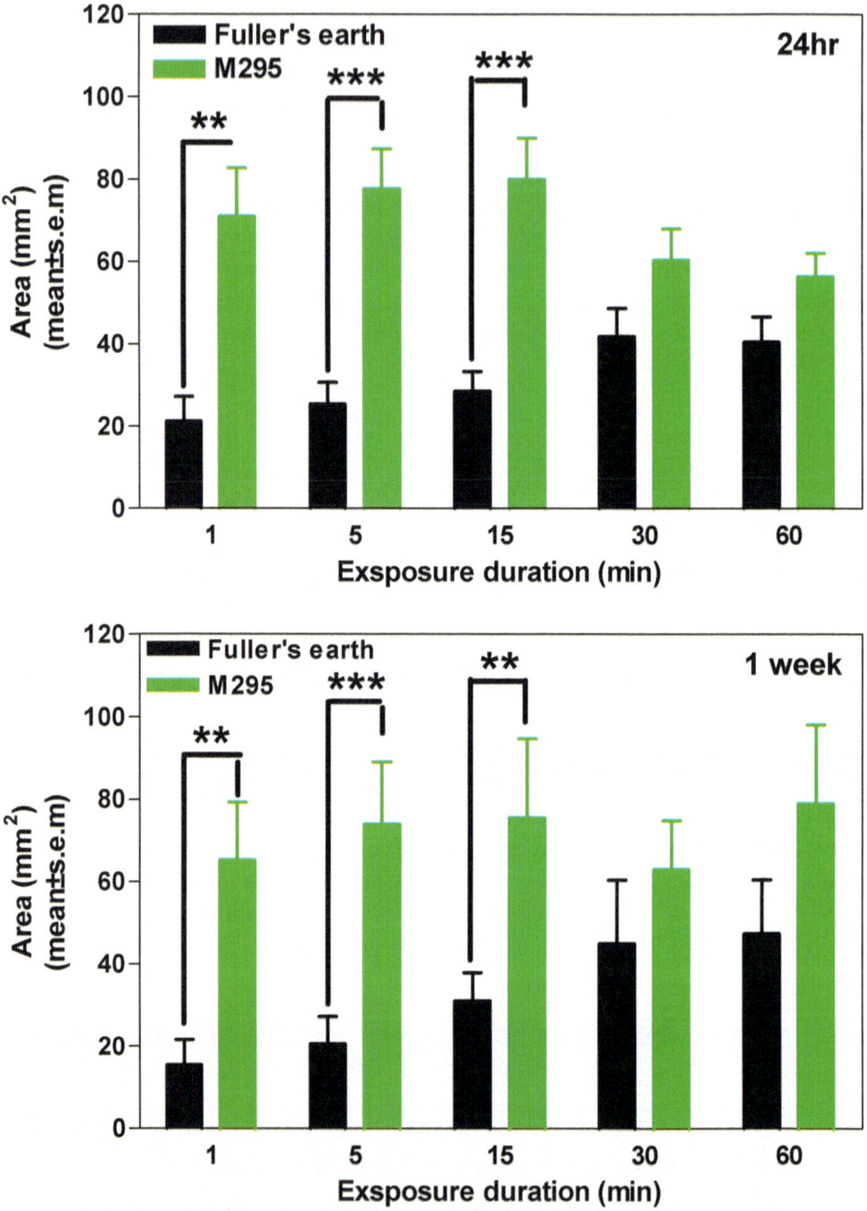

Fig. 7.6 Area of skin lesions 24 hours and 1 week following exposure to 1-μl droplets of HD and decontamination with Fuller's earth or M295 kit. Pigs were exposed for the duration of 1, 5, 15, 30, and 60 minutes ($n = 4$). There is a significant difference in the efficacy of the two decontamination methods. Area of lesions is significantly larger following M295 kit ($*p < 0.03$, $**p < 0.001$, $***p < 0.0001$, $n = 12$ exposed sites on four pigs)

lesions after 1-minute exposure was similar to that developed after 30- or 60-minute exposure (Fig. 7.6).

Even at long-exposure durations such as 30 and 60 minutes, when the lesions are severe and the efficacy of any decontamination method is very limited, still the lesions developed after decontamination with M295 were somewhat larger (Fig. 7.6). The severe exacerbation of the damage following M295 decontamination indicates that this decontamination kit that was initially developed for the decontamination of equipment is not suitable for use on skin.

The Efficacy of Fuller's Earth Compared to RSDL

RSDL is a Reactive Skin Decontaminant Lotion that was developed by the Canadian Department of Defense in the 1980s offering an effective nonirritating skin decontamination system (NSN: 6505–01–507-5074, Canada). RSDL was approved by the US Food and Drug Administration in 2003 for the removal and neutralization of vesicants and nerve agents. This product was selected as the Joint Service Personnel Decontamination System in March 2007.

RSDL is a mixture of potassium 2,3-butanedione monoximate (KBDO) referred to as Dekon 139 and a small amount of 2,3-butanedione monoxime (DAM) in a solvent of polyethylene glycol monomethyl ether (MPEG) and water. This solvent system promotes the decontamination reaction by actively desorbing, retaining, and sequestering the chemical agent, while the active ingredient (Dekon 139) chemically reacts with and rapidly neutralizes the vesicant chemical or the organophosphate nerve agent. According to the manufacture, the reaction starts immediately upon application and neutralization is usually complete within 2 minutes [4, 5, 22, 23].

The RSDL decontamination kit consists of a sponge impregnated with the active lotion.

Exposure to Liquid HD The efficacy of RSDL was tested against exposure to 1-μl HD droplets ($n = 6$) in the pig model. In each pig, one side of the back was decontaminated with RSDL and the second side was used as a control that was decontaminated with Fuller's earth.

Typical HD lesions developed on all exposed site, demonstrating a close relationship between the lesions area and time of decontamination (Fig. 7.7).

The efficacy of RSDL decontamination was similar to that of the Fuller's earth as the area of the lesions was similar in both treatments. Indeed, it seemed that Fuller's earth decontamination at 1 and 5 minutes after exposure had some advantage over RSDL; however, it was significant only in the areas that were exposed for the short duration of 1 minute ($p < 0.025$) and only at the point of 24 hours post exposure (Fig. 7.8).

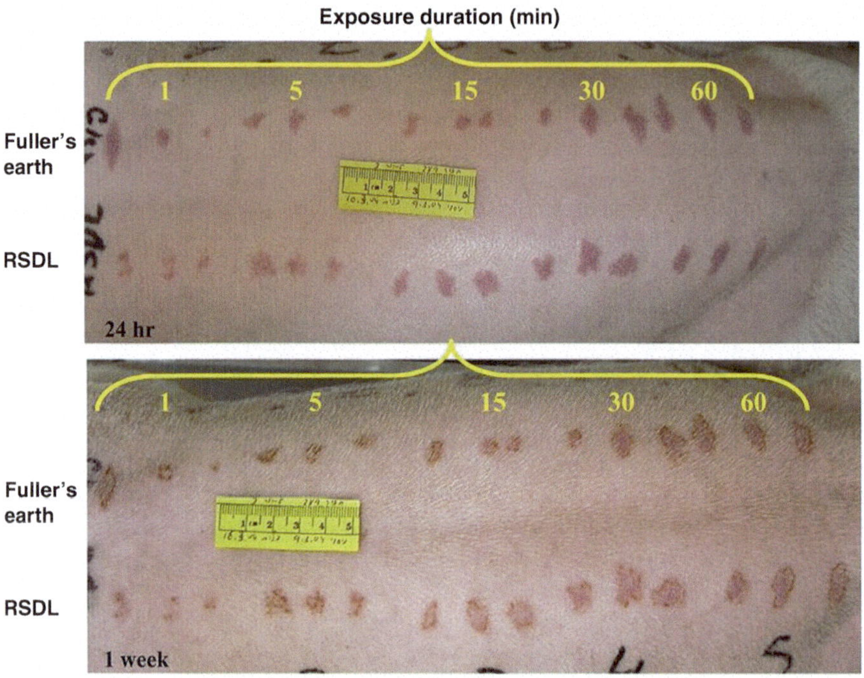

Fig. 7.7 Skin lesions 24 hours and 1 week following exposure to 1-μl droplets of HD and decontamination with RSDL or Fuller's earth at different time points post exposure (1–60 minutes). The effect of the two decontamination systems was very similar

Exposure to VX The efficacy of RSDL (n = 6) was tested against exposure to 2LD50 of VX (1.3 mg/kg), for the duration of 1 and 2 hours. Pigs were monitored for clinical signs of organophosphate (OP) intoxication (fasciculation, salivation, convulsions) and for the inhibition of ChE in whole-blood samples at various time points following exposure. Four additional pigs were decontaminated with Fuller's earth and two were used as control. The control pigs were decontaminated only 12 hours after exposure which can be considered as infinite exposure.

Control Animals These pigs developed severe clinical signs within 3–6 hours following exposure, including substantial salivation, tremors, and convulsions. Their clinical condition deteriorated with time, and one pig died during the night and the second pig died within 24 hours. ChE inhibition in whole blood of the control animals reached 92% within 3 hours of exposure and remained at this level until the end of the experiment (24 hours, Fig. 7.9).

Two-Hour Exposure No clinical symptoms were observed after topical exposure to 2LD50 of VX and decontamination with Fuller's earth. Out of the four pigs that were decontaminated with RSDL 2 hours after VX application, three had no observable clinical signs and one pig exhibited transient symptoms of slight salivation and tremors. At 24 hours, no clinical symptoms were observed in any of the decontaminated pigs.

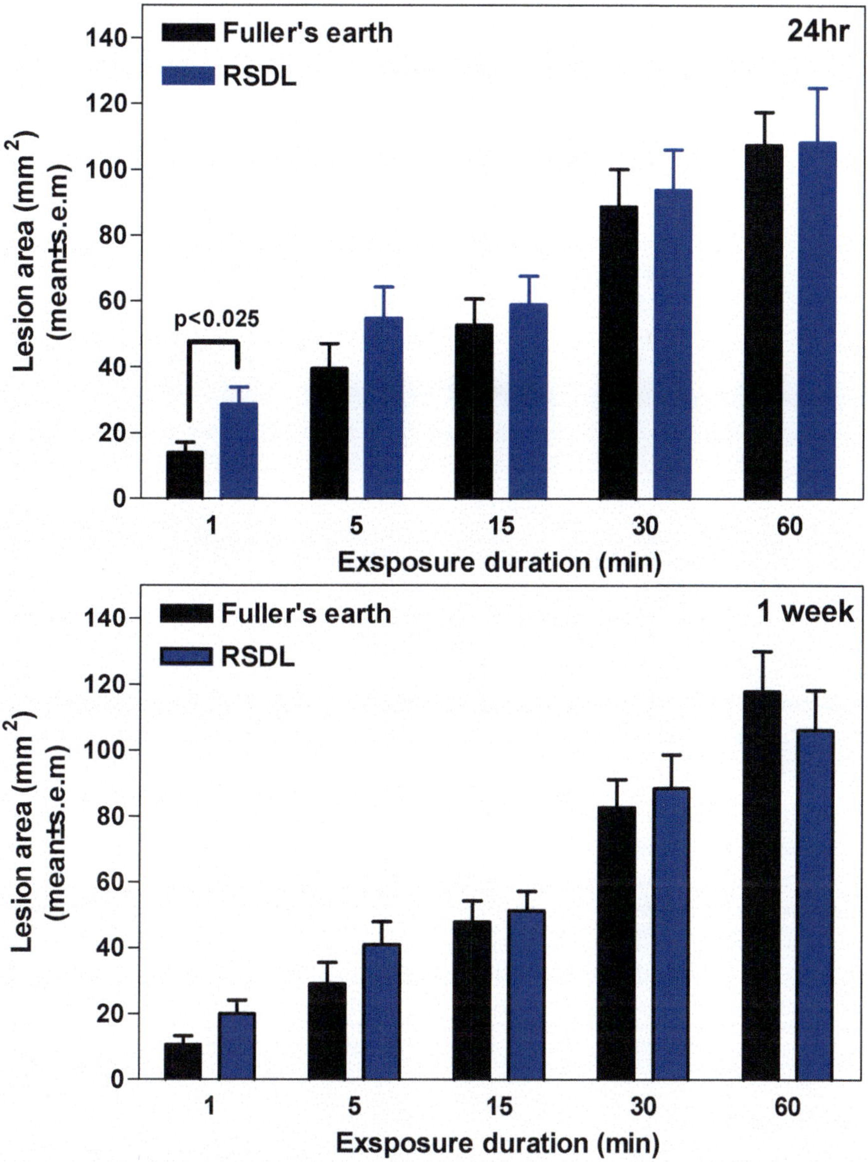

Fig. 7.8 Lesion area 24 hours and 1 week following exposure to HD droplets (1 μl) and decontamination with RSDL and Fuller's earth at various time points post exposure (1–60 minutes). A similar dose–response is found following both decontamination methods ($n = 3$ exposed site on six pigs)

The ChE inhibitions measured in whole blood of animals that were decontaminated with either Fuller's earth or RSDL were similar, and the maximum values were somewhat lower (80%) than those that were measured in the control (92%) animals that were not decontaminated at all (Fig. 7.9). Moreover, there was no indi-

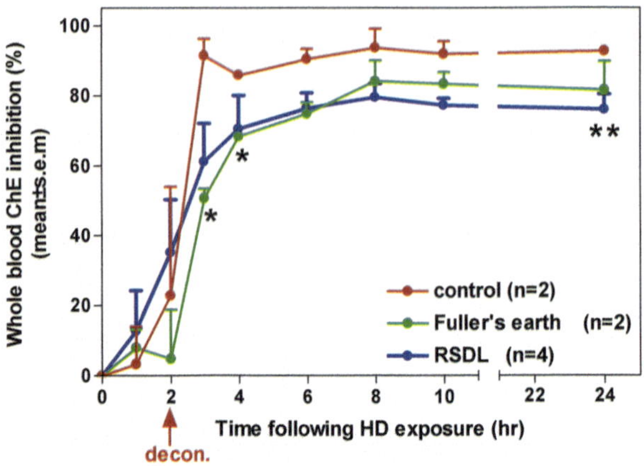

Fig. 7.9 Whole-blood ChE inhibition at various time points following topical exposure of pigs to 2LD50 of VX and decontamination with Fuller's earth or RSDL 2 hours after exposure. Maximal inhibition of about 80% developed around 8 hours after exposure in the decontaminated animals, while in the control animals, a maximal inhibition of 90% developed as early as 2 hours post exposure ($**p < 0.02$ Fuller vs control, $*p < 0.02$ RSDL vs control)

cation to the assumption proposed in the literature (Rolland, 2013) that RSDL neutralized not only the VX that was on the skin but also part of the agent within the epidermis [24] as can be seen in the ChE inhibition curve. The continuous increase in inhibition of ChE after decontamination was similar following both decontamination methods.

Sixty-Minute Exposure In order to elucidate differences between the decontamination methods, if they really exist, an additional experiment was performed. Pigs were exposed to topical VX and decontaminated 1 hour after exposure, and blood samples were collected at narrow time intervals after exposure in order to monitor the first changes in ChE inhibition during the first hours. Similar to the findings in the first experiment, the profile of the development of the ChE inhibition was similar in all pigs and was not related to the decontamination method (Fig. 7.10).

Discussion

The present study demonstrates the high efficacy of Fuller's earth decontamination following percutaneous exposure to HD or VX droplets using the pig model. Fuller's earth was tested against HD and VX that were selected as representatives of vesicants and nerve agents and as the most challenging CWAs in terms of percutaneous toxicity.

Additionally, the importance of decontamination following percutaneous exposure to CWAs even if delayed was shown. For many years, it was accepted that decontamination would be effective only if performed in the first few minutes after

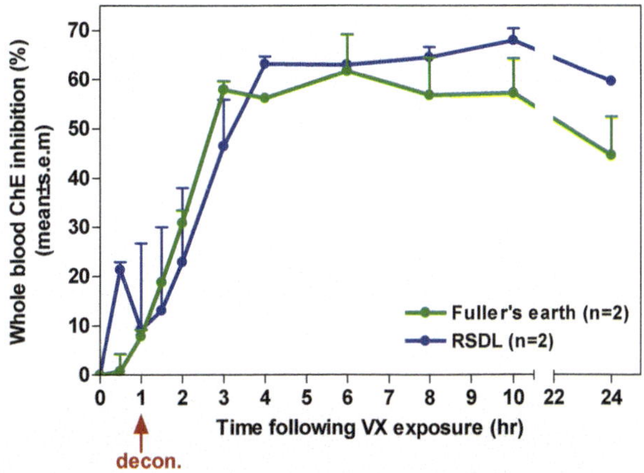

Fig. 7.10 Whole-blood ChE inhibition at various time points following topical exposure of pigs to 2LD50 VX and decontamination with Fuller's earth or RSDL 1 hour after exposure. Maximal inhibition was around 60% in all animals regardless of the decontamination method

exposure. We have shown that decontamination with Fuller's earth can still be effective even if its application is delayed.

The efficacy of decontamination with Fuller's earth was compared to the efficacy of water, M291, M295, and RSDL. None of the decontaminants was found to be more effective than Fuller's earth. While water and M295 were less effective, the M291 (tested up to 5 minutes following HD exposure) and the RSDL yielded similar results.

Our findings are in accordance with results reported by others in the literature, with minor differences in favor of Fuller's earth or RSDL. As discussed below, a comparison between various decontaminants based on efficacy studies is somewhat problematic due to different experimental designs, and this is true also for the comparison between Fuller's earth and RSDL. In general, the effectiveness of a decontaminant is influenced by several factors, such as chemical properties of the contaminant, amount of contaminant on the skin, timing of decontamination, duration of decontamination, the animal model, and anatomical site of exposure [7].

Summarizing the limitations of efficacy studies of decontamination, Braue et al. [4, 5] added that the efficacy of decontamination products can be greatly affected by whether the agent used is neat or diluted. Moreover, if a large amount of agent is present initially, a longer time is needed to completely neutralize it and turn it into a harmless substance. Most studies are carried out under anesthesia which can by itself affect the toxicity. Conscious animals and neat agents like in our experimental setup are preferred as the model mimics a more realistic scenario [4, 5].

The time of decontamination varies between doctrines and studies. The US Army doctrine advises that skin decontamination should be done within the first 2 minutes after exposure [5], and therefore, most studies tested a 2-minute immediate decontamination. In Israel, it is accepted that decontamination should be performed within 15 minutes, considering that 2-minute decontamination is not realistic. In a real-life scenario, warfighters or civilians may not realize that they were contaminated with a toxic agent. Therefore, they might not start the decontamination process within the recommended 2 minutes. Nonetheless, the efficacy of the decontamination (regardless of the type of decontaminant) depends on the time it is performed relative to time of exposure: earlier decontamination increases its efficacy.

The efficacy studies in the literature use different animal models such as rats, guinea pigs, rabbits, pigs, and others. The penetration rate of CWAs through the skin and their toxicity varies widely between species. Most of our studies were performed with pigs which were shown to be the most suitable model for human skin [16, 17]. Additional points to consider, even when the same agent is tested, are as follows: the anatomical site that affects strongly the penetration rate, the dose, the time interval from exposure to decontamination, and the parameters used to assess the efficacy [7, 8, 15].

Few examples that demonstrate these problematics even in the same animal model are given:

Taysee et al. [15] compared the efficacy of RSDL with Fuller's earth in swine challenged with VX or HD. For HD, 8 μl was applied to each site on the back, for 5 minutes and the evaluation was based on degree of erythema and histological measures up to 72 hours after exposure. The authors found that both Fuller's earth and RSDL provided significant reduction in observable tissue damage, yet RSDL was superior in some of the histological parameters at 72 hours (perinuclear vacuoles and infiltration of neutrophils, but similar for necrosis of epidermis, blister formation, and re-epithelialization). For VX, decontamination was performed at 5 minutes after exposure to 9LD50 (1.5 mg/kg) and the evaluation of the efficacy was based only on percent ChE at 6 hours. Both Fuller's earth and RSDL showed a significant effect, yet, clinical signs and mortality rate, which are more relevant measures, were not reported. Nevertheless, based on the histological parameters for HD damage, the authors concluded that RSDL was significantly superior.

Bjarnasson et al. [6] tested the efficacy of RSDL vs Bleach, soapy water, or Fuller's earth in the swine model against VX (5LD50, 79.6 μgr/kg) following decontamination at 30 or 45 minutes, based on ChE inhibition and clinical signs at 6 hours. The results showed that both RSDL and Fuller's earth prevented death following the 45-minute delayed decontamination, but the clinical signs were minor only following decontamination with RSDL. Yet, the number of animals was too few to reach a statistical significance. In our hands, there was no statistical significant difference between Fuller's earth and RSDL against 2LD50 of VX for up to 2-hour exposure duration in both clinical signs and ChE inhibition.

Fuller' Earth: Advantages and Disadvantages

Our studies showed that decontamination with Fuller's earth following exposure to 1-μl droplets of neat HD or VX (2LD50), using the pig model, reduced skin damage following HD when performed up to 30 minutes and severity of clinical symptoms of VX when performed up to 2 hours following exposure. Similar results were obtained with RSDL at the same experimental setup. Nonetheless, the major difference between Fuller's earth and RSDL is the ability of the latter to neutralize the agent.

According to US Army doctrine, the primary objective of an efficient decontamination is to remove the chemical agent from the skin rapidly. Chemical destruction of the agent, although important, is a desirable secondary objective [2].

The advantages of Fuller's earth are as follows:

Rapid Removal of the Agent The main advantage of Fuller's earth use is the rapid and complete physical removal of the agent, even large quantities. In contrast, a complete reactive decontamination takes longer time. This is especially crucial for vesicants that penetrate the skin rapidly, probably even before neutralization, while a complete removal of the chemical by adsorbents will take only few seconds.

Safety Due to its chemical inactivity, the use of Fuller' earth on the skin is safe, and there is a low risk of affecting the victim's health, even when large amount of the decontaminant is used. In contrast, reactive materials require the use of relatively large quantities to neutralize the agent; otherwise, their efficacy is limited, and this, by itself, may be harmful to the skin.

Nonspecificity Fuller's earth works equally well on wide variety of chemical agents. From our experience, it decontaminates efficiently also pesticides such as parathion and toxic industrial chemicals (TICs) such as acrolein [25]. Thus, knowledge of the chemical structure of the specific decontaminated agent is not required.

Easy to Use Reactive products are mostly used by trained professionals and therefore are mainly designated for decontamination of military personnel. In fact, RSDL was developed to address the threat of CWAs in military personnel during wartime, and its role in any civilian mass human-decontamination strategy is unclear [26]. Taking into account that nowadays, mass decontamination is often discussed because of the potential terrorist threat of CWA, Fuller's earth seems to be more user friendly.

Low Price and Long Shelf Life Fuller's earth is relatively cheap and has long shelf life. Recently, we tested the efficacy of old batches of Fuller's earth following years of storage and found that the high efficacy did not change (unpublished results).

Disadvantages of Fuller

Fuller's earth like other dry decontaminants does not change the agent or detoxify it; thus, the sorbent material must be carefully collected in order to prevent from toxic fine dust or particulates to be inhaled or remain adherent to exposed skin when desorption might occur [26]. It should be emphasized that if using water to remove the Fuller's earth, it should be with copious amount of running water.

Conclusion

It is concluded that Fuller's earth is a most efficient universal decontaminant against CWA's vesicants such as HD and nerve agents, such as VX, as well as against pesticides and TICs. The removal of the toxic agents by Fuller's earth is rapid and complete, and it is efficient even if decontamination is delayed.

Based on these results and all the advantages of rapid removal of the agents, safety, ease of use, nonspecificity, low price, and long shelf life, Fuller's earth remains a faithful decontaminant and is recommended as a universal decontaminant for both military personnel and civilians.

References

1. Willems JL. Clinical management of mustard gas casualties. Anna Med Militaris. 1989;3(suppl):1–61.
2. Medical management of chemical casualties hand book. U.S. Army Medical Research Institute of Chemical Defense (USAMRICD), 3rd ed. July, 2000.
3. Yang YC, Baker JA, Ward R. Decontamination of chemical warfare agents. Chem Rev. 1922;92:1729–43.
4. Braue EH, Smith KH, Doxzon BHE, Lumpkin HL, Clarkson ED. Efficacy studies of reactive skin decontamination lotion, M291 skin decontamination kit, 0.5% bleach, 1% soapy water, and skin exposure reduction paste against chemical warfare agents, part 1: guinea pigs challenged with VX. Cutan Ocul Toxicol. 2011;30:15–28.
5. Braue EH, Smith KH, Doxzon BHE, Lumpkin HL, Clarkson ED. Efficacy studies of reactive skin decontamination lotion, M291 skin decontamination kit, 0.5% bleach, 1% soapy water, and skin exposure reduction paste against chemical warfare agents, part 2: guinea pigs challenged with soman. Cutan Ocul Toxicol. 2011;30:29–37.
6. Bjarnason S, Mikler J, Hill I, Tenn C, Garrett M, Caddy N, Sawyer TW. Comparison of selected skin decontaminant products and regimens against VX in domestic swine. Hum Exp Toxicol. 2008;27:253–61.
7. Chan HP, Zhai H, Hui X, Maibach HI. Skin decontamination: principles and perspectives. Toxicol Indus Health. 2012;29(10):955–68.
8. Kadar T, Fishbeine E, Meshulam Y, Sahar R, Chapman S, Liani H, Barness I, Amir A. Treatment of skin injuries induced by sulfur mustard with calmodulin antagonists, using the pig model. J Appl Toxicol. 2000;20:S133–6.
9. Babin MC, Ricketts K, Skvorak JP, Gazaway M, Mitcheltree LW, Casillas RP. Systemic administration of candidate antivesicants to protect against topically applied sulfur mustard in the mouse ear vesicant model (MEVM). J Appl Toxicol. 2000;20:S141–4.
10. Dachir S, Fishbeine E, Meshulam Y, Sahar R, Amir A, Kadar T. Potential anti-inflammatory treatments against cutaneous sulfur mustard injury using the mouse ear vesicant model. Hum Exp Toxicol. 2002;21:197–203.
11. Dachir S, Cohen M, Fishbeine E, Sahar R, Brandies R, Horwitz V, Kadar T. Characterization of acute and long-term sulfur mustard-induced skin injuries in hairless Guinea-pigs using non-invasive methods. Skin Res Technol. 2010;16:114–24.
12. Munro NB, Ambrose KR, Watson AP. Toxicity of the organophosphate chemical warfare agents GA, GB, and VX: implications for public protection. Environ Health Perspect. 1994;102:18–38.

13. Mikler J, Tenn C, Worek F, Reiter G, Thiermann H, Garrett M, Bohnert S, Sawyer TW. Immobilization of Russian VX skin depot by localized cooling: implications for decontamination and medical countermeasures. Toxicol Lett. 2011;206:47–53.
14. Joosen MJA, van den Berg RM, de Jong AL, van der Schans MJ, Noort D, Langenberg JP. The impact of skin decontamination on the time window for effective treatment of percutaneous VX exposure. Chem Biol Interact. 2016;267:48–56.
15. Taysse L, Daulon S, Delamanche S, Bellier B, Breton P. Skin decontamination of mustards and organophosphates: comparative efficiency of RSDL and Fuller's earth in domestic swine. Hum Exp Toxicol. 2007;26:135–41.
16. Simon GA, Maibach HI. The pig as an experimental animal model of percutaneous permeation in man: qualitative and quantitative observations – an overview. Skin Pharmacol Appl Ski Physiol. 2000;13:229–34.
17. Sullivan TP, Eaglstein KWH, Davis SC, Mertz P. The pig as a model for human wound healing. Wound Rep Reg. 2001;9:66–76.
18. Taysse L, Dorandeu F, Daulon S, Foquin A, Perrier N, Lallement G, Breton P. Cutaneous challenge with chemical warfare agents in the SKH-1 hairless mouse (II): effects of some currently used skin decontaminants (RSDL and Fuller's earth) against liquid Sulphur mustard and VX exposure. Hum Exp Toxicol. 2010;30:491–8.
19. Johnson CD, Russel RL. A rapid simple radiometric assay for cholinesterase, suitable for multiple determinations. Anal Biochem. 1975;64:229–37.
20. https://www.ncjrs.gov/pdffiles1/nij/189724b.pdf.
21. luxfermagtech.com/m295-decontamination-kit.
22. https://chemm.nlm.nih.gov/countermeaure_RSDL.htm.
23. Elsinghorst PW, Worek F, Koller M. Detoxification of organophosphorus pesticides and nerve agents through RSDL: efficacy evaluation by 31(P) NMR spectroscopy. Toxicol Lett. 2015;233:207–13.
24. Rolland P, Bozinger MA, Cruz C, Josse D, Briancon S. Hairy skin exposure to VX *in vitro*: effectiveness of delayed decontamination. Toxicol In Vitro. 2013;27:358–66.
25. Kadar T, Eisenkraft A, Barness I, Dachir S. Dermostyx (IB1) – high efficacy safe topical skin protectant against percutaneous toxic agents. In: Proceedings of the 2014 medical defense bioscience review; U.S. Army Medical Research Institute of Chemical Defense; Maryland.
26. Schwartz MD, Hurst CG, Kirk MA, Reedy SJD, Braue JREH. Reactive skin decontamination lotion (RSDL) for the decontamination of chemical warfare agent (CWA) dermal exposure. Cur Pharmaceu Biotech. 2012;13:1971–9.

Chapter 8
Comparison of Four Different Fuller's Earth Formulations in Skin Decontamination

Short Title: Fuller's Earth Efficiency in Skin Decontamination

Annick Roul, Cong-Anh-Khanh Le, Marie-Paule Gustin, Emmanuel Clavaud, Bernard Verrier, Fabrice Pirot, and Françoise Falson

As part of this work has been collected during my PhD work, I would like to thank my supervisors Prof Françoise Falson and Prof Fabrice Pirot for their help and the University of Lyon (University Claude Bernard Lyon1) for their continuous guidance, support and encouragement.

Abbreviations

4-CP	4-Cyanophenol
ATR-FTIR	Attenuated total reflectance Fourier transform infrared
CWA	Chemical warfare agents

A. Roul (✉)
Université de lyon 1, UMR 5305-CNRS/UCBL1; LBTI Lyon and Direction générale de la Sécurité civile et de la gestion des crises Ministère de l'interieur, Paris, France

Laboratoire de galénique industrielle ISPB UCBL1 Lyon, Lyon, France

Cong-Anh-Khanh Le · F. Pirot · F. Falson
Université de lyon 1, UMR 5305-CNRS/UCBL1; LBTI Lyon and Direction générale de la Sécurité civile et de la gestion des crises Ministère de l'interieur, Paris, France

Laboratoire de galénique industrielle ISPB UCBL1 Lyon, Lyon, France

M.-P. Gustin
Université Lyon 1, CNRS UMR 5308,- Inserm U1111 /UCBL1, ENS Lyon, Lyon, France

E. Clavaud
Service départemental d'incendie et de secours de la Savoie, Saint Alban-Leysse, France

B. Verrier
Université de lyon 1, UMR 5305-CNRS/UCBL1; LBTI Lyon and Direction générale de la Sécurité civile et de la gestion des crises Ministère de l'interieur, Paris, France

H. Zhu, H. I. Maibach (eds.), *Skin Decontamination*,
https://doi.org/10.1007/978-3-030-24009-7_8

FE Fuller's earth
SC *Stratum corneum*
TIC Toxic industrial chemicals
TS Tape stripping
UV Ultraviolet

Introduction

The first chemical warfare occurred during First World War with the use of chemical warfare agents (CWA) causing dramatic short-term health effects and long-term effects in survivors. Worldwide disasters are always relevant with the potential use of chemical, biological, radiological and nuclear agents.

CWA include (i) haemoglobin-binding agents (i.e. blood agents), (ii) choking agents (e.g. chlorine) [8], (iii) vesicating agents (e.g. sulfur mustard) [26] and (iv) organophosphorous compounds (COP) (i.e. nerve agents) [24]. Furthermore, toxic industrial chemicals (TIC) can be released such as in the world's worst industrial disaster [3], at Union Carbide, Bhopal, in December 1984, involving the poisonous methyl-isocyanate (MIC), causing thousands of deaths and abysmal long-term consequences after exposure [2]. After a chemical explosion on July 10, 1976, in Seveso, Italy, 2,3,7,8-tetrachlorodibenzo-para-dioxin (TCDD), a widespread contamination induced increased cancer incidence in the exposed population more than 30 years later [39]. Toxicity of CWA and TICs is associated with (i) acute epithelial reactions and (ii) long-term morbidity depending on exposure time. Acute effects including irritation, inflammation, oxidative stress and necrosis especially affect respiratory tract, skin, eyes and upper digestive tract mucosa causing dramatic damage.

Oxidative stress in skin injuries, caused by vesicating agents, such as sulfur mustard, a highly reactive alkylating agent, and subsequent DNA lesions are leading to the acute toxicity producing massive inflammation in case of skin contact as well as to the long-term carcinogenicity [1]. Similar long-term effects have been described for other CWA. Acute exposure to organophosphorous compounds involves an acute cholinergic crisis in addition to signs of neurotoxicity that could develop neurocognitive deficits and structural brain damage over the long term. Although [25] cancer incidence after industrial accidents such as Seveso continues to be investigated, chloracne appears to be the only effect linked with sufficient certainty to dioxin exposure [14].

Whereas inhalation of toxics may be harmful for the breathing system, skin is the most external and relatively large (~ 2 m^2) organ primarily exposed to toxic or harmful chemical [18, 19].

Skin decontamination in victims is thus an essential phase of action aimed to (i) prevent the local damage, transcutaneous absorption and subsequent local and systemic toxicity, (ii) limit skin damage and (iii) facilitate skin repair.

At present, water is largely proposed for mass decontamination [7], for it is easily provided, e.g. from fire trucks. The alternative to such "wet" decontamination is "dry" decontamination based on adsorptive properties of powders, e.g. talcum, flour or clays [21].

Fuller's earth (FE) [23], an alumina silicate, chemically inert, abundant in nature, known for its adsorptive properties, provides decontamination opportunities for chemical, biological, radiological and nuclear agents [22, 36]. FE, currently used in firefighter decontamination processes in France [34], is provided as powder in container and prefilled gloves. In the present study we investigate the FE as furnished by our official supplier (i) in its original form, (ii) dispersed in water, in order to optimize the skin decontamination process after short exposure to water-soluble chemicals.

Therefore, 4-CP [33] ranged in aqueous solutions is used as tracer model to assess adsorption capacity of the fuller's earth in vitro and its efficiency on porcine skin decontamination ex vivo. The 4-CP was used as a model contaminant for several reasons: (i) its IR signal allows a rapid and noninvasive quantification of uptaken chemical agent onto the skin; (ii) it has been used to model cutaneous absorption of chemical both in vitro and in vivo [28] and (iii) it possesses a similar hydrophobicity to most CW agents and TICs, as indicated by its $\log P_{oct/water}$ (table 0 supplement data) while its toxicity is much lower, thus allowing simple, safe and short-duration studies with diverse possible exposure scenarios.

Firstly, Fuller's earth adsorption capacity is carried out in vitro for three 4-CP aqueous solutions in function of time ensuring that the resulting benefits have taken into account constraints challenging operational realities (i.e. time from 5 min to 120 min).

The first study is performed with a fixed amount of FE (1 g) in function of contact time ranging from 5 to 120 min, whereas we assessed the impact of amount of FE on adsorption capacity for the 4-CP after both contact times 15 and 60 min.

Then, contamination is designed ex vivo by exposing porcine skin to 4-CP in aqueous solution during a short time exposure followed by water showering or by FE's application (i) as free powder, (ii) loaded on adhesive tape, (iii) on powdered glove or (iv) as a suspension. Extent of 4-CP skin penetration and subsequent efficiency of FE-based decontamination methods are investigated by tracking skin 4-CP content using attenuated total reflectance Fourier transform infrared spectroscopy (ATR-FTIR). Fifteen-minute exposure was defined (i.e. minimal delay expected in case of a real-life incident before initiation of the decontamination procedure).

Materials and Methods

Materials

FE ($\rho = 0.7$ kg.m^{-3}) is presented as a free powder (stored in bottle) with adsorptive properties available for firefighter decontamination process (NBC-Sys 42,408; St-Chamond, France) [17]. 4-Cyanophenol (4-CP) [MW 119.1 g.mol^{-1}, Log P 1.6, water solubility 8.98 g.L^{-1}], with purity of 95%, was purchased from Aldrich (St-Quentin-Fallavier, France). Aqueous solutions of 4-CP were extemporaneously prepared with purified water (0.055 μS.cm^{-1}) produced by PURELAB Option before each set of measurements at 24–25 °C and sonicated for 5 min to ensure 4-CP total dissolution.

Instrumentation

UV spectrophotometer (Jasco V-630 spectrophotometer) was used to measure 4–CP absorbance at the wavelength 246 nm with specific disposable cuvettes (7591 50) of 1.5 mL (BRAND GMBH, 97861 Wehrheim, Germany). Quantitative analysis data were treated by software Spectramanager2.

Centrifuge sigma 3-16P (Fisher Scientific, Illkirch, France), ultrasonic equipment 89878 (Biobloc scientific, Illkirch, France), pH meter HI 991002 (Hanna ORP Meter, Sigma-Aldrich, France), magnetic stirrer (RH Basic 2 IKA, Brumath, France).

ATR-FTIR analyses were conducted from 400 to 4000 cm^{-1} using an infrared spectrometer (Perkin Elmer UATR Spectrum two, Waltham, MA 02451, USA) equipped with a triglycine sulfate (TGS) pyroelectric thermic mid-detector. The sample compartment is a horizontal internal reflection accessory holding a diamond crystal ($\theta = 42°$) with a refractive index 2.4. Therefore, an evanescent wave at the reflective surface was entering for a path of 1–2 μm into the sample in contact with the diamond producing a spectrum collected on database. This mono reflection system requires a spectrum acquisition time of 2 min [38].

Methods

Kinetic Adsorption Studies (In Vitro)

Kinetic studies were performed in vitro to assess the adsorption capacity of the Fuller's earth in function of three parameters: the concentration of the 4-CP aqueous solutions, the amount of FE and contact time. 10 mL of each of the three 4-CP aqueous solutions, C_0 (10, 100, 500 mg. L^{-1}) were treated by (i) fixed or (ii) various amounts of FE.

(i) 4-CP aqueous solutions C_0 (10 mg.L^{-1}, 100 mg.L^{-1}, 500 mg.L^{-1}) were treated by 1 g of FE and left in contact (t = 5, 15, 30, 45, 60, 90 and 120 min).
(ii) The 4-CP aqueous solution (C_0 = 10 mg. L^{-1}) was treated by (0.01, 0.1, 1) g of FE, whereas (C_0 = 100 mg. L^{-1}) and (C_0 = 500 mg. L^{-1}) by (0.1, 1) g of FE (t = 15, 60 min).

These obtained suspensions were agitated by magnetic stirrer for a determined time t (min) ranging from 5 to 120 min, taken into microcentrifuge tubes (02 681-291,

10 mL, Fisher Scientific, Illkirch, France), centrifuged at 3000 g for 12 min, in which supernatant was filtered (pores ∅ 0,1 μm, ANOTOP™ 10 filter; Whatman GmbH Dassel, Germany). Absorbance of residual 4-CP in the filtered supernatant (C_L) was measured by UV spectrometer at 246 nm at 25 °C and pH 7. Calibration was established for 4-CP aqueous solutions ranged from 2.5 to 12.5 mg.L^{-1} [31]. The tests were performed in triplicate.

C_L (mg. L^{-1}) measured in function of time was used to determine the adsorbed amount of 4-CP (mg) per gram of FE in real-time kinetic and at equilibrium (C_{FEmax} mg.g^{-1}), whereas the impact of FE's amount on adsorption capacity was assessed by percentage removal of 4-CP (%) for each treated solution for both times 15 and 60 min [37].

Furthermore, the data were tested to fit the rate constant of adsorption (k_1, k_2) of 4-CP onto FE, with the first-order kinetic model of Lagergren [40] and the second-order kinetic model of Ho and Mac Kay [11].

Porcine Skin, Contamination: Decontamination

Unscalded porcine ears, obtained from a local slaughterhouse, were washed with purified water, softly wiped and stored in sealed plastic bags at − 20 °C within 12 hours after animal sacrifice. On the day of experiment, porcine ears were slowly thawed at 4 °C, and hair were clipped; 1.54 cm^2 explants were cut with a biopsy punch. Porcine skin is advantageously easily prepared and the whole skin structure is conserved, as the skin is not detached from the subcutaneous tissues, which helps maintain skin hydration. All experiments were performed on appropriate laboratory equipment, easy to clean and anti-slip (silicone holder).

Contamination by 4-CP Aqueous Solution

Preliminary calibration, for reference 4-CP, powder (depot, 50 mg; 8 scans) and its aqueous solutions (21–105 mM, depots 100 μL; 8 scans) were analysed by ATR-FTIR spectroscopy.

Then, accuracy of 4-CP detection method in the skin was tested by applying 100 μL of 4-CP aqueous solutions (21–105 mM) onto porcine skin explants (skin area, 1.54 cm^2; $n = 4$). The volume of 100 μL allowed adequately covering skin disc surface (1.54 cm^2) with contaminant. In most cases, solution remained on the skin surface and, if any liquid run off the skin, the experiment was reconducted with a new specimen. After 15 min of contact unabsorbed 4-CP solution was gently wiped from the skin surface and skin explants were immediately analysed by ATR-FTIR (8 scans). ATR-FTIR spectroscopy was successfully exploited for 4-CP tracking within the SC layers by integration of the cyanyl (C ≡ N) stretching vibration absorbance peak (i.e. 2231 cm^{-1}), as in this spectral region (2250 and 2200 cm^{-1}.), low interference with SC enables accurate evaluation of skin 4-CP content [28, 35].

Next, 100 μL of 105 mM 4-CP saturated solution was applied onto porcine skin explants (skin area, 1.54 cm^2; $n = 4$) for 1, 5 and 15 min, in order to appreciate 4-CP penetration as a function of time as described previously [20].

Finally, after 15 min of skin exposure to 105 mM 4-CP aqueous solution, the profile of 4-CP penetration was assessed by successive tape stripping ($n = 4$) (pre-cut tape strips, 19 mm × 50 mm; Scotch 3M, Cergy, France) and concomitant ATR-FTIR analysis of skin surface (8 scans) [15, 32]. SC at the treated site was progressively removed by repeated adhesive tape stripping (time 5 seconds). Adhesive layer of the tape was applied uniformly with the same low pressure for each strip by the same trained operator. The adhesive tape carefully adhered to the disc surface (1.54 cm^2) covering the treated surface, and the application pressure was uniform on this small area completed by a constant velocity for removal (duration 5 seconds).

Porcine Skin Decontamination

Decontamination methods were performed in the same conditions as those used in firefighter processes and five different decontamination methods were investigated at room temperature (25 °C) and compared with each other. In method I, FE powder (0.16 g. cm^{-2}) was applied onto skin explant contaminated with 4-CP ($n = 30$) for 1 min and then gently removed from the skin surface by using absorbent paper (Precision Wipes Kimtech Science, Surrey, UK). In method II, FE powder (0.03 g.cm^{-2}) was stuck onto adhesive tapes. FE loaded adhesive tapes were applied for fifteen seconds and then stripped from the contaminated skin explant surface ($n = 30$). In method III, FE powder (0.02 g.cm^{-2}) was stuck onto the palmar face of cotton wash gloves (14 × 21 cm; GT-1000, LCH medical products, Paris, France) by using glue spray (BI2L, Villeneuve-d'Ascq, France). FE powder loaded on the palmar face of a glove was applied to a contaminated skin explant ($n = 30$) for 30 seconds; after that skin surface was cleaned with the posterior face of the glove. In method IV, FE suspension was prepared by dispersing 10 g of FE in purified water (100 mL) and was applied (0.65 g.cm^{-2}) onto 4-CP-contaminated skin explants ($n = 30$) for 1 min, and then skin surface was gently dry-wiped. In method V, water decontamination by the rinsing of contaminated skin explants (1.54 cm^2; $n = 30$) was performed with 3 mL of demineralized water for 15 seconds (23 mL.cm^{-2}.min^{-1}) using pipette Pasteur(Fontenay-sous-Bois, France).

In methods I–V, residual 4-CP content within the SC was assessed after decontamination by integration of cyanyl stretching vibration absorbance peak obtained with ATR-FTIR (8 scans), as described in the previous section.

Statistical Analysis

Statistical analysis was performed to study the effect of decontamination methods on percentage of decontamination. Percentage of decontamination distribution normality was checked by normality AGOSTINO test for the four decontamination methods. Homoscedasticity of data across the four decontamination method groups was investigated with Bartlett test. In case of heteroscedasticity (i) multiple pairwise comparisons between variances were performed with Fisher test to compare the variability of results between groups and (ii) non-parametric Kruskal-Wallis tests was used to evidence a potential effect of decontamination methods on percentage of decontamination. In the case of a significant method effect on percentage of decontaminating six pairwise comparisons between means for the four methods were conducted with the Welch test to take into account heteroscedasticity.

A significant level of 5% was selected for single comparison. The p-value was adjusted for multiple comparisons with Bonferroni method.

Statistics were performed using the R language, version 3.0.2., available on the website http://cran.r-project.org/ [17 December 2015].

Results

Results highlight adsorption capacity of the fuller's earth for 4-CP from aqueous solutions; therefore, quantification is analysed by both kinetic studies.

Decontamination efficiency of four FE's methods has been performed ex vivo on contaminated porcine skin and compared with water decontamination.

Adsorption Capacity of the Fuller's Earth

The preliminary study was dedicated to the calibration by UV spectrophotometer where the absorbance (A) of residual 4-CP concentration in the supernatant (C_L), expressed in mg.L^{-1}, was measured for the 4-CP aqueous solutions (2.5–12.5 mg. L^{-1}) in which linear regression equation is:

$$A = 0.149 C_L + 0.013; R^2 = 0.99 \tag{8.1}$$

Adsorption Capacity of 1 g Fuller's Earth for the 4-CP from Aqueous Solution

Absorbance (A) of residual 4-CP in the supernatant was measured for the three 4-CP aqueous solutions (10, 100, 500 mg. L^{-1}), respectively, after 5, 15, 30, 45, 60, 90 and 120 min of contact time with 1 g of FE. Based on Eq. 8.1, residual 4-CP concentration in the supernatant (C_L) was calculated. The amount of 4-CP adsorbed within 1 g of FE, C_{FE} [mg.g^{-1}], was calculated, according to Eq. 8.2:

$$C_{FE} = \frac{(C_0 - C_L) * V}{m * 1000} \tag{8.2}$$

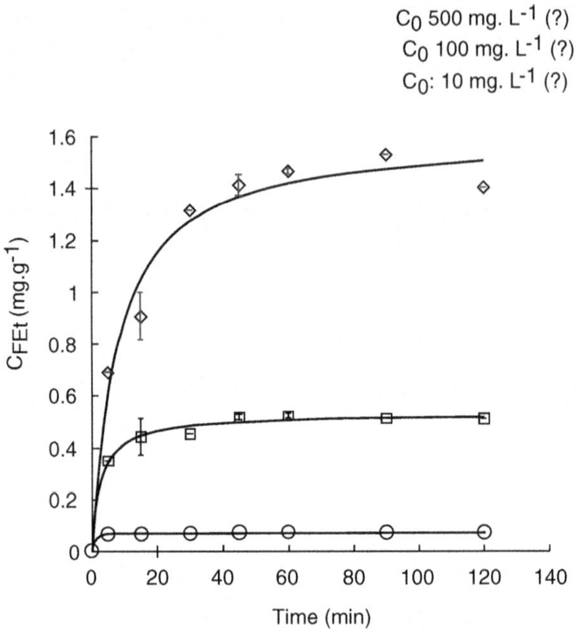

Fig. 8.1 Effect of time on the 4-CP adsorption by FE for three C_0 4-CP concentrations: 10 mg.L^{-1} (○), 100 mg.L^{-1} (□), 500 mg.L^{-1} (◇). Data is fitted with the second-order kinetic model (—)

where C_0 (mg.L^{-1}) is the initial concentration of 4-CP in solution, V (mL) the solution volume and m (g) the weight of FE.

Results highlight the increase of the adsorbed amount of 4-CP by FE, in function of time for the three 4-CP aqueous solutions, 10 mg.L^{-1} (○), 100 mg.L^{-1} (□) and 500 mg.L^{-1} (◇), as illustrated in Fig. 8.1. Adsorption started immediately after contact between FE and the 4-CP aqueous solutions (5–15 min), to reach a plateau phase between 45 min and 60 min with an apparent steady state at 60 min. As observed, the equilibrium time depends on the initial concentration of 4-CP as it is reached faster for the lower concentrations. Beyond 60 min, for contact time 90 and 120 min, adsorption values (C_L, C_{FE}) were not significantly different from those obtained at 60 min.

The experimental values and the correlation coefficient fit the rate constant of adsorption, k_1 (min^{-1}) and k_2 (min.g.mg^{-1}) of 4-CP onto FE, with the first-order kinetic model of Lagergren (Eq. 8.3) and the second-order kinetic model of Ho and McKay (Eq. 8.4) for the lowest concentration in 4-CP as presented in Table 8.1:

$$\log\left(C_{\mathrm{FE}} - C_{\mathrm{FEt}}\right) = \log C_{\mathrm{FE}} - k_1 t / 2.303 \tag{8.3}$$

$$t / C_{\mathrm{FEt}} = 1 / \left(k_2 C_{\mathrm{FE}}^{\ 2}\right) + t / C_{\mathrm{FE}} \tag{8.4}$$

The modelling results confirmed that the adsorption rate constant decreases with an increase in 4-CP concentration.

Table 8.1 First- and second-order kinetic models for adsorption of 4-CP from aqueous solution by FE (estimation made using KaleidaGraph 3.6)

Parameters		First-order kinetic model $\log(C_{FE} - C_{FEt}) = \log C_{FE} - k_1t/2.303$			Second-order kinetic model $t/C_{FEt} = 1/(k_2C_{FE}^2) + t/C_{FE}$			
C_0	C_{FE} (exp)	C_{FE} (cal)	k_1(min^{-1})	r^2	C_{FE}	k_2 (min.g.mg^{-1})	r^2	t plateau phase (min)
10	0.0729	0.0722	0.8314	0.9868	0.0723	24.851	0.9972	14
100	0.5129	0.4884	0.2101	0.9479	0.5233	0.6106	0.9805	37
500	1.5225	1.4653	0,0779	0.9584	1.6278	0.0735	0.9637	58

C_0 (mg.L^{-1}): initial concentration of 4-CP in solution

C_{FE}, C_{FEt} (mg.g^{-1}): mg of 4-CP adsorbed by 1 g of FE at equilibrium and at time t (min), respectively

k_1, k_2: rate constant of adsorption for first- and second-order kinetic models, respectively

cal calculated, *exp* experimental

Percentage Removal of 4-CP from Aqueous Solution Depends on FE's Amounts

Recovery of 4-CP from initial aqueous solutions (C_0) by FE was assessed by measuring the absorbance of residual 4-CP in the supernatant (C_L) in function of time. We focused our analysis on 4-CP recovery at 15 and 60 min with three amounts of FE (0.01, 0.1, 1) g for low 4-CP concentration (10 mg.L^{-1}) and (0.1, 1) g for FE or medium (100 mg.L^{-1}) and high (500 mg.L^{-1}) 4-CP concentrations using Eq. 8.5:

$$\text{percentage removal}(\%) = 100 * \frac{C_0 - C_L}{C_0} \tag{8.5}$$

Results show that percentage of removal of 4-CP from aqueous solutions by FE correlates with its amount, 4-CP initial concentration and contact time (Table 8.2). We observed that the 4-CP amount adsorbed by FE was higher after 60 min of contact than after 15 min. The difference between values obtained after 15 and 60 min is ranged from 40% to 93% depending on C_0, residual concentration of 4-CP in the supernatant C_L.

Porcine Skin Contamination and Decontamination Efficiency

Porcine skin explants were contaminated to evaluate the efficiency of decontamination methods. Furthermore, decontamination methods were assessed by ATR-FTIR allowing fast and easy-to-handle 4-CP tracking within the *stratum corneum*.

Table 8.2 Comparative analysis of 4-CP adsorbed from aqueous solutions by FE after contact time 15 and 60 min

Results are expressed in percentage removal $(\%) = 100 * \frac{C_0 - C_L}{C_{0.}}$

C_0 (mg. L^{-1})	FE (g)	C_L (mg. L^{-1}) 15 min	Percentage removal (%) 15 min	C_L (mg. L^{-1}) 60 min	Percentage removal (%) 60 min
10	1.00	3.11	68.87	2.60	74.04
10	0.10	6.04	39.55	5.49	45.11
10	0.01	9.88	1.23	9.81	1.94
100	1.00	55.91	44.09	47.89	52.11
100	0.10	91.53	8.47	81.04	18.96
500	1.00	409.37	18.13	358.77	28.25
500	0.10	481.03	3.79	453.25	9.35

C_0 initial concentration of 4-CP in solution
C_L residual concentration of 4-CP in solution

Contamination with the Validated Model Molecule 4-CP

Porcine skin was exposed to the saturated 4-CP aqueous solution for 15 min (relevant time maximized for this study). Beforehand the ATR-FTIR spectra of (A) 4-CP powder, (B) 4-CP aqueous 105 mM solution, (C) untreated porcine skin surface and (D) skin contaminated skin by 4-CP aqueous solution (105 mM) for 15 minutes were recorded (Fig. 8.2a–d). Typical cyanyl peak area (2250–2200 cm^{-1}) was observed in 4-CP-contaminated skin as reported in earlier studies [29].

Furthermore, a linear relationship was evidenced in both cyanyl peak area in the skin (treated by 4-CP aqueous solutions (21–105 mM) for 15 min) [$y = 10^{-3}.(4.3x - 70.1)$; $R^2 = 0.972$] (●) and 4-CP concentration in aqueous solutions (21–105 mM) [$y = 10^{-3}.(0.6x - 6.8)$; $R^2 = 0.976$] (○) (Fig. 8.2e). 4-CP tracking in the skin was effective after a very short exposure time (i.e. 1 min). Burst of 4-CP penetration (0–5 min) was clearly evidenced followed by a slow plateau phase (5–15 min) confirming 4-CP as relevant model compound for experimental skin contamination. Furthermore, skin surface tape stripping was performed to evaluate 4-CP diffusion within the *stratum corneum*. The cyanyl peak area in successive tape strips ($n = 3$) decreased evidencing depth-dependant 4-CP concentration within the SC and therefore validating the contamination protocol (Fig. 8.2f).

Decontamination Efficiency: Comparing FE and Water Methods

In order to evaluate the efficiency of porcine skin decontamination by FE, residual 4-CP content in the assayed skin was determined by measuring cyanyl absorbance peak area on the skin explants by ATR-FTIR. The spectra recorded just after applying one of the four decontamination methods based on the FE are shown in Fig. 8.3: method I (Fig. 8.3a), method II (Fig. 8.3b), method III (Fig. 8.3c) and method IV (Fig. 8.3d), highlighting the efficiency of the last method, FE in suspension.

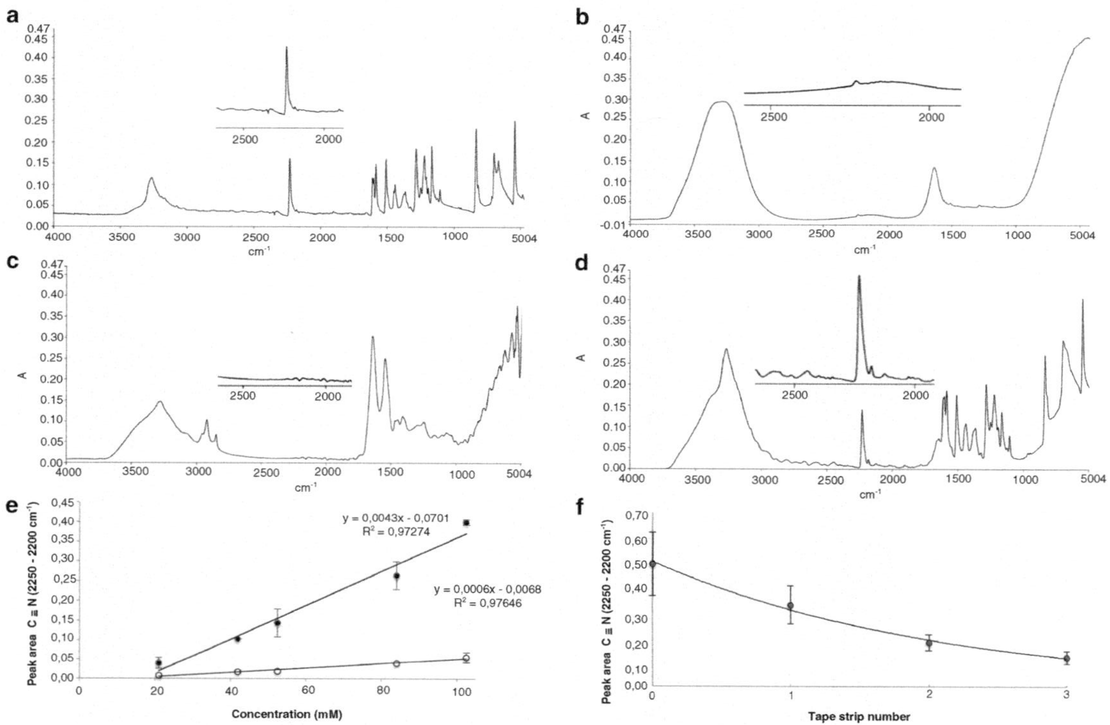

Fig. 8.2 ATR-FTIR spectra of 4-CP powder (**a**), 4-CP aqueous solution (105 mM) (**b**), uncontaminated porcine explant (**c**), porcine explant after contamination by 4-CP aqueous solution 105 mM for 15 min (**d**). (**e**) Relationship between cyanyl peak area in skin (treated by 4-CP aqueous solutions for 15 min) [$y = 10^{-3}.(4.3x - 70.1)$; $R^2 = 0.972$] (●) and 4-CP concentration in aqueous solution (21–105 mM) [$y = 10^{-3}.(0.6x - 6.8)$; $R^2 = 0.976$] (○). Each data is the mean ± standard deviation of four experimental measurements. (**f**) Mean [skin surface contaminated by 105 mM 4-CP aqueous solution; tape stripped ($n = 3$)] of C ≡ N peak area measured by ATR-FTIR. Each data is the mean ± standard deviation of three experimental measurements

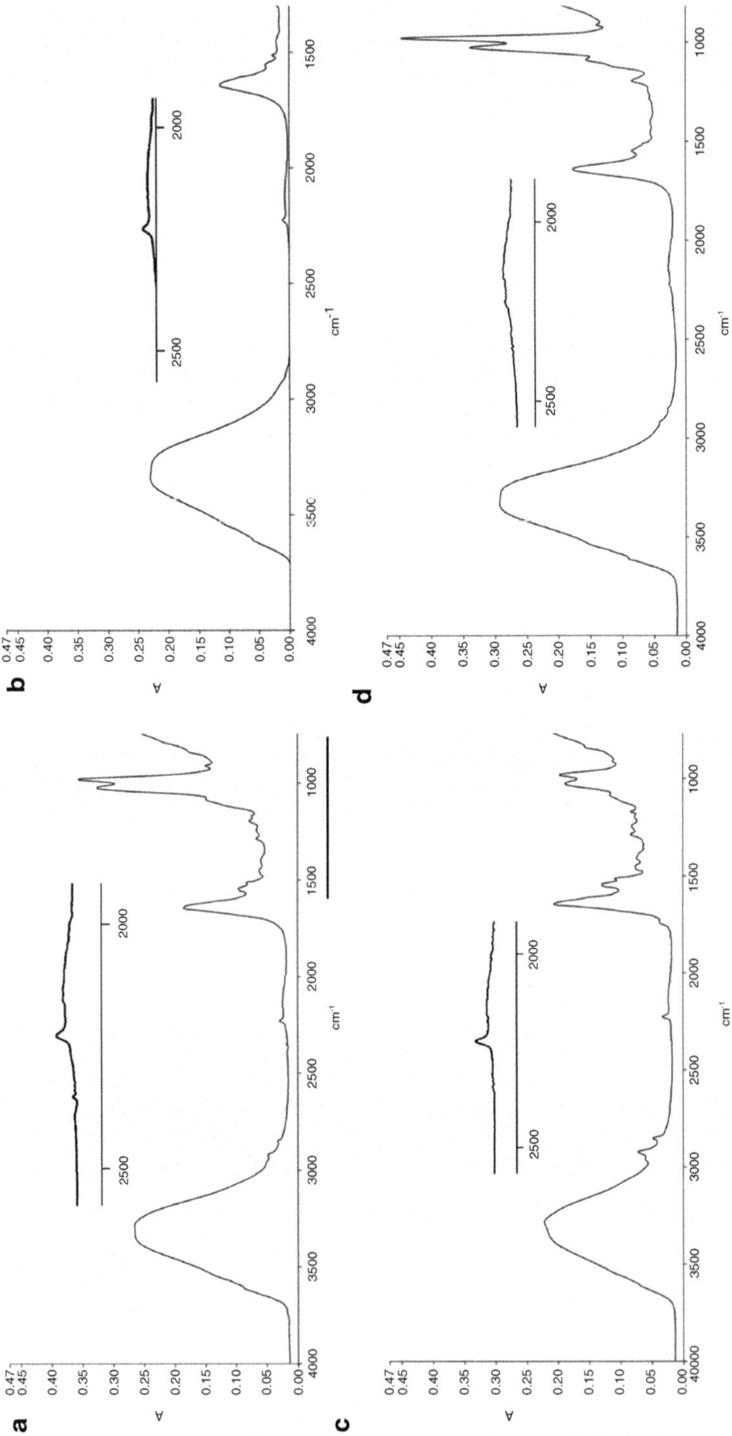

Fig. 8.3 ATR-FTIR spectra of porcine specimen after decontamination by one of the four methods: method I (**a**) free FE, method II (**b**) FE loaded on adhesive tape, method III (**c**) FE loaded on a single-use glove, method IV (**d**) FE's suspension

Decontamination efficiency (DE) of each method was calculated as the percentage of 4-CP recovered from the contaminated skin as follows:

$$\mathrm{DE}(\%) = 100 \bullet \frac{4\text{-CP peak area}_{\text{after contamination}} - 4\text{-CP peak area}_{\text{after decontamination}}}{4\text{-CP peak area}_{\text{after contamination}}} \quad (8.6)$$

Results, according to methods with standard deviation (method I, DE (71% ± 20,3); method II, DE (72% ± 14,3); method III, DE (60,8% ± 22,1); method IV, DE (88,1% ± 8,3); method V, DE (53,58% ± 10,15)), are detailed in Table 8.3 and presented in Fig.8.4. Percentage of decontamination distribution was not different from normal distribution for the four decontamination methods (Suppl Table IV). Percentage of decontamination was heteroscedastic according to decontamination methods ($p < 10^{-5}$, Bartlett test). Results obtained with FE suspension method were significantly less variable than those with the three other FE's methods (Suppl Table V). The method of decontamination showed a significant effect on percentage of decontamination efficiency (DE %) ($p < 10^{-6}$, Kruskal-Wallis rank sum test). Decontamination rate obtained with method IV was significantly different than those with the other methods (suppl Table VI).

Discussion

Decontamination after chemical exposure, mainly based on wet methods (i.e. water) may be alternatively carried out with adsorptive powders (i.e. talcum, flour, fuller's earth) as called dry decontamination [6, 16]. In our study we have investigated fuller's earth's adsorptive properties in vitro in function of the three parameters: (i) time, (ii) FE's amount and (iii) 4-CP concentration in aqueous solutions. Then we compared decontamination efficiency (DE) of the FE (powder or suspension) with water rinsing on ex vivo porcine skin. 4-CP was selected as validated and appropriated molecular model to perform the studies in vitro and ex vivo as shown with the results.

In vitro, 4-CP may be adsorbed from aqueous solution onto the FE. The relationship adsorbent (FE) adsorbate (4-CP) calculated for C_{FE} with Eq. 8.2 was plotted in function of time underlying that the higher the 4-CP concentration, the longer it takes to reach the plateau as shown in Fig. 8.1. Besides, the adsorption profile of 4-CP was shown to fit with the second-order kinetic model exhibiting a higher R^2. Nonetheless, the validity of this model correlates for low (10 mg.L^{-1}) and medium (100 mg.L^{-1}) 4-CP concentrations with respective R^2 (0.99, 0.98) pointing out that boundary conditions should be set up to optimize the adsorption profile. Our results confirm a stabilization of 4-CP adsorption by the FE after 30 min contact time for the low and medium 4-CP concentrations and 60 min of contact time for the highest 4-CP concentration (500 mg.L^{-1}) [22]. The plateau phase appears to be stable until at least 120 min indicating that 4-CP adsorbed from aqueous solutions by FE is not desorbed in the same conditions of adsorption. This objective criterion could impact

Table 8.3 Comparison of four decontamination methods on contaminated porcine skin (area, 1.54 cm^2) [100 μL by 105 mM 4-CP aqueous solution]

	Porcine explant	Method I	Method II	Method III	Method IV	Method V
Description	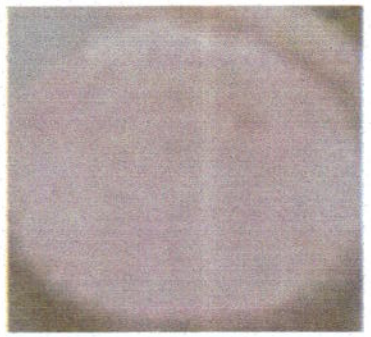	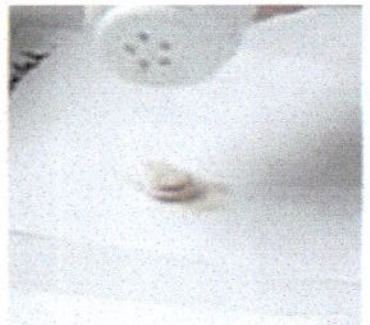	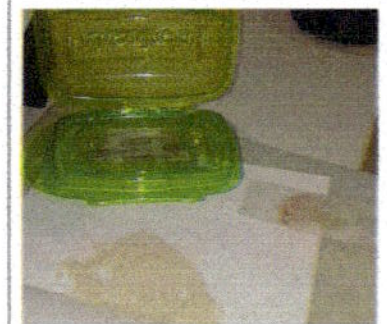	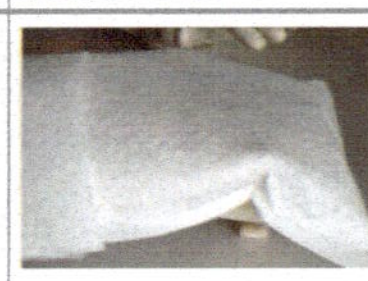	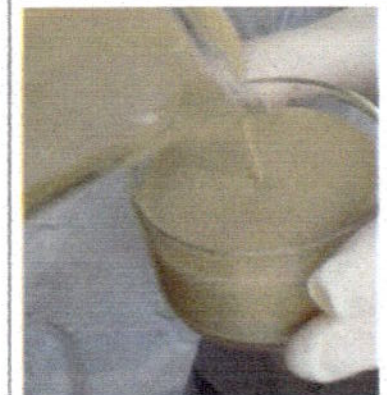	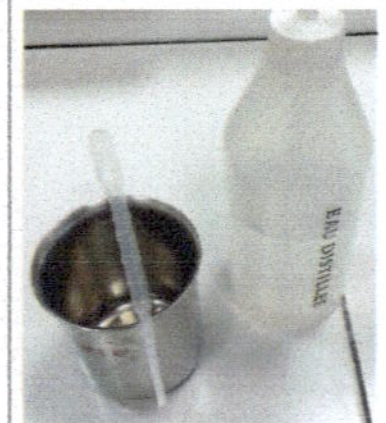
	Decontaminant	FE dry, free powder	FE loaded on adhesive strip	FE loaded on palmar face of single-use wash glove	FE (10 g) soaked in 100 mL of purified water as suspension	Demineralized water press with Pasteur pipette (3 mL)
	Depot of FE	0.15 g.cm^{-2} Possible occlusion	0.03 g.cm^{-2}	0.02 g.cm^{-2}	0.65 g.cm^{-2}	–
	Method of decontamination	Full coverage of area with free powder	Full coverage of area with adhesive strip applied with finger pression	Full coverage of area with palmar face glove	Full coverage of area with the suspension	Showering with a direct water stream (23 mL.cm^{-2}. min^{-1})
	Time	1 min	15 seconds	30 seconds	1 min	15 seconds
	DE (%)	71.0 ± 20.3	72.0 ± 14.3	60.8 ± 22.1	88.1 ± 8.3	53.6 ± 10.2

DE decontamination efficiency (mean ± SD, n = 3)

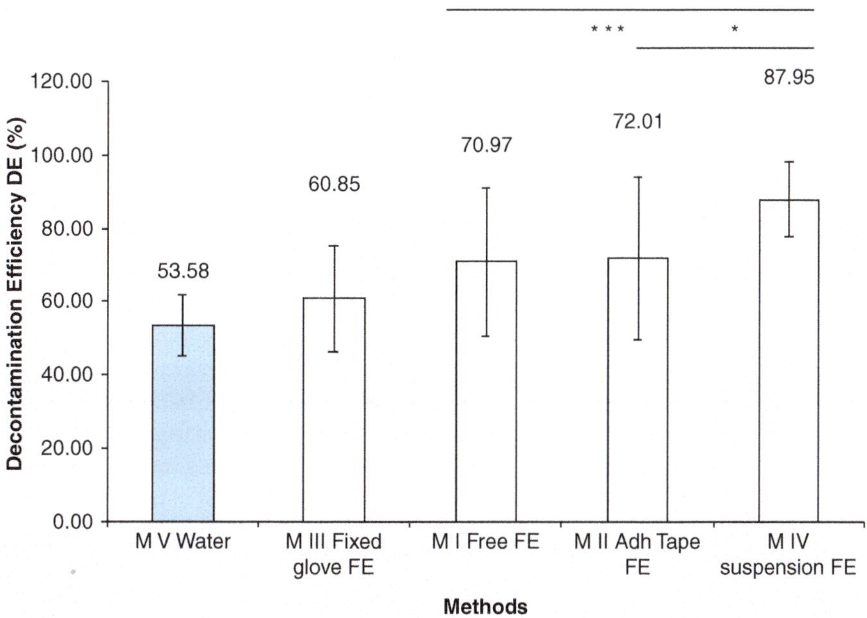

Fig. 8.4 Mean percentage of decontamination according to methods with standard deviation *** adjusted p-value for multiple pairwise comparisons by Bonferroni method $<10^{-3}$ for the three pairwise comparisons between method IV (FE's suspension) with the three other methods involving FE free (method I) or loaded on a support as adhesive tape (method II) or a glove (method III). Horizontal bars indicate significant difference between treatments ($p < 0.05$). FE's methods are compared with water decontamination

operational protocols increasing then contact time skin-FE to improve adsorption rate for water-soluble chemicals. In further studies, other 4-CP concentrations will be tested to plot the ratio FE to 4-CP against % removal. One objective is to prepare an operational abacus useful for skin decontamination.

Ex vivo, 4-CP was chosen as the model because of its amenability to analysis by ATR-FTIR after brief exposure (15 min) on porcine skin. Then, to track the decontamination efficiency, it was relevant to work with 4-CP saturated aqueous solution (105 mM) because the cyanyl (C ≡ N) peak area was significant by ATR-FTIR. Decontamination efficiency was directly calculated as the ratio of the peak area absorbance before and after decontamination *since absorbance is related to quantity* [35]. Elsewhere, to estimate and predict the dermal/transdermal absorption in humans [10, 13], excised porcine skin was used, as animal model. The concentration profile, absorbed through the skin, provided by this type of experiment, is easily translated into parameters of human SC diffusion [30]. In the five methods carried out by dry FE, loaded FE (adhesive tape or single-use glove), FE's suspension and water rinsing, it is assumed that decontamination efficiency is potentially higher with FE compared to water and can be boosted further when FE is used as suspension. The apparent increase in decontamination efficiency seen with the suspension may be due, at least in part, to the re-dissolution of 4-CP back into solution or back into the aqueous phase of FE suspension and passive diffusion of 4-CP in the SC layers has to be explored. Further investigations should be undertaken to elucidate the partitioning of chemicals during decontamination steps as previously discussed by Phuong and Maibach [27].

Whereas dry FE sprayed directly onto the skin is an effective decontamination method I (DE $\approx 71\%$), the compact crust created when applied on wet or humid skin is a major drawback, while unintended consequences due to the secondary contamination of victims, e.g. via inhalation, can occur when directly sprayed from container or manufactured prefilled glove. In this concept of application a serious risk of suffocation [9] and corrosive effects on vitreous humour may occur if inadvertently sprayed into the eyes. The alternative to prevent drawbacks of volatility of sprayed FE could be an appropriate protection of the nose, mouth and eyes with an adapted device without worsening the cutaneous and mucous penetration. Contaminated FE should be kept on surface and filtered to protect pipes and the environment.

It might also be pointed out that two other methods involving an adhesive tape loaded with FE (method II) and a loaded single-use glove created in our lab (method III) give different results (DE, 72% and 61%) even though it involves FE fixed on adhesive for both methods with a performance gap $\approx 10\%$. One of its benefits consists in its capacity to be prepared ahead of time, which could be included in a manufacturing program, not only for accidental or criminal decontamination but also for detoxification after environmental exposition. Additionally, the other side of the glove removes all unused powder from the skin. Even if the results are irregular, it may be suggested to stabilize FE fixed on an adhesive, to increase the shelf life of this device. This process could be extended to treat many people, distributing a single-use device to each person, thus reducing spreading of generated sludge and improving the self-decontamination.

Finally, the extemporaneous suspension preparation of FE with water (method IV; DE 88%) results in a smooth and viscous paste. The preparation allows *in situ* high volume ready for use by dispersing the FE's powder in water (ratio 1/10), therefore increasing the adsorption surface. It is relevant to mention that fuller's earth provided by NBC-SYS was readily dispersible in water. FE suspension should be easy to apply and allows a clean and safe use of raw material giving an attractive alternative to dry decontamination. Based on our results, method IV with FE suspension is by far the most effective and the most reproducible and presents key advantages. First, its low variance makes it the most attractive in large operational applications of cutaneous decontamination. Second, covering the skin with this suspension offers a double advantage, adsorbing chemicals as well as protecting from further external contamination.

Health risk assessors may therefore find this prompt and safe methodology useful in decontamination by FE [5], in order to prevent potentially dangerous transdermal absorptions [36].

Skin decontamination after chemical exposure must be performed as fast as possible, to limit skin penetration and avoid secondary contamination by transfer [6, 12]. Considering that victims on the crime scene could be contained for a lengthy period due to restriction imposed by managing operational response, results of kinetic studies highlight the feasibility to treat and protect them by the application of the FE's suspension for up to 120 min.

Compared to the water-based decontamination method initially proposed in firefighter processes [4], FE seems to be more interesting to work with and gives promising results when mixed with water as suspension. After testing on 4-CP aqueous solution, further work is required to establish the decontamination efficiency performance of the FE suspension on neat or diluted hydrophilic and lipophilic chemicals. FE aqueous suspension is efficient to remove hydrophilic liquid or solid contaminant. Both water and FE are advantageous and give additive effect. We think that water favours close contact between the particles of the FE and the agent. Decontamination step was tested for a short application time of the suspension. Therefore enhanced, skin absorption of toxic agents by water-based decontamination system like FE suspension due to long contact time will not occur.

Conclusion

The straightforward experimental methods described here provide practical and predictive assessments to extrapolate to human decontamination either after accidents, after criminal attacks or after the spread of raw or artificial chemicals, which impact human health. Adsorptive properties of FE investigated in vitro and ex vivo for the validated 4-CP model allow us to validate fuller's earth for skin decontamination process further boosted in the suspension form when compared to water showering or dry application.

In vitro studies have shown the importance of contact time on chemical adsorption observing solid performance for adsorption parameters tested in a time range 15–120 min.

Ex vivo studies have demonstrated that decontamination efficiency is higher with FE as powder (60–72%) than with water alone (54%), but reaches ~ 90% with FE suspension. In the light of this performance it is necessary to accurately determine the protocols of its operational use.

Based on this study, FE may be prepared as suspension and applied by covering skin for a contact time ranging from 15 to 60 min. Beyond 60 min, 4-CP desorption from FE is not observed. Removing FE suspension from the skin is easy either with water showering or single-use soft wipes.

This alternative to the current firefighter processes based on water or FE either sprayed or applied with manufactured prefilled gloves can be particularly appropriate for disabled victims and developed for self-decontamination.

Moreover, the abundance and availability of these materials and their relatively low cost guarantees their continued utilization in the future. The added value appears to come from the suspension extemporaneously prepared by mixing FE and water. This safe and reliable suspension method may emerge as a new trend to decontaminate after chemical exposure for firefighter processes.

Acknowledgments and Disclosures Cong-Anh-Khanh LE was supported by Explo'RA Sup region Rhône-Alpes.

References

1. Batal M, Boudry I, Mouret S, Cléry-Barraud C, Wartelle J, Bérard I, Douki T. DNA damage in internal organs after cutaneous exposure to sulphur mustard. Toxicol Appl Pharmacol. 2014;278:39–44. https://doi.org/10.1016/j.taap.2014.04.003.
2. Bose P, Bathri R, Sajal De K. CD14 C-159T polymorphism and its association with chronic lung diseases: a pilot study on isocyanate exposed population of Central India. Indian J Hum Genet. 2013;19:188. https://doi.org/10.4103/0971-6866.116124.
3. Bowonder B. The Bhopal accident. Technol Forecast Soc Chang. 1987;32:169–82.
4. Burgess JL, Kirk M, Borron SW, Cisek J. Emergency department hazardous materials protocol for contaminated patients. Ann Emerg Med. 1999;34:205–12. https://doi.org/10.1016/S0196-0644(99)70230-1.
5. Carretero MI. Clay minerals and their beneficial effects upon human health. A review. Appl Clay Sci. 2002;21:155–63. https://doi.org/10.1016/S0169-1317(01)00085-0.
6. Chilcott RP. Managing mass casualties and decontamination. Environ Int. 2014;72:37–45. https://doi.org/10.1016/j.envint.2014.02.006.
7. Cox RD. Decontamination and management of hazardous materials exposure victims in the emergency department. Ann Emerg Med. 1994;23:761–70.
8. Gaskin S, Pisaniello D, Edwards JW, Bromwich D, Reed S, Logan M, Baxter C. Chlorine and hydrogen cyanide gas interactions with human skin: in vitro studies to inform skin permeation and decontamination in HAZMAT incidents. J Hazard Mater. 2013;262:759–65. https://doi.org/10.1016/j.jhazmat.2013.09.040.
9. Gibbs A, Pooley F. Fuller's earth (montmorillonite) pneumoconiosis. Occup Environ Med. 1994;51:644–6.
10. Herkenne C, Naik A, Kalia YN, Hadgraft J, Guy RH. Pig ear skin ex vivo as a model for in vivo dermatopharmacokinetic studies in man. Pharm Res. 2006;23:1850–6. https://doi.org/10.1007/s11095-006-9011-8.
11. Ho YS, McKay G. Kinetic models for the sorption of dye from aqueous solution by wood. Process Saf Environ Prot. 1998;76:183–91. https://doi.org/10.1205/095758298529326.
12. Joosen MJA, van der Schans MJ, Kuijpers WC, van Helden HPM, Noort D. Timing of decontamination and treatment in case of percutaneous VX poisoning: a mini review. Chem Biol Interact. 2013;203:149–53. https://doi.org/10.1016/j.cbi.2012.10.002.
13. Jung EC, Maibach HI. Animal models for percutaneous absorption. In: Shah VP, Maibach HI, Jenner J, editors. Topical drug bioavailability, bioequivalence, and penetration. New York: Springer New York; 2014. p. 21–40.
14. Kerger BD, Leung H-W, Scott P, Paustenbach DJ, Needham LL, Patterson DG Jr, Gerthoux PM, Mocarelli P. Age-and concentration-dependent elimination half-life of 2, 3, 7, 8-tetrachlorodibenzo-p-dioxin in Seveso children. Environ Health Perspect. 2006;114:1596–602. https://doi.org/10.1289/ehp.8884.
15. Mak VHW, Potts RO, Guy RH. Percutaneous penetration enhancement in vivo measured by attenuated total reflectance infrared spectroscopy. Pharm Res. 1990;7:835–41. https://doi.org/10.1023/A:1015960815578.
16. Matar H, Larner J, Kansagra S, Atkinson KL, Skamarauskas JT, Amlot R, Chilcott RP. Design and characterisation of a novel in vitro skin diffusion cell system for assessing mass casualty decontamination systems. Toxicol In Vitro. 2014;28:492–501. https://doi.org/10.1016/j.tiv.2014.01.001.
17. McKay G, Otterburn MS, Aga JA. Fuller's earth and fired clay as adsorbents for dyestuffs. Water Air Soil Pollut. 1985;24:307–22. https://doi.org/10.1007/BF00161790.
18. Mircioiu C, Voicu VA, Ionescu M, Miron DS, Radulescu FS, Nicolescu AC. Evaluation of in vitro absorption, decontamination and desorption of organophosphorous compounds from skin and synthetic membranes. Toxicol Lett. 2013;219:99–106. https://doi.org/10.1016/j.toxlet.2013.03.005.
19. Moore CA, Wilkinson SC, Blain PG, Dunn M, Aust GA, Williams FM. Percutaneous absorption and distribution of organophosphates (chlorpyrifos and dichlorvos) following dermal

exposure and decontamination scenarios using in vitro human skin model. Toxicol Lett. 2014;229:66–72. https://doi.org/10.1016/j.toxlet.2014.06.008.
20. Moser K, Kriwet K, Naik A, Kalia YN, Guy RH. Passive skin penetration enhancement and its quantification in vitro. Eur J Pharm Biopharm. 2001;52:103–12. https://doi.org/10.1016/S0939-6411(01)00166-7.
21. Okumura T, Seto Y, Fuse A. Countermeasures against chemical terrorism in Japan. Forensic Sci Int. 2013;227:2–6. https://doi.org/10.1016/j.forsciint.2012.11.008.
22. Oubagaranadin JUK, Sathyamurthy N, Murthy ZVP. Evaluation of Fuller's earth for the adsorption of mercury from aqueous solutions: a comparative study with activated carbon. J Hazard Mater. 2007;142:165–74. https://doi.org/10.1016/j.jhazmat.2006.08.001.
23. Parsons CL. Fuller's earth. US Government Printing Office; 1913.
24. Pereira EF, Aracava Y, DeTolla LJ, Beecham EJ, Basinger GW, Wakayama EJ, Albuquerque EX. Animal models that best reproduce the clinical manifestations of human intoxication with organophosphorus compounds. J Pharmacol Exp Ther. 2014;350:313–21. https://doi.org/10.1124/jpet.114.214932.
25. Pesatori AC, Consonni D, Bachetti S, Zocchetti C, Bonzini M, Baccarelli A, Bertazzi PA. Short-and long-term morbidity and mortality in the population exposed to dioxin after the "Seveso accident". Ind Health. 2003;41:127–38.
26. Pesonen M, Vähäkangas K, Halme M, Vanninen P, Seulanto H, Hemmilä M, Pasanen M, Kuitunen T. Capsaicinoids, chloropicrin and sulfur mustard: possibilities for exposure biomarkers. Front Pharmacol. 2009;1:140. https://doi.org/10.3389/fphar.2010.00140.
27. Phuong C, Maibach HI. Recent knowledge: concepts of dermal absorption in relation to skin decontamination. J Appl Toxicol. 2016;36:5–9. https://doi.org/10.1002/jat.3222.
28. Pirot F, Kalia YN, Stinchcomb AL, Keating G, Bunge A, Guy RH. Characterization of the permeability barrier of human skin in vivo. Proc Natl Acad Sci. 1997;94:1562–7.
29. Potts RO, Golden GM, Francoeur ML, Mak VHW, Guy RH. Mechanism and enhancement of solute transport across the stratum corneum. J Control Release. 1991;15:249–60. https://doi.org/10.1016/0168-3659(91)90116-U.
30. Potts RO, Guy RH. Predicting skin permeability. Pharm Res. 1992;9:663–9.
31. Rafatullah M, Sulaiman O, Hashim R, Ahmad A. Adsorption of methylene blue on low-cost adsorbents: a review. J Hazard Mater. 2010;177:70–80. https://doi.org/10.1016/j.jhazmat.2009.12.047.
32. Reddy MB, Stinchcomb AL, Guy RH, Bunge AL. Determining dermal absorption parameters in vivo from tape strip data. Pharm Res. 2002;19:292–8. https://doi.org/10.1023/A:1014443001802.
33. Richards S, Bouazza A. Phenol adsorption in organo-modified basaltic clay and bentonite. Appl Clay Sci. 2007;37:133–42. https://doi.org/10.1016/j.clay.2006.11.006.
34. Secrétariat général de la défense nationale. 2008. Circulaire n° 700/SGDN/PSE/PPS du 7 novembre 2008 relative à la doctrine nationale d'emploi des moyens de secours et de soins face à une action terroriste mettant en œuvre des matières chimiques.
35. Stinchcomb AL, Pirot F, Touraille GD, Bunge AL, Guy RH. Chemical uptake into human stratum corneum in vivo from volatile and non-volatile solvents. Pharm Res. 1999;16:1288–93.
36. Taysse L, Daulon S, Delamanche S, Bellier B, Breton P. Skin decontamination of mustards and organophosphates: comparative efficiency of RSDL and Fuller's earth in domestic swine. Hum Exp Toxicol. 2007;26:135–41.
37. Toor M, Jin B. Adsorption characteristics, isotherm, kinetics, and diffusion of modified natural bentonite for removing diazo dye. Chem Eng J. 2012;187:79–88. https://doi.org/10.1016/j.cej.2012.01.089.
38. Touitou E, Meidan VM, Horwitz E. Methods for quantitative determination of drug localized in the skin. J Control Release. 1998;56:7–21. https://doi.org/10.1016/S0168-3659(98)00060-1.
39. Warner M, Mocarelli P, Samuels S, Needham L, Brambilla P, Eskenazi B. Dioxin exposure and cancer risk in the Seveso Women's Health Study. Environ Health Perspect. 2011;119:1700. https://doi.org/10.1289/ehp.1103720.
40. Yuh-Shan H. Citation review of Lagergren kinetic rate equation on adsorption reactions. Scientometrics. 2004;59:171–7. https://doi.org/10.1023/B:SCIE.0000013305.99473.cf.

Chapter 9
The Mass Decontamination Paradigm: Response Relating to Gas Phase Exposures and Skin Decontamination

Christina Baxter, Sharyn Gaskin, Michael Logan, and Dino Pisaniello

The Problem

The accidental or intentional releases of toxic gases or vapors[1] are the most common occurrence in hazardous material (HAZMAT) incidents that result in human injuries [1, 2]. Such atmospheric releases are typically associated with industrial accidents. (e.g., chlorine gas release after a train derailment in South Carolina [29]) and terrorism-related events. (e.g., Tokyo subway nerve agent sarin attack [3]). Historically, deliberate acts using hazardous materials and chemical agents have been sparse. Nonetheless, in the last few years, deliberate releases dispersing chlorine, mustard agent, and sarin in Iraq and Syria have occurred illustrating ongoing national and terrorist groups' interest.

---

[1] Here, the terms gas and vapor are used interchangeably. A vapor refers to the gaseous form of a substance that is a liquid or solid at room temperature.

C. Baxter
Department of Defense, Combating Terrorism Technical Support Office, CA, Virginia, USA
e-mail: christina.baxter@cttso.gov

S. Gaskin (✉)
Department of Occupational & Environmental Health, School of Public Health, University of Adelaide, Adelaide, SA, Australia
e-mail: sharyn.gaskin@adelaide.edu.au

M. Logan
Research and Scientific Branch, Queensland Fire and Emergency Services, Brisbane, QLD, Australia
e-mail: Michael.logan@qfes.qld.gov.au

D. Pisaniello
Adelaide Exposure Science and Health Laboratory, School of Public Health, University of Adelaide, Adelaide, SA, Australia
e-mail: dino.pisaniello@adelaide.edu.au

H. Zhu, H. I. Maibach (eds.), *Skin Decontamination*,
https://doi.org/10.1007/978-3-030-24009-7_9

These releases of hazardous materials have significant consequences on public health and impose significant demands on HAZMAT response resources [4, 5]. During and following HAZMAT incidents, there are four main groups of people affected: (a) exposed and deceased, (b) exposed and symptomatic, (c) exposed and asymptomatic, and (d) unexposed and asymptomatic. Groups (a) and (b), usually acutely affected by inhalation exposure, are the most clearly recognized, with group (b) being able to be triaged and evacuated to hospital or treated at the scene. However, the onsite management of group (c) is problematic as it may be numerically large and potentially resource-intensive. Group (d), also known as the 'worried well', may self-present to first responders at the scene, or at nearby hospitals, or medical facilities, placing further demands on valuable resources and adding to the potential delay in identifying and treating those who need more urgent attention.

The established approach globally is, by default, to decontaminate the skin of all exposed persons using field portable shower systems. Jurisdictions have invested hundreds of millions of dollars establishing and extending their field deployable mass decontamination resources. Nonetheless, a significant incident will likely rapidly overwhelm the available field deployable HAZMAT mass decontamination capacity.

Is this approach consistent with the nature of the exposure incurred by the affected persons? Is it always appropriate for the skin interactions between the contaminant and the exposed persons? There is little if any published work investigating these interactions and their implication on the subsequent approaches that should be applied during a HAZMAT emergency. Most published works have focused on the mechanics of decontamination rather than whether decontamination is necessary, and what, if any, type and extent of decontamination should be applied before medical care. Decontamination modeling estimates show that if the number of persons undergoing decontamination can be reduced by 80%, then the available resource demand is reduced by 63% and the times required by 77% [6]. This has a significant impact on the efficiency of a HAZMAT response and saving the lives of those who were affected.

There is a limited evidence base describing skin absorption of toxic gases and vapors in HAZMAT exposure scenarios, which tend to be relatively brief compared with traditional test periods for skin absorption studies. In order to address this gap, there is a need for a testing strategy that encompasses the relevant kinetics and equilibria of skin deposition, absorption and penetration of gases and vapors, and the moderating effects of environmental factors. (e.g., temperature, humidity), clothing, and other factors. This is a complex multicompartment system, and any protocol should also take into account typical short-term exposures of less than 1-h duration and subsequent periods of off-gassing. Investigations within this period (sometimes termed as the "golden hour") are of particular relevance to HAZMAT incidents [1].

From the first responder perspective, a number of key questions arise: (1) how much gas gets on, in, or through the skin in this first hour following contact, (2) what are the modifying influences of environmental factors and street clothing worn, and (3) what are the off-gassing rates from skin and clothing.

Relevant toxicological testing should aim to generate data and provide advice. These empirical data and advice relate only to the specific chemical exposures and are not intended to support recommendations regarding dissimilar HAZMAT chemicals for which alternative individual data must be gathered.

Nature of Gas Exposure

Compared with liquid or aerosol exposure scenarios, gas concentrations in gas-only scenarios are often low, i.e., typically less than 1% v/v. Following toxic gas exposure, it is often assumed that isolation from the source and removal of clothing is typically all that is needed to prevent further exposure or injury [1, 7, 8]. Levitin et al. [1] and Houston et al. [7] suggest removal and double-bagging of the victim's clothing can eliminate 80% to 90% of the contaminant and minimize the risk of spreading the toxic agent to others. This percentage may depend on amount/type of clothing worn and the duration of exposure. Bagged clothing should be left at the scene and managed by emergency responders so as to minimize risk of exposure to hospital personnel [7, 8]. However, accident scene management and victim care varies throughout the world and is based primarily on personal judgment and dogma rather than on scientific evidence. Ill-informed decisions about the management of exposed individuals and groups during chemical releases have the potential to cause a significant drain on resources as well as a variety of undesired outcomes among those affected. In particular, decisions about mass decontamination following suspected or known chemical exposure should be risk-based and supported by suitable empirical evidence.

Following a review of toxic gas exposure literature, there appears to be limited specific advice for first responders regarding skin decontamination. As mentioned, the current generally accepted approach to mass-casualty decontamination is that all exposed individuals must "strip and shower", regardless of the mechanism or likely form of exposure (liquid versus gas/vapor). This advice could be seen as inconsistent with ATSDR studies from 13 US states for 7 years, which determined that in 90% of cases, only six or fewer human casualties required care after chemical exposures [1, 9]. The Chemical Weapons Improved Response Program projects at least a 5:1 ratio of unaffected to affected casualties [10]. These "worried well" noninjured victims comprise the largest group in mass-casualty events (80–90% of survivors in most cases). These victims will wait for care at the scene, transport themselves to the closest medical facility for care, or leave the scene and not seek care. While evacuation from the area of chemical release will decrease their level of primary exposure, secondary exposure can potentially occur from the amount of gas/vapor remaining in their clothing. By the time showers can be set up, any trapped gas/vapor in victims' clothing may have dispersed, making decontamination unnecessary. In this regard, Markel et al. [11] supports a "scoop and run" evacuation approach rather than onsite decontamination. Little has been done to investigate the degree and duration of trapped gas/vapor released from different types of street clothing. Furthermore, sunscreen and cosmetics may enhance, buffer or reduce dermal exposure or act as a chemical reservoir [12, 13]. In practice, emergency personnel need practical guidance about ongoing exposure potential and decontamination advice [4].

Nature of Gas/Vapor Interactions with Skin

There is a limited evidence base for the extent and kinetics of skin absorption in HAZMAT scenarios involving toxic gases and vapors [5, 14]. Much of the preplanning has generally been based on knowledge of the basic physicochemical properties of the released chemical such as volatility/vapor pressure, water and oil solubility, molecular mass, density and other routine information. However, this information may do little to inform a dynamic or evolving risk assessment process under the variable environmental conditions that may exist during an incident.

It is well recognized that vapors, aerosols, and liquids deposit onto the skin from the atmosphere. If sufficient vapor is deposited onto the skin, condensation may occur and a liquid-like phase formed. A proportion of these absorbed molecules also evaporate. The molecules will either physically interact (absorption) or chemically interact (adsorption) with the surface. The transport of chemicals through the skin [17, 18] is either active (mediated transport requiring energy) or passive (diffusion requiring no energy). Often, the kinetics of skin absorption of gases/vapors (and their dissociation products) is slow, with competing processes of absorption and desorption more evident than that of liquid exposures.

The literature indicates that a variety of factors can play a significant role in the dermal absorption of chemicals. These include skin thickness and lipid content, occlusion, clothing, temperature and humidity, and skin damage/disease.

Clothing may serve to initially protect and buffer the skin from toxic chemicals, depending on the material, thickness, cover, and yarn twist. A tightly woven fabric using a high twist yarn gives the most protection against penetration and in conjunction with a thick fabric gives a high protection factor. However, significant skin uptake of chemical may occur if contaminated clothing is in contact with, or occludes, the skin. There do not seem to be any systematic studies of the chemical protection afforded by street clothing or personal skin products.

Personal products applied to the skin and hair, such as cosmetics and sunscreen, may enhance, buffer or reduce dermal exposure. They may also act as a chemical reservoir. The ability to enhance or reduce skin uptake depends primarily on whether the product is oil- or water-based [12], although some active ingredients can enhance penetration [13]. Indeed, it is only recently that the community usage of personal products has been studied for risk assessment purposes [15, 16].

Current Experimental Approaches to Gas Interaction Studies

The best models for understanding dermal exposures during CBR incidents would be human volunteer skin exposure studies, either whole body, or segmental, or limb exposures. These exposures may be authentic in that the chemicals may have been applied via surface sprays, droplets, spills, immersion, deposition, or from gas and vapor contact. They may be further modified under varying conditions of temperature and humidity, clothing coverage, occlusion, vehicle, and all other parameters that may be imagined or predicted for 'real-life' exposures. However, these methods cannot be applied for highly toxic materials, or for other materials at concentrations that may be toxic. Individuals are highly variable in their absorption, and the small number of trials that may be performed limits statistical interpretation. Also, the measures that indicate the extent of absorption may be limited to blood concentrations, urine concentrations or other such estimates that, being markers of systemic absorption, may not fully inform investigators about localized concentrations and effects. However, tape-stripping applications, in which the stratum corneum may be removed by successive applications and removal of adhesive tape, have been performed to identify the localizations of dermally applied chemicals in the stratum corneum or to demonstrate altered rates of penetration through skin in the absence of stratum corneum. Recently, confocal Raman spectroscopy has been used to examine chemical concentrations in skin strata [17]. Such approaches, however, have not been nor could easily be applied to gas or vapor exposures.

Whole animal (in vivo) models may suffer from poor extrapolation to human circumstances because of significant interspecies variation. These are also relatively expensive, especially in large, statistically justified investigations. Ex-vivo systems, including the isolated perfused pig ear, have also been used to examine the uptake of chemicals through a system whose blood circulation (through arteries, arterioles, capillaries, venules, and veins) remains intact.

In vitro models, using either animal- or human-derived tissue, remain the most common methods used for a wide range of assessments of dermal absorption of chemicals. The Organization of Economic Cooperation and Development (OECD) approach has gained widespread acceptance and adoption for in vitro testing for dermal absorption (OECD 2004) [18]. While these models suffer from the handicap of being remote from real-life situations (with consequent reduction in direct validity to human exposure scenarios), they are reliable, generally reproducible, and allow at least the rank comparison of different chemicals under similar exposure parameters. At best, they can provide quantitative comparisons, enabling some numeral risk assessments to be extrapolated.

Rat dorsum, pig ear, human cadaver skin, or viable human skin (commonly obtained from cosmetic reduction surgery) may be used in chambers with an upper application well and a lower receptor well, containing a receptor fluid to mimic cutaneous blood. This may be a simple static diffusion type (such as the Franz cell) or a dynamic, or flow-through cell. The static-type cell requires any media removed from the lower receptor chamber to be replaced at each sampling time point. The flow-through cell has a reservoir of fresh receptor fluid that is pumped through the receptor chamber and collected downstream. The tissues may be full thickness (stratum corneum, epidermis and sometimes partial dermis), split thickness (stratum corneum and epidermis only), or some defined fraction of the skin layer (sometimes dermatomed to a specified standard thickness). Each of these approaches yields different results that may not be directly comparable between methodologies. Furthermore, there are currently no test cells commercially available with a modified donor chamber to allow for gas/vapor delivery to the skin surface. This methodological challenge may in part account for the limited number of published studies on skin exposure to gases. Gaskin et al. [19]) describe a bespoke static diffusion cell with a modified donor chamber to allow for gas delivery, and appear to be one of the only research group assessing dermal exposure to toxic gases and vapors [5, 14, 19, 20].

Recent work has focused on emerging technologies to produce skin substrates that are more consistent, reliable or in other ways considered advantageous for dermal absorption experiments. These include human cell line models (growing sheets of keratinocytes of uniform or near-uniform characteristics) and partial culture (such as using viable human skin, seeded with human stem cells that form a uniform upper skin surface devoid of accessory structures and flaws).

Fresh human skin, from cosmetic reduction surgery, is the most convenient and reliable substrate available, notwithstanding the variations between donor skin characteristics. It usually provides sufficient skin for several diffusion chambers to be set up, allowing manipulation of key parameters in a controlled experiment that is internally consistent and comparable. Skin is usually from breast or abdomen, reducing the extent of site-specific variations that have been identified with skin sourced from varying anatomical sites. Skin can be used in a variety of modes (full thickness, split thickness) to satisfy the needs of the experimental approach.

Dermatomed split-thickness skin is considered by some to be superior to skin split by other methods (heat or chemical treatment), but this has been seen predominantly in studies in which maintenance of metabolic capacity of skin was desirable. For simple diffusion studies, heat-treated, split-thickness skin has been found be effective and reproducible. Integrity of skin is checked by visual inspection under a dissecting microscope prior to mounting in the diffusion cell, and by transdermal resistance (with electrical probes placed on the skin surface and in the lower receptor chamber), following mounting. This is usually sufficient to establish whether the skin sample has defects or perforations that may affect results.

Tape stripping prior to mounting or following chemical exposure can allow examination of the role of the stratum corneum as a barrier or a chemical reservoir, but is methodologically challenging. Skin washing is a common contaminant removal technique (post-exposure), and is appropriate for chemicals that have low rates of dermal absorption.

Keratinocyte culture is currently unproven and may generate a model that is more similar to the stratum corneum than to the integrated structure of the skin.

Similarly, the partial culture/stem cell methods have been developed predominantly for medical applications (for treatment of skin injuries such as burns) and have not been used for dermal absorption models.

Although the use of human skin represents the most robust approach, a multispecies study has suggested that pigskin can be a very useful model for in vitro percutaneous absorption studies, provided that the skin integrity is checked prior to skin exposure, and in-house electrical resistance cut-off values are adhered to.

Systematic In Vitro Approach

The approach by Gaskin et al. represents a modification of the OECD experimental protocol for skin absorption of chemicals by specifically aligning with the context of HAZMAT incidents in which exposures occur by vapor or gas for relatively brief periods [19]. It also allows examination of the influence of fabrics and other potential barriers or reservoirs on the secondary exposure and need for decontamination. Supplementary fabric off-gassing experiments may also be conducted under variable conditions. The use of the human in vitro model allows repeatable studies to gauge variation in contributions of the various environmental conditions. Observations may then be summarized and translated into a format that guides emergency personnel in public health management at HAZMAT incidents.

The experimental approach addresses the kinetics and equilibria of skin absorption and penetration, and the moderating effects of environmental factors. (e.g., temperature, humidity), and clothing. An overview of the technique can be described in three steps: (1) Substrate (skin sample) preparation, (2) Gas challenge, and (3) Post-exposure analysis of absorption and penetration. Figure 9.1 is a block diagram of the equipment setup.

Test Cell

Jacketed 9 mm Static Franz diffusion cells housed in a stirrer unit (PermeGear, Hellertown, PA) may be used. Cells have a diffusion-available surface area of 0.64cm^2 and utilize appropriate receptor fluid. (e.g., physiological saline, pure water or 50% ethanol). A modified donor compartment of the cell has been described for flow-through gas delivery to the surface of the skin [5]. Of note, the central bar is positioned to ensure turbulence is created in the neck of the donor chamber and allows even distribution of gas flow over the surface of the skin/substrate. The side arm may be enlarged to accommodate real time monitoring of the receptor fluid, e.g., pH/ISE probe. Prepared skin epidermis may be mounted between the donor compartment and the receptor compartment, in this way acting as a barrier for the

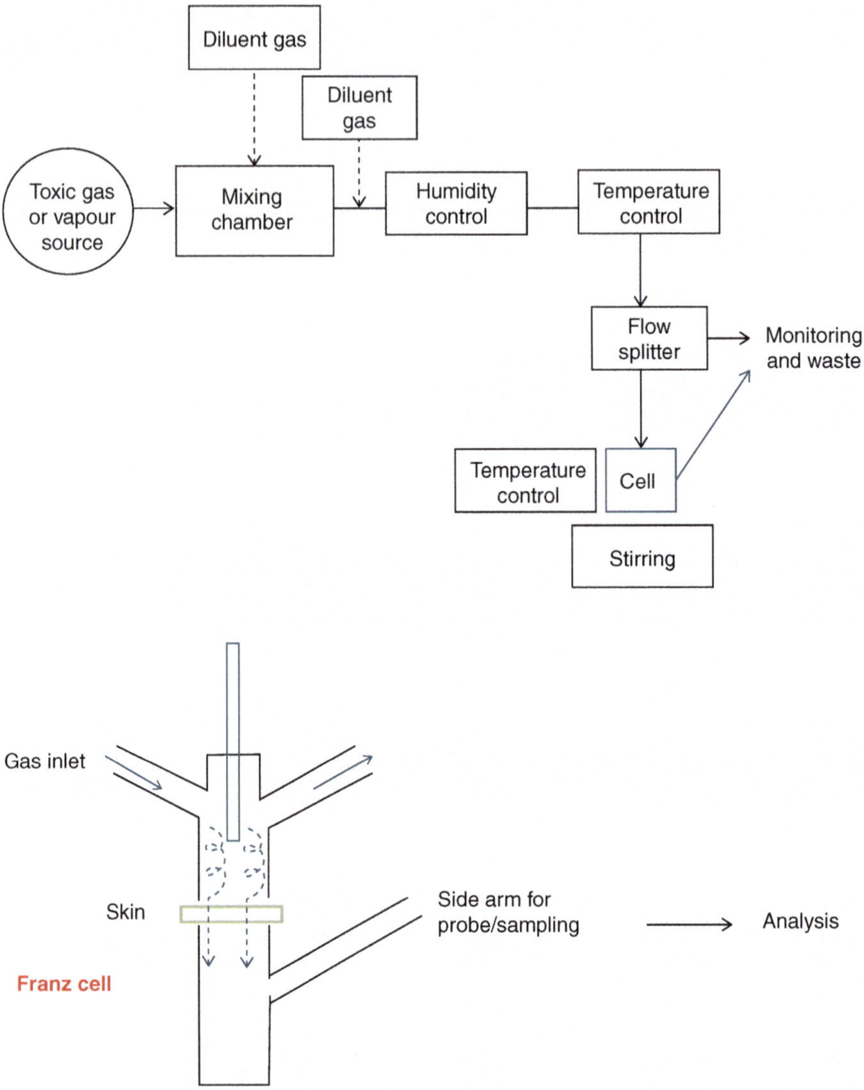

Fig. 9.1 Block diagram of apparatus

applied test chemical to permeate into the receptor fluid. Receptor fluid is kept in contact with the skin under-surface and continuously stirred with a Teflon-coated magnetic stirring bar. After the set exposure period, the Franz cell can be dismantled and the skin and complete volume of receptor fluid used for measurements of contaminant concentration in and through skin.

Substrate Preparation

Various skin substrates may be used. However, the use of human skin samples is usually preferred for in vitro studies of dermal absorption [21] as it provides data more appropriate to human in vivo conditions. Freshly excised human abdominal skin obtained from cosmetic reduction surgery is used. In this approach, epidermis is harvested from full thickness skin within 1 h of excision from the donor. Subcutaneous tissue is removed, and the epidermal layer harvested from full thickness skin by heat treatment [17, 22, 23]. Pre-exposure skin electrical impedance (EI) testing is performed to provide a rapid assessment of barrier integrity in vitro [23–25]. For this purpose, a Tinsley LCR Databridge 6401 [26] is used set in Resistance (R), Parallel Equivalent (PAR) and 100 Hz modes. Skin EI may also be assessed post-exposure to toxic gas in order to assess changes in barrier integrity resulting from exposure.

Gas Challenge

Toxic gases and vapors may be delivered directly from the source, for example, a certified gas mixture cylinder. More commonly, it is diluted to test concentrations as required using a bespoke dynamic atmosphere generator and a diluent gas stream, typically purified air [27]. For HAZMAT scenarios, challenge gas concentrations should be physiologically relevant and appropriate for first responder guidance, for example, the lowest lethal concentration (LCLo), the concentration immediately dangerous to life and health (IDLH), or other relevant concentrations. (e.g., eye irritation). Short-term exposure times of 5, 10, 20, and 30 min are used, simulating HAZMAT incident exposures [5, 14]. A minimum of four replicates for each variable at each exposure time should be gained. For some experiments, a post-exposure open-to-atmosphere ventilation period is used to read at 60 min (i.e., 5 min exposure with 55 min ventilation, 30 min exposure with 30 min ventilation etc.). In all experiments, a method of destructive sampling is applied to make determination of contaminant concentration IN, ON and THROUGH skin possible.

Experimental variables such as temperature and relative humidity may be accommodated using auxiliary components [27]. For elevated temperatures, electrical heating tape wrapped around Teflon tubing can be used in order to maintain an injected gas stream temperature of 30 °C to 60 °C. The system minimizes thermal losses by the use of foam insulation around the Teflon tubing. The heating tape temperature is controlled by a simmerstat or voltage regulator. For lower temperatures of 10–20 °C, a refrigeration unit circulates chilled water around jacketed glass fittings (for the gas stream and also the cell). Humidification of the diluent gas is achieved by using a split stream saturator [27]. Temperature, humidity and pressure are monitored in the final gas stream, which is typically reduced from 10 L/min to 500 mL/min over the exposed substrate. The whole assembly is mounted in a fume cupboard.

Post-exposure Analysis of Absorption and Penetration

Quantification of skin absorption and penetration requires a suitable analytical method. Chemical interactions with skin could be studied, and suitable detection techniques were identified and utilized for a range of toxic gases, using standard calibration curves and relevant blanks. Receptor fluid could be analyzed to determine gas penetration, and following exposure, the amount of gas absorbed was assessed by rapid dismantling of the cell and extraction of the skin substrate in a vial.

Chemicals of Interest

In Australia, using a combination of intelligence assessments, hazardous materials properties and use a list of materials was created, often referred to as the COAG (Council of Australian Governments) list of hazardous materials [28]. Similar lists have been complied by other nations [29, 30]. These lists are applied as a basis to assist communities in focusing their efforts to prevent the misuse of such materials and prepare to manage the consequence of attacks using hazardous materials. The materials are a mixture of solids, liquids and gases and range from toxic chemicals like parathion (organophosphate) to corrosive toxic gases like hydrogen chloride. They are generally toxic and/or corrosive materials.

The toxicity of the chemical is a crucial factor. Toxicity and classification criteria are described in the United Nations recommendations on the transport of dangerous goods. The toxic effect of a material is dependent on several factors, including the route of entry. Materials most toxic by inhalation find favor for deliberate use. The most effective materials to be dispersed are selected on a combination of their toxicity and physicochemical properties, such as volatility, state, and reactivity.

The prioritization of chemicals to be included in the skin decontamination studies should be based on the national lists combined with their intrinsic properties. Toxic and/or corrosive chemicals naturally found in the gaseous state are highest priority. In order to contaminate mass numbers of people, the threat material would likely be a gas or vapor.

For an initial study by the authors, ten chemicals of high priority were addressed. Based upon the way in which the chemicals interact with skin, they were divided into categories of reactive gases, biochemical degradation gases, and fumigant gases.

Reactive Gases

Chlorine

Inhalation is the most significant route of exposure, with approximately 1000 ppm being rapidly fatal, but exposures at half this concentration will be fatal after some delay (over 30 min). This is a deep lung irritant resulting in delayed chemical pneumonitis at lower concentrations. Skin exposure to the gas results in significant irritation, and at higher concentration, blisters and chemical burns, although there are no reports of serious systemic effects following skin exposure only, suggesting poor dermal uptake. Occupational standards do not suggest a skin notation.

Ammonia

A potent upper respiratory tract irritant, ammonia has excellent warning properties for inhalational exposure, resulting in severe lacrimation and irritation on exposures to relatively low concentrations. The physiological response to ammonia is a reduced depth of tidal breathing, limiting the extent of penetration of ammonia into the deeper lung. Short durations of inhalational exposure may be tolerated in this way, although this breathing pattern is not sustainable for extended duration exposures. Skin is a target for toxic effects, with erythema, irritation and chemical burns seen after exposure to ammonia gas, although this has most often been associated with direct exposure to releases from pressurized containers. Skin damage occurs from anhydrous ammonia gas at over 10,000 ppm (a concentration rapidly fatal by inhalation), although this may relate to the lower concentration of ammonium ion. Ammonia (ammonium) in aerosol form may exhibit a different (possibly higher) dermal toxicity.

Hydrogen Chloride

Deleterious effects of gaseous hydrogen chloride exposure are predominantly by the inhalation route, but lower concentrations result in severe irritation and corrosion of skin. Toxicity appears to be limited to the site of application, with physiologic pH buffering systems providing protection from severe systemic exposures, although there are few human studies that reliably examine the systemic characteristics of dermal exposures. Ocular damage is likely at exposures likely to be significant for skin.

Sulfur Dioxide

Sulfur dioxide may enter the body via the respiratory tract or, following dilution in saliva, it may be swallowed and enter gastrointestinal tract in form of sulfurous acid. Due to its high solubility, SO_2 is rapidly distributed throughout the body. In the blood, sulfuric acid is metabolized to sulfates which are excreted in the urine [30]. Most people can smell sulfur dioxide at levels of 0.3 to 1 ppm [31].SO_2 is very soluble in, and reactive with, water. In the moist pulmonary environment, SO_2 produces sulfurous acid (H_2SO_3), a severe irritant, in addition to H+, bisulfate (HSO_3-), sulfite (SO_3=), which in turn affect the smooth muscles and nerves involved in bronchoconstriction [31–33]. There are no available studies addressing dermal absorption of sulfur dioxide.

Biochemical Degradation Gases

Hydrogen Cyanide

Rapidly fatal by inhalation but lower airborne concentrations are associated with moderate dermal absorption, shown in a few anecdotal reports and in in vitro skin absorption studies [34–36]. Hydrogen cyanide is a relatively unreactive, small molecule with skin permeation outcomes likely to be related to solubility and ionization. In animal investigations and in vitro cases, exposures are continuous, whereas in the event of an environmental release, the duration of exposure may be likely to be short, resulting in a lower total absorption of CN.

Hydrogen Sulfide

Pungent with strong olfactory warning properties initially (prior to olfactory fatigue), and with significant respiratory toxic effects, hydrogen sulfide is a deep lung irritant capable of causing delayed chemical pneumonitis. Absorption through skin is possible although the toxic sequelae have not been reported (other than death within hours in animals with dermal exposure). For example, historic animal in vivo dermal exposure studies indicate some potential for H_2S gas to be absorbed through skin but only at very high concentrations and long experimental time frames [35, 37]. No skin notation is recorded for occupational standards. The corneal surface appears sensitive to hydrogen sulfide, with eye symptoms reported with extended duration exposures.

Nitrogen Dioxide

A deep lung irritant, NO_2 has been associated with significant respiratory symptoms with acute exposures and long term respiratory damage with repeated exposures at lower levels. While skin effects have been reported (linked to dissolution of nitrogen dioxide in sweat to generate nitric acid) there is little evidence to suggest a significant systemic toxicity associated with dermal exposure [38].

Fumigant Gases

Phosphine

Phosphine is a deep lung irritant with effects by the respiratory route dominating its toxicity. Phosphine does not have a skin notation for occupational standards. No dermal exposure studies for phosphine gas in humans or animals have previously been reported in the literature.

Methyl Bromide

Direct dermal contact with methyl bromide can lead to severe injury to the skin [39] Symptoms usually do not appear immediately, but develop a few hours after exposure. Early signs typically include a burning or itching sensation, with erythema, edema, and large blisters that resemble second-degree burns developing somewhat later. In the presence of moisture, methyl bromide breaks down to methanol and bromide ion. This may be pH- and temperature-dependent (alkaline conditions increases bromide ions). The published human dermal exposure data for methyl bromide are principally associated with occupational accidental exposures [40, 41]. Methyl bromide has been assigned a "skin notation" in the context of workplace exposure standards, suggesting the potential for skin absorption [42].

Sulfuryl Fluoride

Sulfuryl fluoride is noncorrosive and not very reactive; it does not hydrolyze in water but is hydrolyzed by aqueous sodium hydroxide solution [42]. Based on its low boiling point and high vapor pressure, sulfuryl fluoride is expected to remain a gas over a wide range of ambient temperatures, thus dermal and oral exposure to surface residues are expected to be insignificant. Although no available studies address dermal absorption of sulfuryl fluoride, mucous membrane and dermal permeability are expected to be very low based upon sulfuryl fluoride's relative insolubility in water and low octanol/water partition coefficient [43].

Detection Methodologies

Table 9.1 shows the detection techniques used for each chemical interaction assessed.

Table 9.1 Detection techniques used to assess chemical interactions with skin

Test gas	Analyte/s assessed; detection method (reference)
Ammonia	pH; expressed as equivalent mg/L NH_4^+ [5]
Chlorine	pH; expressed as equivalent mg/L Cl^- [14]
Hydrogen chloride	pH; expressed as equivalent mg/L Cl^-
Hydrogen cyanide	CN-; ion selective electrode (adjusted to pH 11) [14]
Hydrogen sulfide	Total-S; inductively coupled plasma emission spectrometry [19]
Methyl bromide	Br-; ion chromatography
Nitrogen dioxide	NOx; UV-spectrophotometry
Phosphine	Total-P; UV-spectrophotometry [19]
Sulfur dioxide	Total-S; inductively coupled plasma atomic emission spectrometry [19]
Sulfuryl fluoride	F- and SO_4^{2-}/SO_3^{2-}; ion chromatography [44]

Findings

The detailed results are presented in Tables 9.2, 9.3, and 9.4 for gases grouped together in the following way:

- Reactive gases (skin destruction, oxidize and/or ionize)
- Gases which interfere biochemically (redox, methylation, oxygen transport)
- Fumigant gases

Inferences for Other Chemicals

Many chemicals exhibit similar physicochemical properties and solution chemistry, hence other chemicals may be inferred from the results of chemicals tested. Where possible, tests may performed to support or refute inferences about other chemical.

Inference of Phosphine and Ammonia Data for Arsine

Arsine cannot be inferred from phosphine and ammonia based on physicochemistry and speciation on skin in published studies. Arsine and phosphine have similar physicochemical properties including little water solubility and acidity. Arsine is a slightly bigger molecule, but slightly more polarizable and fat soluble. It is likely that arsine will penetrate marginally more. The Henry's law constants for phosphine or arsine ($8E^{-3}$ mol/(L-atm)) are vastly different from ammonia ($5E^{1}$), suggesting that the former gases do not readily dissolve in liquids –i.e., tend to prefer the gas phase. It seems that hydration and protonation are not easy for phosphine, based on the thermodynamics.

Inference of Hydrogen Sulfide Data for Hydrogen Selenide and Hydrogen Telluride

Hydrogen selenide and hydrogen telluride can be inferred from hydrogen sulfide experimental results. As hydrogen selenide and hydrogen telluride are (1) more water soluble; (2) more acidic; and (3) larger molecules than hydrogen sulfide, one could be reasonably confident that H_2Se and H_2Te would be less capable of penetrating the skin than H_2S. Although H_2Se is very toxic, no literature is available of reported fatalities from skin exposure, possibly because H_2Se is easily oxidized to red selenium on the surface of mucous membranes of the nose and throat.

Table 9.2 Results for chemicals which interfere with skin as reactive gases

	Ammonia IDLH = 300 ppm LC_{lo} = 2000 ppm	Chlorine IDLH = 10 ppm LC_{lo} = 500 ppm	Hydrogen chloride IDLH = 50 ppm LC_{lo} = 3000 ppm	Sulfur dioxide IDLH = 100 ppm LC_{lo} = 3000 ppm
Concentration	No penetration at LC_{Lo} Negligible absorption only at LC_{Lo}	No penetration at LC_{Lo} Absorption at LC_{Lo} for >10 min exposures	No penetration at LC_{Lo} No absorption at LC_{Lo}	No penetration at LC_{Lo} No absorption at LC_{Lo}
Post-exposure ventilation	Absorbed component released to atmosphere	Increased penetration for ≥30 min exposures Increased absorption for ≥30 min exposures	No effect	No effect (except where clothing present, see below)
High temperature, humidity	No effect	(Further) Increased penetration for >10 min exposures Increased absorption for >10 min exposures	No effect	No effect
Clothing	Initial barrier (< 10 min exposures), then reservoir especially when wet	Enabled penetration at LCLo	No effect	Denim on skin marginally increased absorption for 20 + min exposures at LCLo, and ventilation did not reduce
Speciation	NH_3, NH_4^+	Cl_2, $HClO^-$, OCl^-, Cl^-, H^+, HCl	H_3O^+, Cl^-	SO_2, HSO_3^-, H^+, H_2SO_4,H_2SO_3,SO_3^-
Suggested decontamination protocol	At concentrations greater than 700 ppm: If clothing is damp, remove immediately; if clothing is dry, remove outer layer; and, decontaminate with enhanced ventilation or washing with water. Otherwise, move to fresh air	At concentrations greater than 30 ppm, remove all clothing and decontaminate with enhanced ventilation. When contact time is greater than 30 min and concentration exceeds LC_{Lo}, decontaminate with water. Otherwise, move to fresh air	If concentration is greater than LC_{Lo}, consider decontamination with water to minimize potential skin irritation. Otherwise, move to fresh air	At concentration exceeding IDLH remove outer layer of clothing and decontaminate with enhanced ventilation or washing with water. Otherwise, move to fresh air

Table 9.3 Results for chemicals which interfere with the skin biochemically via redox, methylation, or oxygen transport

	Hydrogen cyanide IDLH = 50 ppm LC_{Lo} = 300 ppm	Hydrogen sulfide IDLH = 100 ppm LC_{Lo} = 800 ppm	Nitrogen dioxide IDLH = 20 ppm LC_{Lo} = 200 ppm
Concentration	No penetration at LC_{Lo} No absorption at LC_{Lo}	No penetration at LC_{Lo} No absorption at LC_{Lo}	No penetration at LC_{Lo} Absorption at LC_{Lo}
Post-exposure ventilation	No effect	No effect	No effect
High temperature, humidity	No effect	No effect	No effect
Clothing	No effect	No effect	Fabric an ongoing "sink"
Speciation	HCN, CN^-	H_2S, HS^-, S_2^-	NO_2, NO_3^-, NO_2^-, HNO_3, NO
Suggested decontamination protocol	Move to fresh air	Move to fresh air	Above LC_{Lo}, remove outer layer of clothing and consider decontamination with enhanced ventilation or washing with water. Otherwise, move to fresh air

Table 9.4 Results for fumigant gases

	Phosphine IDLH = 50 ppm LC_{Lo} = 1000 ppm	Sulfuryl fluoride IDLH = 200 ppm LC_{Lo} = 5000 ppm	Methyl bromide IDLH = 250 ppm LC_{Lo} = 60,000 ppm
Concentration	Negligible penetration at LC_{Lo} Negligible absorption at LC_{Lo}	No penetration at LC_{Lo} No absorption at LC_{Lo}	No penetration at LC_{Lo} No absorption at LC_{Lo}
Post-exposure ventilation	No effect	No effect	No effect
High temperature, humidity	No effect	No effect	No effect
Clothing	No effect	No effect	No effect
Speciation	PH_3, H_2PO_4, HPO_4^{2-}, PO_4^{3-}, $H_2PO_3^-$, HPO_3^{2-}	SF_2O_2, SO_4^{2-}, F^-, H^+	CH_3Br, CH_3OH, Br^-
Suggested decontamination protocol	Move to fresh air	Move to fresh air	Above LC_{Lo}, remove outer layer of clothing and consider decontamination with enhanced ventilation or washing with water. Otherwise, move to fresh air

Inference of Hydrogen Chloride Data for Hydrogen Bromide, Hydrogen Iodide, and Hydrogen Fluoride

Hydrogen bromide and hydrogen iodide can be inferred from hydrogen chloride data, but hydrogen fluoride cannot be inferred. Molecules that dissociate and/or are ionized may behave differently. Molecules that ionize may not be fat soluble, which tends to explain why ammonia and hydrogen chloride do not penetrate so easily. HCl, HBr, and HI will all ionize completely, therefore one would expect little penetration through the lipid skin layer. HF is not fully ionized and as a small, partly fat soluble molecule (based on its log Kow), it is able to pass through the skin. On exposure to HF, the fluoride anion (F-) will dissociate from its hydrogen counterpart and be readily absorbed through the skin, penetrating through the epidermal and dermal layer causing tissue damage and systemic injury.

Limitations

The main limitations to the application of this test protocol can be related to the test substrate (human skin), the chemical entities used for challenge, and the quantitative analysis of chemical on skin, in skin and penetration through skin. The system does not represent functional skin, but rather the barrier properties of the epidermis. While one may simulate physiological circumstances, such as the presence or absence of sweat by the hydration film of saline solution, this may not adequately represent the physiological events that occur in exposed individuals. In particular, the model uses skin at a high level of hydration, whereas exposed skin may present a more-dry surface. The relative humidity of challenge chemicals is also practically limited to approximately 80%. Similarly, the available temperature range in these experiments can be restricted unless gas delivery lines are not all jacketed. The nature of challenge chemical may restrict the range of concentrations available to be investigated, for example, the corrosive nature of strongly acidic and alkaline gases would disrupt the skin structure and lead to perforation. Some gases or vapors may be degraded under the conditions of humidity and temperature appropriate to maintain the integrity of the skin.

Ideally, measurements of skin absorption and flux should be specific to the parent chemical. This is not always possible. For reactive challenge chemicals, there may be complex skin interactions and degradation. In these cases, more sophisticated techniques such as GC-MS, or integrative techniques, such as radioactivity monitoring, may be used [45].

Implications for Skin Decontamination in HAZMAT Incidents

One underlying uncertainty is whether there has been enough penetration through skin to induce systemic effects in the short or long term. Therefore, the experimental design allowed for an understanding of what remains on skin, the amount within the epidermis and the proportion that has passed through the epidermis. These chemical processes will be modified by clothing, sunscreen, moisture and temperature. Supplementary fabric off-gassing experiments were also conducted under variable conditions. Knowledge of the independent and combined interactions with the chemical, allows for selective interventions that are cost-effective. This knowledge can be integrated into decision-making tools, e.g., a decision to remove clothing or not remove clothing once direct exposure has ceased.

In the case of ammonia (up to 2000 ppm, and exposure for short durations), the results suggest that the barrier function of unabraded skin is supplemented by clothing and oil-based sunscreen. However, wet and or thicker clothing may act as a reservoir for secondary exposure. In general removal of heavy and/or wet clothing that may have been worn at the time of exposure is recommended. Otherwise our data do not support the need for onsite decontamination of nonsymptomatic potentially exposed individuals.

For someone wearing a cotton shirt and exposed to ammonia gas, a decision not to remove the shirt may be justifiable. In this study, the observed skin flux of toxic gas in the tested range seems too low to affect normal pH or circulating levels of ammonium ion. However, evidence of some absorption into skin is demonstrated. Effects were noted for the influence of clothing and other barriers (oil-based sunscreen) and these have remedies in terms of decision-making in HAZMAT incidents. There appears to be no other literature to demonstrate a significant effect in terms of percutaneous penetration for ammonia gas at the concentrations tested. Based on findings observed for different concentrations of ammonia, environmental conditions, and clothing parameters a set of practical guidelines can be derived for emergency responders. These are diagrammatically represented (Fig. 9.2) as actions corresponding to different concentrations (similar diagrams are available for all studied chemicals). By changing the current approach, a focus can be placed on those individuals/groups requiring assistance, and can minimize the number of people requiring decontamination thereby reducing logistical and resource burdens on emergency services. Actions are based on gas exposures only to unabraded skin, and in the absence of reports or visual evidence of signs/symptoms.

The results suggest that exposures to concentrations below 500 ppm of chlorine for less than 30 min exposure, and 800 ppm of hydrogen cyanide do not warrant skin decontamination, but that removal of clothing and ventilation is sufficient. Concentrations of chlorine above 500 ppm and hydrogen cyanide above 800 ppm require consideration and treatment on a case by case basis. These data provide a basis for rational decision-making by first responders dealing with potential casualties in the event of a chemical release incident.

Based on the outcomes of the acid gas chemicals at the IDLH and LC_{Lo} concentrations and based on consensus that there is absence of reports/visual evidence for signs/symptoms, removal of clothing and skin decontamination is not essential. The hazard of hydrogen chloride and hydrogen sulfide at the LC_{Lo} concentration for 30 min is predominantly a respiratory concern therefore natural ventilation is always beneficial.

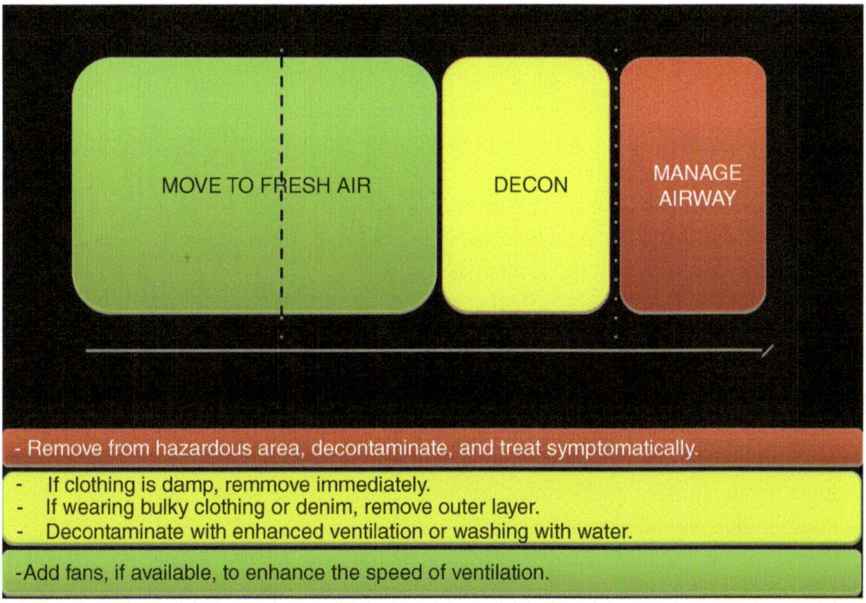

Fig. 9.2 Suggested risk-based approach for decontamination decision-making for ammonia release incidents.

Overall, our results may challenge the current dogma requiring mass personal decontamination by strip and shower for two of the three tested fumigants (sulfuryl fluoride and phosphine) up to LCLo concentrations for up to 30 min exposures (for undamaged skin). The removal of bulky outer layer of clothing. (e.g., denim) to minimize secondary exposure, and ventilation is sufficient. In contrast, dermal absorption and penetration outcomes for methyl bromide, along with relevant published exposure studies, endorse the continued adoption of personal decontamination by strip and shower.

The in vitro human skin absorption profile for sulfur dioxide at LC_{Lo} and IDLH concentrations (3000 ppm and 100 ppm, respectively) demonstrates inconsequential absorption and penetration of the gas via the dermal route. The influence of temperature and relative humidity on skin absorption and penetration was negligible. The application of heavier fabric had some influence on absorption, marginally increasing absorption for 20 + min exposures (~3 mg/L), and ventilation did not reduce.

In conclusion, we describe here an in vitro testing protocol suitable for toxic gases and short-term exposure scenarios typical of HAZMAT incidents. The data gathered may be useful for risk-based decision-making by first responders, particularly with regard to skin decontamination [5, 14, 18, 19]. Mass decontamination is established when large numbers of people need to be decontaminated at the scene of a HAZMAT emergency. The general goal is to provide the greatest good to the greatest number of people in the shortest amount of time [46]. Mass decontamination is a gross decontamination process that typically relies on the use of water or soap and water solutions to flush the majority of the contaminant from individuals. Removing clothing is also an initial form of decontamination, and reportedly removes up to 90% of the contaminant [1]. Once clothing has been removed, flushing a victim with a low pressure/high volume of water will remove additional amounts of the contaminant.

In practice, rather than use an unwieldy mass approach to all potentially contaminated individuals during a HAZMAT incident, the emergency services may use a triage approach in which those identified as having relatively low exposures, without significant risk of adverse effects, may be advised to shower and change clothing at home, whereas those in need of expert support may be prioritized for decontamination at the scene. To make decisions during this triage phase, emergency responders must have information regarding the likely levels of exposure, the potential for dermal contact and uptake and the likely effects arising from that exposure. They will be then able to use this information to exclude lightly exposed individuals from further processing, as well as advising some individuals about managing their own decontamination.

References

1. Levitin HW, Siegelson HJ, Dickinson S, Halpern P, Haraguchi Y, Nocera A, Turineck D. Decontamination of mass casualties—re-evaluating existing dogma. Prehosp Disaster Med. 2003;18(3):200–7.
2. Kirk MA, Deaton ML. Bringing order out of chaos: effective strategies for medical response to mass chemical exposure. Emerg Med Clin North Am. 2007;25(2):527–48.
3. Okumura T, Suzuki K, Fukuda A, et al. The Tokyo subway sarin attack: disaster management, Part 2: hospital response. Acad Emerg Med. 1998;5:618–24.
4. Edwards J, Pisaniello D, Barton R, et al. Hazardous materials emergency incidents in South Australia, 1997–2000. Appl Env Sci Public Health. 2003;1:63–7.
5. Gaskin S, Pisaniello D, Edwards JW, Bromwich D, Reed S, Logan M, Baxter C. Application of skin contamination studies of ammonia gas for management of hazardous material incidents. J Hazard Mater. 2013a;252:338–46.
6. Baxter C. Skin Decontamination, Presentation to the Executive Committee of the Memorandum of Understanding Concerning Combating Terrorism Research and Development between the Depart of Defense of the United States of America and the Department of Defence of Australia. 2008.
7. Houston M, Hendrickson R. Decontamination. Crit Care Clin. 2005;ll:653–72.
8. Makarovsky I, Markel G, Dushnitsky T, Eisenkraft A. Ammonia – when something smells wrong. Isr Med Assocl J. 2008;10:537–43.
9. Agency for Toxic Substances and Disease Registry. Hazardous substances emergency events surveillance. Annual Report. Atlanta, GA; 2007.
10. Feldman R. Chemical agent simulant release from clothing following vapor exposure. Acad Emerg Med. 2010;17:221–4.
11. Markel, G., Krivoy, A., Rotman, E. et al. 2008. Medical management of toxicological mass casualty events. 10, pp. 761–766.
12. Bronaugh RL, Congdon ER, Scheuplein RJ. The effect of cosmetic vehicles on the penetration of *N*-Nitrosodiethanolamine through excised human skin. J Invest Dermatol. 1981;76(2):94–6.

13. Pont AR, Charron AR, Brand RM. Active ingredients in sunscreens act as topical penetration enhancers for the herbicide 2,4-dichlorophenoxyacetic acid. Toxicol Appl Pharmacol. 2004;195:348–54.
14. Gaskin S, Pisaniello D, Edwards JW, Bromwich D, Reed S, Logan M, Baxter C. Chlorine and hydrogen cyanide gas interactions with human skin: in vitro studies to inform skin permeation and decontamination in HAZMAT incidents. J Hazard Mater. 2013b;262:759–65.
15. Loretz LJ, et al. Exposure data for cosmetic products: facial cleanser, hair conditioner, and eye shadow. Food Chem Toxicol. 2008;46:1516–24.
16. Loretz LJ, et al. Exposure data for cosmetic products: lipstick, body lotion, and face cream. Food Chem Toxicol. 2005;43:279–91.
17. Bonnist EY, Gorce JP, Mackay C, Pendlington RU, Pudney PD. Measuring the penetration of a skin sensitizer and its delivery vehicles simultaneously with confocal Raman spectroscopy. Skin Pharmacol Physiol. 2011;24(5):274–83.
18. Organization for Economic Co-operation and Development (OECD) 2004. Guidance document for the conduct of skin absorption studies. OECD series on testing and assessment. Number 28. Joint meeting of the chemicals committee and the working party on chemicals, pesticides and biotechnology.
19. Gaskin S, Pisaniello D, Edwards JW, Bromwich D, Reed S, Logan M, Baxter C. In-vitro methods for testing dermal absorption and penetration of toxic gases. Toxicol Mech Methods. 2014;24(1):70–2.
20. Gaskin S, Heath L, Pisaniello D, Evans R, Edwards JW, Logan M, Baxter C. Hydrogen sulphide and phosphine interactions with human skin in vitro application to hazardous material incident decision making for skin decontamination. Toxicol Ind Health. 2016:1–8.
21. Byford T. Environmental health criteria 235: dermal absorption. Int J Environ Stud. 2009;66:662–3.
22. Bronaugh RL, Stewart RF, Simon M. Methods for in vitro percutaneous absorption studies VII: use of excised human skin. J Pharm Sci. 1986;75(11):1094–7.
23. Davies DJ, Ward RJ, Heylings JR. Multi-species assessment of electrical resistance as a skin integrity marker for in vitro percutaneous absorption studies. Toxicol In Vitro. 2004;18(3):351–8.
24. Diembeck W, Beck H, Benech-Kieffer F, Courtellemont P, Dupuis J, Lovell W, Paye M, Spengler J, Steiling W. Test guidelines for in vitro assessment of dermal absorption and percutaneous penetration of cosmetic ingredients. Food Chem Toxicol. 1999;37(2):191–205.
25. Lawrence JN. Electrical resistance and tritiated water permeability as indicators of barrier integrity of in vitro human skin. Toxicol In Vitro. 1997;11(3):241–9.
26. Fasano WJ, Hinderliter PM. The Tinsley LCR Databridge model 6401 and electrical impedance measurements to evaluate skin integrity in vitro. Toxicol In Vitro. 2004;18(5):725–9.
27. Pisaniello D. The generation of test atmospheres for occupational hygiene laboratory evaluation of organic vapor monitoring devices. Report prepared for the Occupational Health and Radiation Control Branch, South Australian Health Commission. 1988. Available online: www.adelaide.edu.au/oeh/research/testatmon88.pdf.
28. Council of Australian Governments List of Security Sensitive Materials. Available online: https://www.nationalsecurity.gov.au/ChemicalSecurity/Pages/default.aspx.
29. UK Home Office Poisons and Precursors Lists. Available online: https://www.gov.uk/government/consultations/precursors-and-poisons-consultations.
30. US Department of Homeland Security. Chemicals of Interest List. Available online: https://www.dhs.gov/publication/cfats-coi-list.
31. Agency for Toxic Substances and Disease Registry (ATSDR). Toxicological profile for sulfur dioxide. Atlanta: U.S. Department of Health and Human Services, Public Health Service; 1998.
32. Gunnison AF, Jacobsen DW, Schwartz HJ. Sulfite hypersensitivity. A critical review. CRC Crit Rev Toxicol. 1987;17(3):185–214.
33. Du Z, Meng Z. Effects of derivatives of sulfur dioxide on transient outward potassium currents in acutely isolated hippocampal neurons. Food Chem Toxicol. 2004;42(8):1211.

34. Dugard P. The absorption of cyanide through human skin in vitro from solutions of sodium cyanide and gaseous HCN. In: Marrs T, Ballantyne B, editors. Clinical and experimental toxicology of cyanides. Bristol: John Wright; 1987. p. 127–37.
35. Walton C, Witherspoon M. Skin absorption of certain gases. J Pharmacol Exp Ther. 1925;26:315–24.
36. Fairley A, Linton E, Wild F. The absorption of hydrocyanic acid vapour through the skin: with notes on other matters relating to acute cyanide poisoning. J Hyg. 1934;34:283–94.
37. Schutze W. Deleterious action through the skin of poisonous gases at high concentrations (carbon monoxide, hydrogen sulfide, hydrocyanic acid, and aniline). Arch Hygiene. 1927;98:70.
38. Eberlein-Konig B, Przybilla B, Kuhnel P, et al. Influence of airborne nitrogen dioxide or formaldehyde on parameters of skin function and cellular activation in patients with atopic eczema and control subjects. J Allergy Clin Immunol. 1998;101:141–3.
39. Agency for Toxic Substances and Disease Registry (ATSDR). Toxicological profile for Bromomethane. Atlanta: US Public Health Service; 1992.
40. Jordi AU. Absorption of methyl bromide through the intact skin; a report of one fatal and two non-fatal cases. J Aviat Med. 1953;24(6):536–9.
41. Hezemans-Boer M, Toonstra J, Meulenbelt J, Zwaveling JH, Sangster B, van Vloten WA. Skin lesions due to exposure to methyl bromide. Arch Dermatol. 1988;124(6):917–21.
42. American Conference of Governmental Industrial Hygienists (ACGIH), 2011. Documentation of the Threshold Limit Values and Biological Exposure Indices, 7th Edition, 2011 Supplement, Document number 0100DocS11, ACGIH.
43. US EPA. Sulfuryl Fluoride (Vikane®) RIisk Characterisation Document,Volume II, Exposure Assessment, Worker Health and Safety Branch, Department of Pesticide Regulation California Environmental Protection Agency.
44. American Public Health Association (APHA). Standard methods for the examination of water and wasterwater 4110B: determination of anions by ion chromatography. 18th ed. Washington, DC: APHA; 1992.
45. te Brake L, Gaskin S, Pisaniello D, Edwards J, Bromwich D, Reed S, Scheepers P. Effects of street clothing, sunscreen, and temperature on skin absorption of organophosphate pesticides–a review and case study of diazinon. J Health Safety Res Pract. 2012;4:10–8.
46. Noll GG, Hildebrand MS, Rudner G, Schnepp R. Hazardous materials: managing the incident: New York, USA: Jones & Bartlett Publishers; 2012.

Chapter 10
Binding Affinity and Decontamination of Dermal Decontamination Gel (DDGel) to Model Chemical Warfare Agent (CWA) Simulants

Yachao Cao, Akram Elmahdy, Hanjiang Zhu, Xiaoying Hui, and Howard I. Maibach

Introduction

Chemical absorption into and through skin is important in dermato-pharmacology and dermato-toxicology. Stratum corneum (SC), the outermost skin layer, constitutes a main rate-limiting barrier to transport of most chemicals across the skin [11, 29, 30, 38]. The chemicals first partition into the SC before penetrating the remaining epidermal layers, dermis, and vascular system to gain access to system circulation. Chemical partitioning proceeds much faster than complete diffusion through whole SC, and the partitioning process quickly reaches equilibrium [31]. In partitioning, chemicals may bind to components of the SC and be retained by SC, which serves as a reservoir [44]. Therefore, understanding the processes behind chemical partitioning into the SC is essential to gaining insight into the barrier properties of the SC and chemical transport across skin.

Human SC has been used as an in vitro model to explore percutaneous absorption and local or systemic risks associated with dermal exposure to toxic chemicals [24, 32]. Driven by applications in transdermal drug delivery and safety assessment, there has been a continuous interest in revealing a chemical's partition and binding to the SC. Studies on chemical partitioning into SC lipids were broadly published [2, 5, 14, 18, 21, 24]. A good correlation exists between overall partitioning of

Yachao Cao and Akram Elmahdy are contributed equally to this work.

Y. Cao · A. Elmahdy · H. I. Maibach (✉) · H. Zhu · X. Hui
Department of Dermatology, University of California San Francisco, San Francisco, CA, USA
e-mail: Howard.Maibach@ucsf.edu

H. Zhu, H. I. Maibach (eds.), *Skin Decontamination*,
https://doi.org/10.1007/978-3-030-24009-7_10

chemicals into SC and chemical partitioning into SC lipids. But evidence shows that chemicals diffuse into SC corneocytes and also bind to SC proteins [1, 2, 19, 25]. A two-phase partitioning model has been proposed for analysis of the heterogeneous structure of the SC [2, 22, 25].

Penetrant's binding to SC components can lead to differences in the effective and true diffusion and partition coefficients, a retardation of the absorption process, and a sustained presence of the bound compound. Therefore, accurate estimates of binding coefficients become essential to improve understanding of binding mechanisms to the major stratum corneum components. Stratum corneum study shows the relative role of lipids and proteins and thus provides a mechanistic insight into the relationship between the SC lipids and proteins as well as dermal penetration, absorption prevention, and skin decontamination.

An effective skin decontaminant should: (i) decrease the quantity of contaminant absorbed into skin (from stratum corneum to receptor fluid), (ii) significantly delay absorption time (if overall absorption could not be significantly decreased (holding), and/or (iii) have an ability to degrade the contaminant present on and/or in the skin. The nonabsorbed fraction (total quantity of chemical present on the skin surface) is the fraction considered as the removable amount from the skin surface. On the other hand, the absorbed fraction (i.e., sum of the quantities from the stratum corneum to receptor fluid) is the quantity of chemical which can potentially move into the blood. This is why, for each decontamination experiment, quantities of chemical in the nonabsorbed fraction and in the absorbed fraction have been compared.

Chemical weapons pose significant threats to society. In response to these threats, scientists have long searched for environmentally benign approaches to their decontamination. Knowledge to decontaminate chemical warfare agents (CWAs) such as distilled mustard, lewisite, tabun, sarin, soman, and VX is thus important. However, it is often necessary to conduct studies examining chemical agent behavior using simulants due to the toxicity of the agents and usage restrictions [4]. An ideal chemical agent simulant would mimic all relevant chemical and physical properties of the agent without its associated toxicological properties. Although many chemicals have been used as simulants, no individual compound is perfect because a single simulant cannot satisfactorily represent all properties of a given CWA. Thus, many chemicals have been used as simulants, depending on the physical–chemical properties of interest. Mustard gas (HD) simulates include DEA, DMA, CEMS, CEPS; yet TMP and DES are used as G-agents and VX simulants, respectively. The volatility of CWAs and their simulants are different. HD and G agents have high volatility and VX has a relatively low volatility. There are no experimental volatility data for these simulants; most are volatile; TMP is the most volatile [9, 16, 33, 36].

A successful skin decontamination strategy, for example, should not only remove CWAs from the skin surface, but also back-extract chemicals from the SC reservoir and reduce further penetration and systemic absorption. A dermal decontamination gel (DDGel) has shown excellent decontamination efficiency in removing, and more importantly, back-extracting topically applied chemicals such as chemical warfare simulants and other model chemicals.

Here, we use human stratum corneum as an in vitro model to assess relationship between physicochemical properties of simulants and their perspective partition mechanisms that govern partitioning between (a) the SC and water and (b) DDGel and water. Then we determined whether or not the partition coefficient of $PC_{DDGel/w}$ correlated to $PC_{sc/w}$ and/or to $PC_{o/w}$. These values were further correlated with SC protein and SC lipid binding rates, desorption rates (off-rates), and skin decontamination efficiencies of those simulants. Also, skin decontamination experiments were performed to test decontamination efficacy of DDGel with these chemicals using in vitro human skin models. Those studies serve to verify the theoretical estimation of the relationship between chemical penetration and SC domains of lipid, protein, and water [41].

Materials and Methods

Test Chemicals and Reagents

Radiochemical purities of all carbon-^{14} labeled chemicals (hot) were greater than 95%. [C^{14}]-trimethyl phosphate (TMP) (50 mCi/mmol), [C^{14}]-dimethyl adipate (DMA) (50 mCi/mmol), [C^{14}]-2-chloroethyl methyl sulfide (CEMS) (55 mCi/mmol), [C^{14}]-diethyl adipate (DEA) (50 mCi/mmol), [C^{14}]-chloroethyl phenyl sulfide (CEPS) (50 mCi/mmol), and [C^{14}]-diethyl sebacate (DES) (100 mCi/mmol) were custom synthesized by American Radiolabeled Chemicals, Inc. (St. Louis, MO, USA). Reagent grade ethanol was purchased from Fisher Scientific (Pittsburg, PA, USA). Soluene-350® tissue solubilizer and ULTIMA GOLD™ scintillation cocktails were manufactured by PerkinElmer Life and Analytical Sciences (Boston, MA, USA). Nonradiolabeled (cold) trimethyl phosphate, dimethyl adipate, 2-chloroethyl methyl sulfide, diethyl adipate, chloroethyl phenyl sulfide, and diethyl sebacate were obtained from American Radiolabeled Chemicals, Inc. (St. Louis, MO, USA). Dosing solutions were prepared in ethanol with radiolabeled compounds and 20 mg/ml of nonradiolabeled chemicals to achieve 0.05 m/Ci/ml specific radioactivity. Receptor fluid was 0.01mole/liter phosphate-buffered saline (PBS) aqueous solution containing 6% (v/v) polyethylene glycol prepared using PBS tablets obtained from Diagnostic BioSystems (Pleasanton, CA, USA) and polyethylene glycol from Sigma-Aldrich (St. Louis, MO, USA).

Preparation of DDGel

DDGel is a gel-quickly-dried-film formulation prepared with polymers (Kollidon SR, lutrol, and carboxymethyl cellulose), absorbent clay (Fuller's earth and bentonite), and solvents (ethanol and water). Weight Kollidon SR (3 g), lutrol (1 g), carboxymethyl cellulose (0.3 g), Fuller's earth (2.5 g), and bentonite (0.5 g) were dissolved with 2 ml of water and 10 ml of ethanol and mixed.

Preparation of Intact Stratum Corneum Membranes and DDGel Sheets for Chemical Binding Experiments

Skin samples were obtained from the thigh of adult human cadavers at the Pathology Department of the University of California, San Francisco School of Medicine. Skin samples at a target thickness of 400 μm were prepared using a Padgett Electrodermatome (Padgett Instruments, Inc., Kansas City, MO, USA), and skin samples were stored at 4 °C until use. Skin sample physical conditions were examined visually to exclude samples with surface damage or abnormal appearance. Skin samples were processed to obtain SC membranes by employing a modified method [43]. After submerging the skin sample in 60 °C water for 1 min, the epidermis was carefully peeled from dermis and placed on a cotton pad soaked with 0.5% (wt/wt) trypsin solution with the dermal side down at 37 °C for 15 to 24 hrs during skin digestion. The pH of the trypsin solution was adjusted to 8.0–8.6 with 5% (wt/wt) sodium bicarbonate. When digestion was completed, SC was thoroughly washed thrice with water and then dried under vacuum overnight at room temperature. Prepared SC membranes were stored at room temperature until use (less than 6 months). Stratum corneum thickness was measured by digital caliper (Marathon Watch Company Ltd., Ontario, CA) before experiments.

DDGels were prepared as a film on glass, then punched into discs of the same size (diameter = 10 mm). Weights of DDGel disc sheets were measured by analytical balances (Sartorius AG, Goettingen, Germany).

Stratum Corneum and DDGel Chemical Binding Experimental Procedures

Five samples were utilized per group for binding assay. Preprepared stratum corneum sheets and DDGel sheet samples were accurately weighed and then placed in dialysis tubing. Dialysis system has two parts: dialysis tubing and dialysate section (Fig. 10.1). SC/DDGel sheets and 50 μl of each of the selected test chemicals (1% v/v) were placed in dialysis tubing and 350 μl PBS (0.01 M, PH 7.0) were added in dialysate section. The dialysis system was incubated with horizontal shaking and allowed to equilibrate at 37 °C for 24 hrs. Weight of skin sample, volume, and initial concentration of test chemical solutions were chosen based on the solute amount present in the incubation system to ensure that a significant depletion of solute would not occur after equilibration. Initial concentration of the solute in solution was selected to determine whether the uptake by SC and DDGel can be described by a constant partition coefficient and is independent of solute concentration [3, 32, 35].

Stratum corneum water uptake capacity was calculated by the increase of the post-equilibrium sample weight.

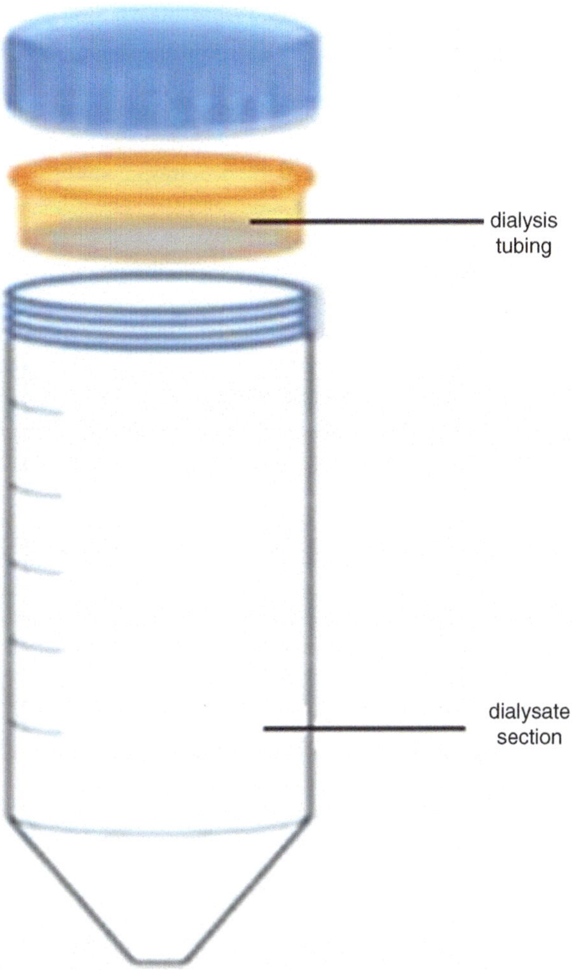

Fig. 10.1 Dialysis system for binding test. This shows the two-part dialysis system

In Vitro Skin Decontamination Efficacy

Adult human cadaver skin samples were stored at −20 °C. On the day of experiment, skin samples were thawed at room temperature and the skin was cut into 6.25 cm^2 circular pieces. Full-thickness unclipped skin was used. Thickness was measured with a digital caliper (Marathon watch company Ltd., Richmond Hill, Ontario, CA). Human skin membrane thicknesses were 300–500 μm. Skin discs were mounted onto Flow-Through diffusion cells and maintained at 37 °C in a water bath in order to obtain a skin surface temperature of 33–34 °C as observed in vivo in humans. Skin samples were divided into groups of six biological replicates from three donors (69, 71, 72 years, White, male). Skin area available for chemical diffusion was 1 cm^2. After 30 min equilibration with receptor fluid, skin integrity was assessed by measuring the Trans-Epidermal Water Loss (TEWL) using a Vapometer (Delfin Technologies, Ltd. Kuopio, Finland) before any drug or chemical dosing. Following the OECD guidelines [23], only skin with TEWL values ranging between 3 and 10 g/h/m were used in the penetration studies. This permeability is comparable to a fresh human skin specimen [10]. The donor compartment of the diffusion cell apparatus remained open during the experiment. An aliquot of 10 μL of a simulant was evenly applied to the center of the unclipped human skin surface, resulting in an applied surface dose of 1 mg/cm^2 [17]. Decontamination procedures were performed at 0.5 hrs post chemical dosing following the procedure as described: An aliquot of 150 mg of DDGel was massaged onto the surface in a circular motion of each skin disc for 5 seconds with a glass rod. DDGel was then peeled off from skin surface after 30 mins from DDGel deposition time. The skin surface was softly wiped one time with a dry cotton ball to remove the residual DDGel. Simulants permeation assay was continued for up to 24 hrs post chemical dosing to ascertain the impact of the skin decontamination process on dermal penetration and percutaneous absorption. Skin samples without any decontamination were used as controls. Receptor fluid (RF) was collected at 30 min, 1 hr, and then every 2 hrs thereafter. RF samples were handled according to established procedures (mixed with liquid scintillation cocktail at volume ratio of 1:100). At the end of the experiment, skin discs were removed from the diffusion cells. The surface of control skin samples was gently wiped two times with a dry cotton ball to recover the fraction of chemical remaining on the skin surface. Stratum corneum was removed by tape stripping for ten times using D-Squame standard sampling disc (Cuderm). The viable epidermis was separated from dermis by heat treatment (in 60 °C water for 45 sec) [28]. Dermis and viable epidermis were cut into small pieces and placed individually into vials with 2 mL of Soluene 350 Tissue Solubilizer (PekinElmer Life and Analytical Sciences, Boston, MA, USA) for total tissue digestion. The test chemical was extracted overnight at room temperature without shaking.

One-hour in vitro skin penetration experiment of CEPS was performed. Skin samples were divided into groups of three biological replicates from one donor (80 years, White, male). The experiment method was the same as for the 24 hrs decontamination experiment. After 30 min exposure, DDGel was applied and then wiped before gel sheet formation (in 5 mins) to avoid DDGel's SC peeling effect so that the back-extracting effect can be demonstrated. RF was collected every 5 mins.

Radioactivity Measurements

Collected test samples were measured for radioactivity with a PerkinElmer Tri-Carb 2900TR liquid scintillation spectrometer (PerkinElmer Life and Analytical Sciences, Inc., Waltham, MA, USA), which was calibrated with background control scintillation cocktail standards.

SC and DDGel samples were mixed with scintillation cocktails for radioactivity quantitation. After binding, the vehicle fluid and surface washes were mixed with scintillation cocktails (Ecolite (+)) for assay. Control and test sample scintillation counts were acquired into, and analyzed by, a computer program which comes with the liquid scintillation spectrometer to generate reportable data.

All in vitro experiments samples were collected and mixed with scintillation cocktail for radioactivity quantitation. Radioactivities in cotton ball and scintillation cocktails were measured.

Accuracy and reliability of liquid scintillation spectrometry were ensured weekly by calibration by running its manufacturer-provided internal quench and calibration standards. Liquid scintillation spectrometer is an automatically calibrated system. Before samples are counted, the system will be normalized and calibrated. Normalization, calibration, and Instrument Performance Assessment (IPA) occurs automatically by leaving the Self Normalization and Calibration (SNC) and IPA cassette (containing the ^{14}C calibration standard, unquenched Tritium standard, and background standard) on the instrument counting deck at all times.

Data Analysis and Regression

1. Partition coefficients of each test chemical between SC and water or between DDGel and water were measured following the method of Hui et al. [13], after a 24-hour incubation period at 37 °C to reach equilibrium. Partition coefficient (PC) of a test chemical between SC and water was calculated as:

$$\mathrm{PC}(\mathrm{SC}/\mathrm{w}) = \frac{\mu Ci(\mathrm{SC})}{\mathrm{mg}(\mathrm{SC})} \div \frac{\mu Ci(\mathrm{i}) - \mu Ci(\mathrm{SC})}{\mathrm{mg}(\mathrm{water})} \tag{10.1}$$

where μCi(i) is the initial chemical radioactivity in vehicle (water), μCi(SC) is the amount (μCi) of chemical absorbed by 10 mg of the SC (expressed in mg (SC in equation 10.1), and mg(water) is the amount (μCi) of chemical remaining in 50 mg of the water post removal of the SC sheet. Since the chemical amount in the SC or in water is proportional to radioactivity counts, the amount of chemical partitioned into the SC equaled the chemical amount calculated from the decrease in the chemical concentration in the vehicle (water).

Similarly, to determine the partition coefficient of DDGel/water, the above formula was applied with μCi (DDGel) and/or mg (DDGel) replacing the corresponding SC parameters as illustrated in Eq. (10.2):

$$\mathrm{PC}(\mathrm{DDGel}/\mathrm{w}) = \frac{\mu Ci(\mathrm{DDGel})}{\mathrm{mg}(\mathrm{DDGel})} \div \frac{\mu Ci(\mathrm{i}) - \mu Ci(\mathrm{DDGel})}{\mathrm{mg}(\mathrm{water})} \tag{10.2}$$

2. Efficacy of a skin decontaminant

Mass balance calculations were performed to ensure data accuracy. Total chemical amount in a given tissue was calculated based on the total sample volume or weight and chemical concentration in that sample. To enhance and ensure best data comparability across treatments (control vs DDGel) and across simulants, the assayed decontamination and absorption data were normalized by total recovery for each diffusion cell and then statistically analyzed and compared.

Amounts of chemical were expressed as percent of dose recovered from receptor fluid, skin surface, stratum corneum, viable epidermis, and dermis. Means of all data are given along with corresponding standard deviations (S.D., $n = 6$ replicates). A normality test (Kolmogorov–Smirnov) was conducted on all data acquired from the in vitro studies: the data were found not normally distributed (non-Gaussian). Because the quantities of chemical in each fraction in a given sample type (receptor fluid, skin surface, stratum corneum, viable epidermis, dermis, total, absorbed fraction, or nonabsorbed fraction) do not follow a normal distribution and variances were not equal, a Student's t-test ($P < 0.05$) was applied to check if decontaminant of DDGel system significantly reduced the chemical amounts in various compartments of the skin and the perfused (mimics the blood in systemic circulation) when compared to the control.

Results

Binding Affinity of SC and DDGel

Figure 10.2 shows partitioning values of the SC and DDGel, expressed as log $P_{sc/w}$ and log $P_{DDGel/w}$, for six CWA simulants. The corresponding data points of log $P_{sc/w}$ and log $P_{DDGel/w}$ are closely colocated at the corresponding log $P_{o/w}$(octanol/water) value of a simulant, which is true across a wide range of log $P_{o/w}$ values representing a diversified group of simulants (see Table 10.1 below). This correlation may explain why DDGel can remove simulants from the skin surface and much more importantly, may back-extract them at least from the SC along with a possibility of removal of the loss surface SC layer. DDGel properties may be similar with properties of the SC in terms of chemical partitioning and may even be more active along with other mechanisms in terms of binding affinity or binding rate. It needs more investigation. DDGel formulation has a similar or higher chemical binding affinity when compared to SC. This finding seems to strongly suggest an opportunity to develop this DDGel formulation into a decontamination platform for much more efficient skin decontamination in military and civilian applications.

Additionally, the data suggest that a simulant's log $P_{sc/w}$ and log $P_{DDGel/w}$ will likely remain relatively consistent within a wide range of log $P_{o/w}$ from −1 to 1.6 (Fig. 10.2), suggesting that the partitioning into DDGel or into the SC are independent of their lipophilicity values of those more water-soluble penetrants. Therefore,

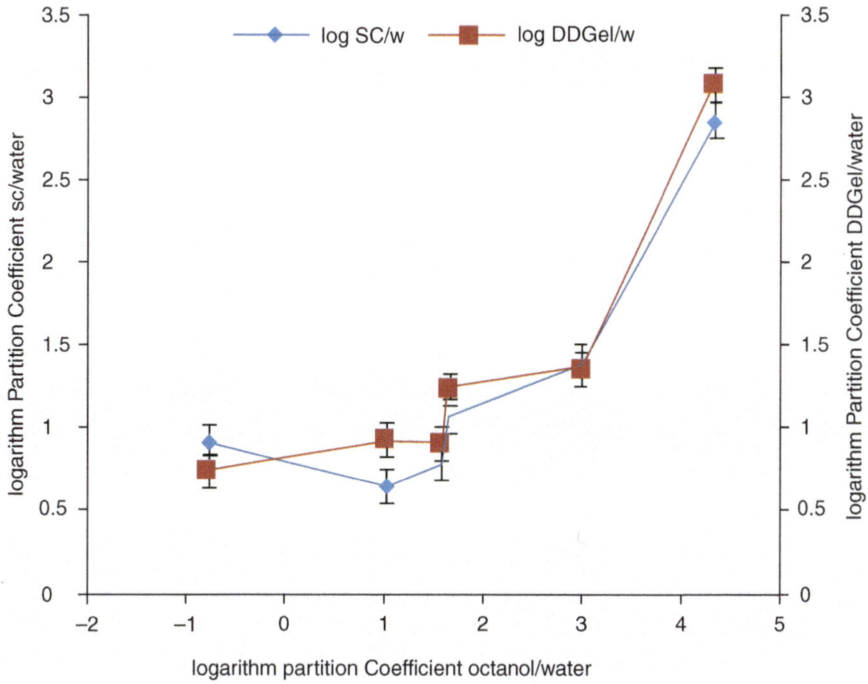

Fig. 10.2 Correlation of log $P_{o/w}$, log $Psc_{/w}$, and log $P_{DDGel/w}$ of six CWA simulants. Data of partition coefficients ($PC_{SC/w}$ and $PC_{DDGel/w}$) of each chemical were the results at equilibrium after a 24-hr incubation. Each logarithm partition coefficient data point in Fig. 10.2 (Log $P_{SC/w}$ or Log $P_{DDGel/w}$) represents the mean ± S.D. (n = 5) of a CWA simulant tested. The corresponding data points of log $P_{sc/w}$ and log $P_{DDGel/w}$ are closely colocated at the corresponding log $P_{o/w}$ (octanol/water) value of a CWA simulant

Table 10.1 Molecular weight (MW), hydrogen-bond (donor and acceptor) counts, log Po/w, log Psc/w, and log PDDGel/w of six CWA simulants tested

		Hydrogen bond		Logarithm partition coefficient				
		Donor	Acceptor	Oct/w	SC/w		DDGel/w	
CWA simulants	MW				Mean	S.D.	Mean	S.D.
Trimethyl phosphate (TMP)	140.07	0	4	−0.78	0.92	0.12	0.74	0.01
Dimethyl adipate (DMA)	174.19	0	4	1.03	0.65	0.16	0.93	0.05
2-Chloroethyl methyl sulfide (CEMS)	110.61	0	1	1.59	0.78	0.08	0.9	0.07
Diethyl adipate (DEA)	202.25	0	4	1.67	1.07	0.05	1.23	0.12
Chlorethyl phenyl sulfide (CEPS)	172.67	0	1	3.01	1.4	0.08	1.35	0.1
Diethyl sebacate (DES)	258.35	0	4	4.33	2.86	0.13	3.08	0.06

Partition coefficient (for $PC_{SC/w}$ or $PC_{DDGel/w}$) values of the CWA simulants started to be sensitive to their lipophilicity, only when the chemicals approach a threshold of organic solvent (very lipophilic) over water partitioning (e.g., Log Ko/w above 3)

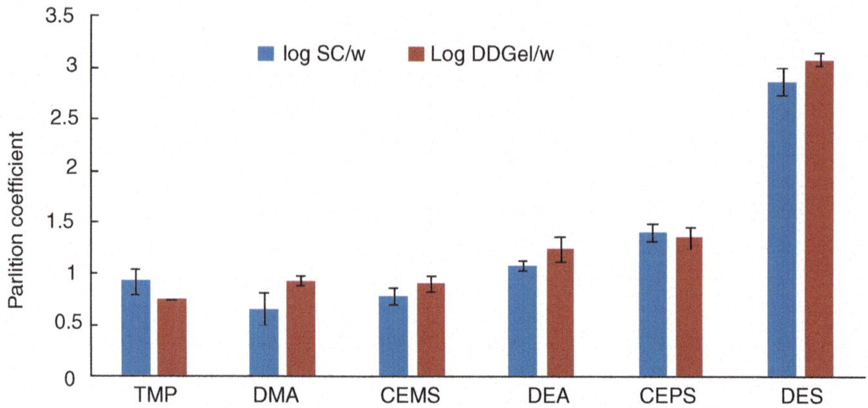

Fig. 10.3 Logarithm partition coefficients of six CWA simulants. This shows partitioning values of the SC and DDGel, expressed as log $P_{sc/w}$ and log $P_{DDGel/w}$, for six CWA simulants. The corresponding data points of log $P_{sc/w}$ and log $P_{DDGel/w}$ are close to each other

little correlation of the partitioning into the SC or DDGel with log $P_{o/w}$ can be expected if the penetrants are less lipophilic.

The logarithm of partition coefficients of six CWA simulants are listed in Table 10.1 and Fig. 10.3.

As shown in Fig. 10.3 and Table 10.1, partition coefficient (for $PC_{SC/w}$ or $PC_{DDGel/w}$) values of the simulants started to be sensitive to their lipophilicity, only when the chemicals approach a threshold of organic solvent (very lipophilic) over water partitioning (e.g., Log Ko/w above 3). For more water-soluble chemicals (those with log ko/w < =3), partition coefficients show less correlation with lipophilicity, and decontamination efficiency of the DDGel is more independent of lipophilicity of a chemical, but if the chemical is very lipophilic with a Log Ko/w over 3, this relationship will likely change. Thus, two types of decontamination approaches were identified: those for lipophilic compounds where partitioning is proportional to their lipid-solubility, and those for hydrophilic compounds, where partitioning appears to be consistent within a certain range of high water solubility. This result demonstrates that the solubility limit of a penetrating compound in the SC is important in determining the degree of partitioning among various domains of the SC and the DDGel formulations. This reveals a mechanism of chemical partitioning and therefore, suggests a strategy to refine skin decontamination technologies.

3.2 In vitro skin decontamination efficacy. All direct assay amounts of simulants quantified in each membrane and subset of tissue/fluid samples are listed in Table 10.2 along with total recovery. Recovery-normalized data were used in plots in Fig. 10.4 to ensure a better data comparability across decontamination methods and simulants.

Figure 10.4 shows the amount of chemical quantified in each skin compartment of DES. Quantity recovered in each compartment for the DDGel can be compared and linked to the decrease in chemical penetration. Skin decontamination with

Table 10.2 DDGel efficacy of decontaminating six CWA simulants from human skin in vitro: Decontamination procedure was performed at 30 min post chemical dosing and the total chemical exposure time in the dermal absorption study was 24 hours. The non-normalized direct assay results are listed here and the values are presented as mean ± SD ($n = 6$)

(% Dose)	TMP		DMA		CEMS	
	Control	DDGel	Control	DDGel	Control	DDGel
Surface removed	7.11±0.92	61.15±1.21	0.17±0.11	85.67±5.85	0.57±0.07	75.91±2.97
Stratum corneum	1.44±0.17	0.75±0.31	0.14±0.06	0.05±0.00	0.27±0.03	0.17±0.05
Viable epidermis	1.03±0.12	0.10±0.08	0.61±0.04	0.15±0.05	0.84±0.01	0.71±0.13
Dermis	1.64±0.05	0.11±0.02	4.09±0.81	0.45±0.08	0.81±0.17	0.80±0.21
Receptor fluid	10.83±1.42	2.36±0.54	38.42±0.25	4.87±1.87	45.42±5.45	2.29±0.38
Total recovery	28.85±2.63	66.25±2.52	55.95±12.36	92.74±8.70	73.72±3.87	106.50±10.37
(%Dose)	DEA		CEPS		DES	
	Control	DDGel	Control	DDGel	Control	DDGel
Surface removed	3.85±0.77	53.53±14.10	31.63±3.38	89.89±0.69	25.24±1.91	76.58±16.55
Stratum corneum	4.14±0.11	0.42±0.08	4.56±0.73	0.24±0.15	9.83±0.65	0.73±0.13
Viable epidermis	0.92±0.25	0.11±0.13	1.86±0.43	0.16±0.04	5.04±3.09	0.28±0.01
Dermis	1.51±0.24	0.19±0.22	1.54±0.11	0.17±0.15	3.05±0.94	0.37±0.10
Receptor fluid	31.03±3.35	5.22±2.65	22.67±1.65	2.13±0.69	8.51±0.14	1.39±0.70
Total recovery	41.40±3.35	68.49±5.89	63.45±11.65	92.83±0.79	59.92±7.17	83.22±13.31

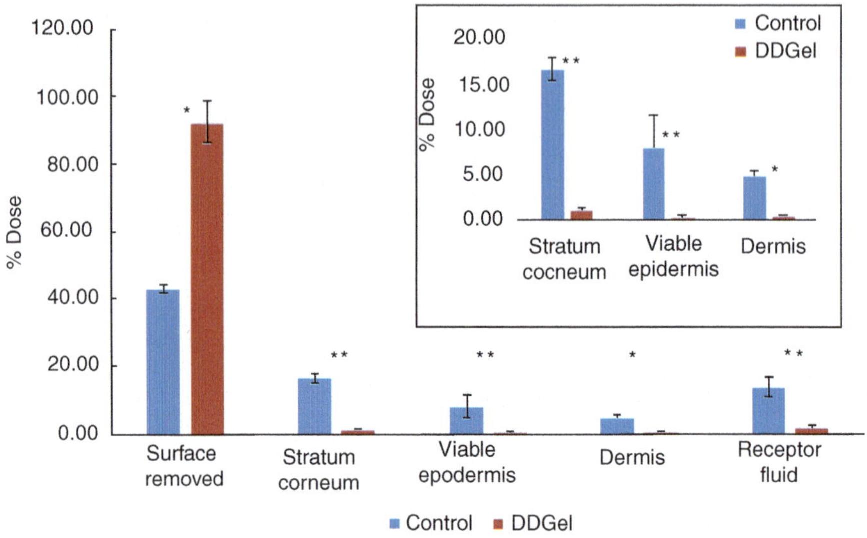

Fig. 10.4 In vitro skin decontamination efficacy of DDGel vs control (non-decontamination) for diethyl sebacate (DES). The % dose amounts of the chemical at 24-hr post chemical exposure were quantified in each sample, except for the RF data as the total chemical amounts in all the collected RF samples during the 24-hr absorption experiment. Surface removed amount including from the skin surface and back-extracting amount from the skin tissue. The direct assay % dose data (Table 10.2) are normalized by total recovery. Values were compared between control and DDGel decontamination groups using the Student's t-test: significant statistical differences are denoted by $*$ at $P < 0.05$ or $**$ at $P < 0.01$. This shows significantly reduced amounts of simulants after skin decontamination with DDGel products in the "skin surface," "Stratum corneum," "viable epidermis," "dermis," and "receptor fluid" compared to control

DDGel products significantly reduced amounts of simulants in the "skin surface" compared to the control.

[C^{14}]-labeled chemical amounts in DDGel, SC (tape strips), epidermis, dermis, and receptor fluid were measured to determine total recovery per mass balance approach (Table 10.2). Total applied dose recovery varied from 28.85% to 106.50% under various dosing and decontamination conditions. The reason for a generally lower and more variable recovery of the control groups may be attributed to volatility, loss during tissue processing, and adherence to apparatus glass components. The total recoveries from DDGel groups were all exceeding 50%. Percutaneous penetration was minimal after DDGel application on the skin surface as a mean of skin decontamination, indicating a much more effective decontamination using DDGel even 30 min after skin exposures to the simulants that have diversified physicochemistry spectrum. This is considered to be very exciting for military and civilian applications as a new platform of skin decontamination.

The amounts of % dose of chemicals removed by DDGel of TMP, DMA, CEMS, DEA, CEPS, and DES were determined to be 61.15, 85.67, 75.91, 53.53, 89.89, and 76.58, with corresponding dermal penetration (including SC, epidermis, dermis, and RF) values of 3.32, 5.52, 3.97, 5.94, 2.70, and 2.77, respectively. Compared to control group, the amount of dermal penetration of TMP, DMA, CEMS, DEA,

CEPS, and DES were decreased more than 45%. The data seem to confirm that the DDGel showed a superior efficiency of removing toxicants from exposed skin surface, SC, and skin tissues beneath as well as percutaneous absorption. Therefore, the local dermal and systemic organ risks from the toxic chemical skin exposures can be significantly reduced by DDGel.

Efficacy of skin decontamination was much higher for all simulants following the DDGel decontamination when compared to control (Table 10.2). Skin decontamination of six simulants by DDGel was more effective in reducing simulants from the epidermis and the dermis than the control. Percent of applied dose in the receptor fluid increased/cumulated with time for all simulants indicating continuous dermal absorption during the 24-hr study period.

From Fig. 10.4, the amounts of chemicals quantified in the SC after decontamination were low. For DEA, CEPS, and DES, the amounts of chemicals in SC decrease from 10%, 7%, and 16%, respectively, to less than 2% (Table 10.2). Total recovery calibrated data showed an even more pronounced efficiency of the DDGel to reduce chemical amount in the skin and in the RF. This means that DDGel can bind to chemicals which possess different hydrophilicities or lipophilicities and then remove the chemicals per the decon procedure. If the chemical agent is relatively water soluble with Log Ko/w of −1 to 3, for example, DDGgel is independent of the lipophilicities of the simulants and thus universally acts as a decontaminant effective for a range of chemicals. This result is consistent with the binding affinity test results. More importantly, DDGel has the ability to back-extract toxic chemicals at least from the SC along with a possibility of removal of the loss surface SC layer and thus reduce further penetration into other epidermal and dermal layers, therefore dramatically reducing dermal absorption into systemic circulation. A 1-hour penetration study of CEPS was performed to verify the back-extracting effect of DDGel. Figure 10.5 shows the amounts of CEPS quantified in each skin compartment. Result showed that the decontamination efficacy of DDGel before sheet formation is higher than soap-water wash as a control treatment. Compared to soap-water wash, chemical remained in SC is reduced from 2.77% to 0.72% (a fourfold reduction). This result suggests DDGel's back-extracting effect. This mechanism of action may deserve further study.

This study evaluated DDGel decontamination potential in removing CWA simulants from the skin surface and back-extracting toxicants from the skin (certainly in the SC and potentially from other deeper layers of the skin that remain to be studied) to reduce systemic toxicity risk of topically exposed chemical warfare agents or other toxicants of public health significance.

Discussion

Chemical partitioning from the dosing vehicle into the SC involves processes in which molecular binding occurs at certain domains/components of the SC, in addition to simple partitioning. Under a given experimental condition (incubation at 37 °C for 24 hours), the concentration required to attain a fixed value of the partition

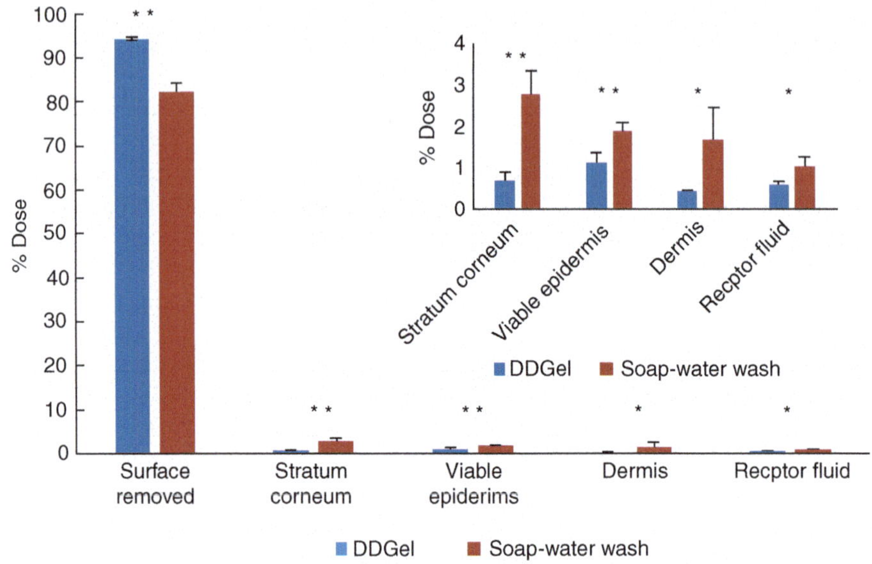

Fig. 10.5 In vitro skin decontamination efficacy of DDGel vs control (soap-water wash decontamination) for chloroethyl phenyl sulfide (CEPS). The % dose amounts of the chemical at 1 hr post chemical exposure were quantified in each sample, except for the RF data as the total cumulative chemical amounts in all the collected RF samples during the 1 hr absorption experiment. Surface removed amount including from the skin surface and back-extracting amount from the skin tissue. The direct assay % dose data are normalized by total recovery to have a more meaningful comparison. Values were compared between soap-water wash and DDGel decontamination groups using the Student's t-test: significant statistical differences are denoted by $*$ at $P < 0.1$ or $**$ at $P < 0.05$. This shows significantly reduced amounts of simulants after skin decontamination with DDGel products on/in the "skin surface," "Stratum corneum," "viable epidermis," "dermis," and "receptor fluid" compared to soap-water wash. This result clearly suggests the DDGel's back-extracting effect

coefficient varied from chemical to chemical. Equilibrium of partitioning largely depends on saturation of chemical binding sites in the SC [26, 32]. Results revealed that, under a given experimental condition, values of partitioning coefficients were compound specific. Because of the protein, lipids, and various substances with widely diversified properties contained in SC, many available binding sites display different selective affinities toward each chemical.

The result demonstrated that the solubility limit of a compound in the SC was important in determining partitioning, as suggested by Potts and Guy [24]. On the basis of the solubility limit of a chemical, the absorption process of water-soluble and lipid-soluble substances was controlled by the protein domain and lipid domain, respectively, or a combination of both [25]. Since lipophilicity of the lipid domain in the SC is much higher than that of water, a lipophilic compound would preferentially partition into the SC over water. Conversely, the protein domain of the SC is significantly more polar than octanol and, therefore, governs the absorption of hydrophilic chemicals [25]. In addition to partitioning into these two domains, some hydrophilic compounds and some lower lipophilic chemicals may be taken into the SC as the result of both the protein domain and water hydration, which was termed as "sponge domain" by Raykar et al. [25].

Partition coefficient reflects a compound's chemical nature. Chemical partitioning proceeds faster than complete diffusion through the whole SC, and the process quickly reaches equilibrium [31]. Time required to reach partition equilibrium varies among chemicals. Partition coefficient as a constant is inherent to the chemical. Time difference in penetration amount may reflect the extent of penetration equilibrium. Over 90% of test chemical amounts can quickly bind to SC protein or other components within less than 30 mins. However, the process is then slowed, needing an additional 2–20 hrs depending upon the tested chemical physicochemical properties to reach full equilibrium. To obtain accurate binding result, we chose a 24-hour incubation period. There may be a small difference in the partition coefficient measured at 30 minutes if it does not reach absolutely full equilibrium at that time. This difference may partially explain why there is no correlation between the decontamination effectiveness and the partitioning data.

Various factors may influence decontamination efficacy including decontaminant characteristics (solubility, molecular weight, volatility), anatomic site, skin pH, volume of decontamination materials, time of removal ratios, and physical enhancements (stripping, rubbing, adhesives) [12, 37, 45]. The result of the in vitro skin decontamination experiment reported here shows that DDGel can simultaneously clean chemical contaminant from the skin surface, decrease the quantity of contaminant available for penetrating into the skin, and reduce chemical penetration and subsequent systemic absorption. The reaction mechanisms of DDGel with a higher decontamination efficiency are not exactly clear now. It looks like competitive affinity to chemicals plays a key role in decontamination efficacy. After a short dermal exposure period, many chemicals either remain in the upper part of the SC or form reservoirs through weak and reversible bonds to SC components or by temporarily retaining in protein, lipids, or water domains. DDGel compete with "bonded" chemical contaminants via desorbing, binding, retaining, and sequestering mechanisms. Some ingredients of the DDGel, such as Fuller's earth play a role of absorbent and can remove the chemical from skin surface. All these effects are related to the physical and chemical properties of the ingredients of the DDGel and the way the gel is formulated.

For DDGels, some ingredients are soluble in water, yet others are not. When mixed together, properties of the DDGel should be affected by the hydrophilicity or lipophilicity of the ingredients. Kollidon® SR, the major component of the DDGel formulation, is a mixture of polyvinyl acetate (PVAc) and povidone (PVP) used as a retardant with universal binding ability. As an emulsion in water, PVAc emulsions are used as adhesives. The insoluble polyvinyl acetate presents a diffusion barrier that slows release of a drug in controlled drug delivery. PVP is soluble in water and other polar solvents, such as various alcohols, including methanol and ethanol [39]. When dry, PVP is a light flaky hygroscopic powder, readily absorbing moisture/water up to 40% of its dry weight from atmosphere. In solution, it has excellent wetting properties and readily forms films. When PVP is mixed with carboxymethyl cellulose (CMC), the mixture can be used as a wound dressing, since the mixture can swell to absorb fluids from blood or other body fluid/discharges from wounds [27]. Water-soluble povidone creates micropores in the framework of the polyvinyl acetate through which water can penetrate through the entire system, thereby dissolving the active drug and allowing its diffusion [34]. Based on the study findings and our new supportive results, possible binding mechanisms for PVAc and PVP to the CWA simulants we tested are considered as the following:

1. Acetate groups on polyvinyl acetate (PVAc) are hydrophobic – thus their high affinity with lipophilic compounds.
2. Positive charges on povidone (PVP) forms chemical complexes with numerous of substances.
3. Diversified characteristics of the two polymers give DDGel its amphipathic character.
4. Lower complexation rate of parathion and CEPS may be caused by higher steric hindrance.

For finite dose in vitro/in vivo experiments, water rinse or soap/water wash is a common skin surface cleaning method as recommended by OCED [23]. Timely use of water, soap, and water or flour followed by wet tissue wipes produced results equal, nearly equal, or in some instances better than those produced by the use of Fuller's Earth, Dutch power, and other compounds. Previous decontamination studies showed that water can reduce 64% of sulfur mustard mass penetrating into guinea pig skin [40] and hair showering led to 72% VX reduction [15]. Soap-water solution can provide modest protection against GD and good protection against VX in the haired guinea pig model [6, 7]. Yet, water with detergent wash may enhance agent transport through garments to skin [8]. After soap-water wash decontamination, considerable chemical mass remained in epidermis and also caused a wash-in chemical effect, which could be accelerated by increasing SC water content [42]. Although soap wash may cause wash-in effect, it does not apply to all chemicals. Compared with water or soap/water wash, DDGel did not show wash-in effect that all have been trying to avoid. "Wash-in" effect [20] was defined as an enhancement of percutaneous absorption elicited specifically by skin decontamination, and simply that as well as washing chemical contaminants off the skin, some chemical is washed into the skin to become bioavailable via the systemic cutaneous blood microcirculation. This DDGel decontamination experiment did not show any "wash-in" phenomenon, and represents a great step forward compared to many traditional skin decontamination products. The reason for the lack of "wash-in" may be related to the physical and chemical properties of decontaminate ingredients, such as Fullers earth, which was utilized as an absorbent to remove chemical from skin surface, and prevent liquid in the DDGel from entering into deep skin layers and thus reduce systemic and local risks. DDGel's back-exacting effect may be weakened when compared to soap/water wash, which may cause wash-in effect. But the data suggest that the DDGel can remove chemicals from skin surface before sheet formation and should not only peel off layers of the SC similar to a D-Squame tape discs. More studies will be performed to verify the back-extracting effect compared to other decontamination products such as Reactive Skin Decontamination Lotion (RSDL) and Fullers' earth.

Conclusion

DDGel is a nano-polymer-based skin decontamination gel formulation, which competitively binds and absorbs chemicals of various physicochemical properties for improved toxicant removal (decon) efficacy from the human skin. DDGel with its major polymers show similar behavior (pattern) as the human stratum corneum in binding and partitioning of chemicals with different hydrophilicity or lipophilicity. More importantly, the DDGel described in this chapter is able to back-extract toxic chemicals from SC, reducing further penetration into other epidermal and dermal layers, and thus reducing absorption into systemic circulation. This result suggests that the DDGel with higher binding affinity and higher decontamination efficacy to chemical toxicants offers a significant opportunity for further development as a NextGen skin decontamination technology against CWAs and other toxicants that possess dermal exposure risk in military and civilian settings.

Taken together, data have revealed some insight into mechanisms of skin decontamination in light of toxicant penetrants' partitioning and binding rates in the skin (including the SC). This is of value for the community dealing with CWAs as well as occupational and environmental toxic chemical skin exposure. In vivo animal/human experimental validation experiments are planned to further demonstrate the clinical relevance of the in vitro observations and the practical applications of the DDGel technology.

Conflict of Interest The authors did not report any conflict of interest.

FundingThis research is supported by Defense Threat Reduction Agency (DTRA) Grant: HDTRA1-14-0005 UCSF (BRBAA11-PerC-9-2-0054-Base).

References

1. Anderson B, Higuchi W, Raykar P. Heterogeneity effects on permeability–partition coefficient relationships in human stratum corneum. Pharm Res. 1988;5:566–73. https://doi.org/10.1023/A:1015989929342.
2. Anderson BD, Raykar PV. Solute structure–permeability relationships in human stratum corneum. J Invest Dermatol. 1989;93:280–6. https://doi.org/10.1111/1523-1747.ep12277592.
3. Anderson RA, Triggs EJ, Roberts MS. The percutaneous absorption of phenolic compounds. 3. Evaluation of permeability through human stratum corneum using a desorption technique. Australian J Pharm Sci NS. 1976;5:107–10.
4. Bartelt-Hunt SL, Knappe DRU, Barlaz MA. A review of chemical warfare agent simulants for the study of environmental behavior. Crit Rev Environ Sci Technol. 2008;38:112–36. https://doi.org/10.1080/10643380701643650.
5. Bunge AL, Cleek RL. A new method for estimating dermal absorption from chemical exposure: 2. Effect of molecular weight and octanol–water partitioning. Pharm Res. 1995;12:88–95. https://doi.org/10.1023/A:1016242821610.
6. Braue EH Jr, Smith KH, Doxzon BF, Lumpkin HL, Clarkson ED. Efficacy studies of reactive skin decontamination lotion, M291 skin decontamination kit, 0.5% bleach, 1% soapy water, and skin exposure reduction paste against chemical warfare agents, Part 1: Guinea

pigs challenged with VX. Cutan Ocul Toxicol. 2011a;30:15–28. https://doi.org/10.3109/15569527.2010.515280.
7. Braue EH Jr, Smith KH, Doxzon BF, Lumpkin HL, Clarkson ED. Efficacy studies of reactive skin decontamination lotion, M291 skin decontamination kit, 0.5% bleach, 1% soapy water, and skin exposure reduction paste against chemical warfare agents, Part 2: Guinea pigs challenged with soman. Cutan Ocul Toxicol. 2011b;30:29–37. https://doi.org/10.3109/15569527.2010.515281.
8. Chang MH, Ciegler A, Crochet R. A survey and evaluation of chemical warfare; 1984. p. AD–A202 525.
9. Clark JH, Hunt A, Topi C, Paggiola G, Sherwood J. Sustainable solvents: perspectives from research, business and international policy. Croydon: Royal Society of Chemistry; 2017.
10. Dennerlein K, Schneider D, Goen T, Drexler H, Korinth G. Impact of storage conditions for excised human skin on percutaneous penetration of chemicals. Paper presented at the 13e Congress PPP. La Grande Motte: France; 2012.
11. Flynn GL, Dürrheim H, Higuchi WI. Permeation of hairless mouse skin II: membrane sectioning techniques and influence on alkanol permeabilities. J Pharm Sci. 1981;70:52–6. https://doi.org/10.1002/jps.2600700109.
12. Hui X, Domoradzki JY, Maibach HI. *In vitro* study to determine decontamination of 3,5-dichloro-2,4,6-trifluoropyridine (DCTFP) from human skin. Food Chem Toxicol. 2012;50:2496–502. https://doi.org/10.1016/j.fct.2012.03.069.
13. Hui X, Wester RC, Magee P, Maibach HI. Partitioning of chemicals from water into powdered human stratum corneum (callus): a model study. In Vitro Toxicol. 1995;8:159–67. https://doi.org/10.1201/9781420009774.
14. Johnson ME, Blankschtein D, Langer R. Evaluation of solute permeation through the stratum corneum: lateral bilayer diffusion as the primary transport mechanism. J Pharm Sci. 1997;86:1162–72. https://doi.org/10.1021/js960198e.
15. Josse D, Wartelle J, Cruz C. Showering effectiveness for human hair decontamination of the nerve agent VX. Chem Biol Interact. 2015;232:94–100.
16. Kondo S, Yamasaki-Konishi H, Sugimoto AI. Enhancement of transdermal delivery by superfluous thermodynamic potential. II. *in vitro-in vivo* correlation of percutaneous nifedipine transport. J Pharmacobiodyn. 1987;10:662–8.
17. Matveev NV, Islam T, Maibach HI. Factors influencing applied amount of topical preparations. In: Wilhelm K-P, Zhai H, Maibach HI, editors. Dermatotoxicology. 8th ed. London: Informa Healthcare; 2012.
18. Mitragotri S. A theoretical analysis of permeation of small hydrophobic solutes across the stratum corneum based on Scaled Particle Theory. J Pharm Sci. 2002;91:744–52. https://doi.org/10.1002/jps.10048.
19. Mitragotri S. Modeling skin permeability to hydrophilic and hydrophobic solutes based on four permeation pathways. J Control Release. 2003;86:69–92. https://doi.org/10.1016/S0168-3659(02)00321-8.
20. Moody RP, Maibach HI. Skin decontamination: importance of the wash-in effect. Food Chem Toxicol. 2006;44:1783–8. https://doi.org/10.1016/j.fct.2006.05.020.
21. Morimoto Y, Hatanaka T, Sugibayashi K, Omiya H. Prediction of skin permeability of drugs: comparison of human and hairless rat skin. J Pharm Pharmacol. 1992;44:634–9. https://doi.org/10.1111/j.2042-7158.1992.tb05484.x.
22. Nitsche JM, Wang TF, Kasting GB. A two-phase analysis of solute partitioning into the stratum corneum. J Pharm Sci. 2006;95:649–66. https://doi.org/10.1002/jps.20549.
23. OECD, Organisation for Economic Co-operation and Development. Guideline for the testing of chemicals. Skin absorption: *in vitro* method. Paris: OECD; 2004.
24. Potts RO, Guy RH. Predicting skin permeability. Pharm Res. 1992;9:663–9. https://doi.org/10.1023/A:1015810312465.

25. Raykar PV, Fung MC, Anderson BD. The role of protein and lipid domains in the uptake of solutes by human stratum corneum. Pharm Res. 1988;5:140–50. https://doi.org/10.1023/A:1015956705293.
26. Rieger M. Factors affecting sorption of topically applied substances. In: Zatz JL, editor. Skin permeation fundamentals and application. Wheaton: Allured Publishing Co; 1993. p. 33–72.
27. Roya N, Sahaa N, Kitanoa T, Sahaa P. Development and characterization of novel medicated hydrogels for wound dressing. Soft Materials. 2010;8:130–48. https://doi.org/10.1080/15394451003756282.
28. SCCS/1358/10. Basic criteria for the *in vitro* assessment of dermal absorption of cosmetic ingredients, adopted by SCCS during the 7th plenary meeting of 22. 2010.
29. Scheuplein RJ. Mechanism of percutaneous absorption. II. Transient diffusion and the relative importance of various routes of skin penetration. J Invest Dermatol. 1967;48:79–88. https://doi.org/10.1038/jid.1967.11.
30. Scheuplein RJ, Blank IH. Permeability of the skin. Physiol Rev. 1971;51:702–47.
31. Scheuplein RJ, Bronaugh RL. Percutaneous absorption. In: Goldsmith LA, editor. Biochemistry and physiology of the skin, vol. 1. Oxford: Oxford University Press; 1983. p. 1255–94.
32. Surber C, Wilhelm KP, Maibach HI, Hall L, Guy RH. Partitioning of chemicals into human stratum corneum: implications for risk assessment following dermal exposure. Fundam Appl Toxicol. 1990;15:99–107. https://doi.org/10.1016/0272-0590(90)90167-I.
33. Teasdale A. Genotoxic impurities: strategies for identification and control. Hoboken: Wiley; 2011.
34. Timmins P, Pygall SR, Melia CD. Hydrophilic matrix tablets for oral controlled release Melia. New York/Heidelberg/Dordrecht/London: AAPS Press/Springer; 2014.
35. Wagner H, Kostka KH, Lehr CM, Schaefer UF. Correlation between stratum corneum/water partition coefficient and amounts of flufenamic acid penetrated into the stratum corneum. J Pharm Sci. 2002;91:1915–21. https://doi.org/10.1002/jps.10183.
36. Wang XW, Liu JF, Yin YG. Development of an ultra-high-performance liquid chromatography–tandem mass spectrometry method for high throughput determination of organophosphorus flame retardants in environmental water. J Chromatogr A. 2011;1218:6705–11. https://doi.org/10.1016/j.chroma.2011.07.067.
37. Wester RC, Hui X, Hewitt PG, Hostynek J, Krauser S, Thomas C, Maibach H. Polymers effect on estradiol partition coefficient between powdered human stratum corneum and water. J Pharm Sci. 2002;91:2642–5. https://doi.org/10.1002/jps.10248.
38. Wester RC, Maibach HI. Cutaneous pharmacokinetics: 10 steps to percutaneous absorption. Drug Metab Rev. 1983;14:169–205. https://doi.org/10.3109/03602538308991388.
39. Wohlfarth C. Thermodynamic properties of polymer solutions. Landolt-Börnstein, new series, group VIII, volume 6D. Berlin, Heidelberg: Springer; 2010. https://doi.org/10.1007/978-3-642-02890-8_752.
40. Wormster U, Brodsky B, Sintov A. Skin toxicokinetics of mustard gas in the Guinea pig: effect of hypochlorite and safety aspects. Arch Toxicol. 2002;76:517–22.
41. Zhu HJ, Jung EC, Hui XY, Maibach HI. Proposed human stratum corneum water domain in chemical absorption. J Appl Toxicol. 2016;36:991–6. https://doi.org/10.1002/jat.3208.
42. Zhu HJ, Jung EC, Phoung C, Hui XY, Maibach HI. Effects of soap–water wash on human epidermal penetration. J Appl Toxicol. 2015;36:997–1002. https://doi.org/10.1002/jat.3258.
43. Zou Y, Maibach HI. Dermal-epidermal separation methods: research implications. Arch Dermatol Res. 2017;310:1–9. https://doi.org/10.1007/s00403-017-1774-8.
44. Zatz JL. Scratching the surface: rationale approaches to skin permeation. In: Zatz JL, editor. Skin permeation fundamentals and application. Wheaton: Allured Publishing Co; 1993. p. 11–32.
45. Zhai H, Chan HP, Hui X, Maibach HI. Skin decontamination of glyphosate from human skin *in vitro*. Food Chem Toxicol. 2008;46:2258–60. https://doi.org/10.1016/j.fct.2008.03.001.

Chapter 11
Dermostyx (IB1): High Efficacy and Safe Topical Skin Protectant Against Percutaneous Toxic Agents

Shlomit Dachir, Izhak Barness, Eliezer Fishbine, Jacob Meshulam, Rita Sahar, Arik Eisenkraft, Adina Amir, and Tamar Kadar

Introduction

Development of a topical skin protectant is aimed to prevent the penetration of toxic agents through the skin and is essential for both military troops and civilian populations. The list of percutaneous toxic agents includes chemical warfare agents (CWAs) and toxic industrial chemicals (TICs) such as pesticides and irritants. The hazard of exposure to TICs has become a realistic threat since many TICs are routinely used in industry, agriculture, and research. Currently, the available therapy is limited and removal of the chemical substances from the body (skin and eyes) is the only way to reduce injury for some of the toxic agents.

A topically applied pretreatment that will act as a skin barrier may prevent the absorption of these toxic agents, as well as their respective toxicity [1].

The topical skin protectant strategy has been adopted by many countries including the USA, UK, and Israel [2]. The requirements from such preparation are to yield a significant protection, to be nontoxic and safe for human use, to remain effective on the skin for a reasonable time following application, to cause minimal discomfort to the user, and to be compatible with decontamination procedures.

We have developed a topical skin protectant that is applied onto the skin before exposure and prevents the penetration of warfare agents such as SM and VX through the skin and thus confers a highly efficient protection against the hazard they pose [2]. The formulation coded IB1 is a hydrophilic water-based solution comprised of magnesium sulfate and glycerin and it was shown to be safe in preclinical and Phase I studies [3]. IB1 was registered and approved by the Israel Ministry of Health as Dermostyx protective solution and is commercially available (Rekah Pharm, Israel).

S. Dachir (✉) · I. Barness · E. Fishbine · J. Meshulam · R. Sahar · A. Eisenkraft
A. Amir · T. Kadar
Department of Pharmacology, Israel Institute for Biological Research, Ness Ziona, Israel
e-mail: shlomitd@iibr.gov.il

H. Zhu, H. I. Maibach (eds.), *Skin Decontamination*,
https://doi.org/10.1007/978-3-030-24009-7_11

The present study aimed to further test the efficacy of IB1 against CWAs, pesticides, and irritants and to elucidate the mechanism of protection/to investigate the role of the ingredients in the protection. The efficacy against the various toxic agents was evaluated in the well-established pig model [4], using clinical, histological, and biochemical monitoring. A representative example from each of these groups was chosen to demonstrate the protection afforded by this unique preparation. The list includes sulfur mustard (SM), VX [O-ethyl-S-(2-diisopropylaminoethyl) methylphosphothiolate], parathion, and acrolein as detailed below.

Sulfur mustard is a potent cutaneous vesicant that penetrates rapidly through the skin, causing severe prolonged injuries. Since its first use in World War I (WWI) and despite vast efforts, only limited success has been attained to find an effective treatment to prevent the injury [5–8]. VX is the most potent nerve agent that due to its low volatility and high persistence penetrates through the skin resulting in cholinergic toxicity and lethality [9]. The pesticide parathion is widely used in agriculture and is known to produce poisoning after dermal exposure in man and animals [10, 11].

Acrolein is a well-known strong irritant that was used by the French during WWI as a warfare agent "Papite" [12]. It is produced commercially worldwide since 1938 and is used mainly as an herbicide in water systems and as an intermediate product in many manufacturing processes [12–14]. According to the EPA reports, about 500 tons of acrolein are sold annually in the USA to use as an herbicide. Therefore, there is a risk of accidental exposure to this chemical. At present, therapy against the deleterious effects of SM and acrolein is only partially effective and for VX and organophosphate pesticides, the efficacy of treatments depends on the dose of the toxicants and on time elapsed from exposure. In addition to the efficacy studies, we hereby present data regarding the mode of protection, focusing on the role of glycerin and magnesium sulfate and their interaction with the stratum corneum.

Material and Methods

Animals

Young female pigs (commercial strain, Institute of Animal Research, Kibbutz Lahav, Israel) weighing 12–13 kg at the beginning of the experiment were used. Animals were housed in individual pens in a ventilated room with artificial lights from 06:00 to18:00 and the environmental temperature was adjusted to 21 ± 1 °C. They were fed with commercially available complete diet for pigs (Kibbutz Lahav) twice a day and had free access to tap water via automatic drinkers (drinking nipples).

All procedures involving animals were in accordance with the Guide for the Care and Use of Laboratory Animals, National Academy Press, Washington, DC, 1996, and were approved by the Institutional Animal Care and Use Committee.

Materials

Toxic agents: Neat sulfur mustard (1250 μg μl^{-1}, purity 95%: MW – 159.08, vapor pressure – 0.11 mmHg at 25 °C, solubility – 0.06% in water at 20 °C, logP – 1.37), neat VX, purity level of at least 95% (using gas chromatography; MW – 265.4, vapor pressure – 0.0007 mmHg at 25 °C, solubility 3% in water at 20 °C, logP – 0.675), Polidol 605E (commercial product, 467 mg/ml ethyl parathion in a diluting and wetting solution, Lidor Chemicals Ltd., Israel), and acrolein (90%, Sigma, Israel: MW –56.06, vapor pressure – 209.4 mmHg at 20 °C, solubility – 208 g/L water at 20 °C, log octanol-water partition coefficient – 0.9) were used for the exposure procedures. Decontamination was conducted using Fuller's Earth powder (Shalon, Israel).

Topical skin protectant (TSP): IB1 – a mixture of magnesium sulfate and glycerin (1:3).

Exposure Procedure

Pigs were restrained on specially made carts and the backs of the pigs were closely clipped. For the exposure of SM and acrolein: 8–10 fields were marked (4–5 fields of 35 cm^2 each on each side) that served as exposure sites. All exposure procedures were performed within a hood at room temperature.

Liquid: SM: Three droplets of 1 μl were applied in each exposure field, VX: a dose of 2LD50 in 1 μl droplets was applied along the back, ethyl parathion: droplets of 20 of 250 μl (for dosing of 40 and 250 mg/kg, respectively) were applied along the back, acrolein: a droplet of 50 μl on each exposure site. All droplets were applied to the pigs' back skin using a digital microliter positive displacement pipette.

Vapor: Toxic agents (5 μl of SM, 50 μl of acrolein) were placed onto filter paper disks (25 mm diameter) within the top inner surface of glass cups that were attached to the animals' back and were sealed for the duration of the exposure (10 glass cups, 5 on each side of the back). At the end of the exposure, procedure pigs were decontaminated with fuller earth. A large amount of powder was applied to the skin to cover the exposed areas and then was removed with a spatula. This was repeated three times and then pigs were rinsed thoroughly with tap water.

Experimental Outline

IB1 (~1 ml/100 cm^2) or water was applied on the skin as a single dose 10 min–12 h before exposure.

SM: Pigs were exposed for the duration of 10, 30, and 60 min (liquid) or 15–60 min (vapor).

VX: Pigs were exposed to $2LD_{50}$ (1.3 mg/kg) for the duration of 1 and 4 h (The LD50 value was determined over a period of 24 h).

Ethyl parathion: Pigs were exposed to 40 mg/kg for 6 h and to 250 mg/kg for 2 h.

Acrolein: Pigs were exposed for the duration of 30 and 60 min (liquid) or 15–60 min (vapor).

Each experimental group consisted of 2–4 pigs.

Quantitative Assessment of Lesions Area

The extent of the damage to the skin following exposure to SM and acrolein was measured using morphometric analysis of the damaged skin area. The exposed sites on the pigs' backs were photographed using a digital camera (Coolpix 950, Nikon, Tokyo, Japan). Pictures were analyzed for the damaged area using an image analysis system (Image-Pro Express 4.0).

Erythema Measurements

The degree of erythema on the skin following exposure to SM or acrolein was measured using a reflectance color meter (Minolta Chroma-Meter Model C-300, Minolta Corporation, Ramsey, NJ), before the exposure (baseline) and at 2, 4, 6, 24, and 48 h following exposure to SM. The chromameter uses reflected light and reads color in a three-dimensional format $L*$, $a*$, and $b*$. The $a*$ coordinate is the balance between red and green and this chromaticity parameter was used as the indicator of the degree of erythema. Three replicate readings were taken on each exposed site and averaged.

Cholinesterase Inhibition in Whole Blood

Blood samples (0.5–0.7 ml) were collected from the jugular vein at various time points following exposure to VX and ethyl parathion. One hundred microliters of blood was immediately transferred into a heparinized tube containing 1.2 double-distilled water and mixed gently to cause hemolysis of red blood cells. Samples were stored at −4 °C until further analyzed.

The inhibition of the enzyme cholinesterase was determined using the radiometric method [15]. The blood samples were incubated with the substrate, H^3-acetylcholine, at a temperature of 25 °C for 30 min. The reaction was ended with a reaction stopper that separated between the radioactive acetate and the choline. Scintillation solution was added and the radioactivity of the acetate in the organic phase was measured using a β counter.

Histology

Skin biopsies were taken at 1 week following exposure for fixation in 4% neutral buffered paraformaldehyde. Six micron paraffin sections were stained with hematoxylin and eosin (H&E) for light microscopy observations.

For studies of the interaction between IB1 and the stratum corneum, skin biopsies were quickly frozen in liquid nitrogen and 12 micron frozen sections were cut and stained for phospholipids by Sudan Black B.

Statistics

Results are expressed as mean ± standard error of the mean (s.e.m.). The quantitative data were subjected to statistical analysis using t-test or two-way ANOVA utilizing GraphPad Prism 4 software. Post hoc comparisons were performed using the Bonferroni test for multiple comparisons.

Results

Protection Efficacy Against SM Liquid and Vapor

Typical SM skin lesions developed on all exposed sites in a dose-dependent manner.

Application of IB1 once, prior to *SM liquid* exposure, provided a significant protection against 1 μl droplets for exposure durations up to 1 h, as demonstrated by the clinical outcome (Fig. 11.1, $p < 0.001$) and by the quantitative analysis of damaged skin area (Fig. 11.2). Over 90% protection was obtained when compared to untreated SM-exposed controls (0% protection = untreated SM lesion).

The protective properties of IB1 were immediate upon application and remained effective for at least 12 h. No change was found in the efficacy of protection whether the protectant was applied 10 min, 1 h, 3 h, 6 h, or 12 h before exposure.

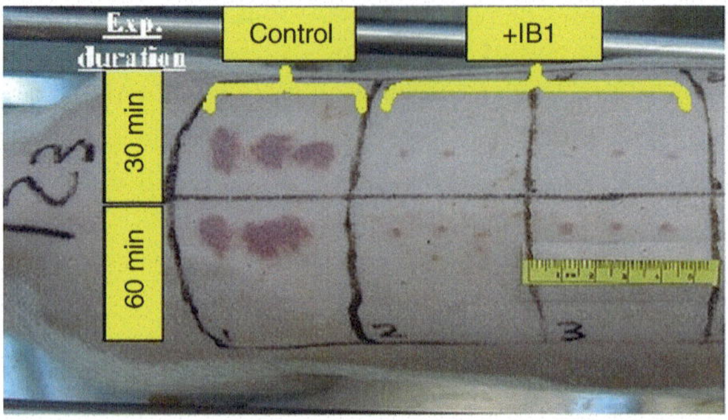

Fig. 11.1 The efficacy of IB1 in pigs, 24 h following exposure to SM (1 μl droplets) for exposure durations of 30 and 60 min. Note the minor damage in the treated skin, compared to the severe lesions in the untreated control areas. IB1 was applied 1 h before exposure

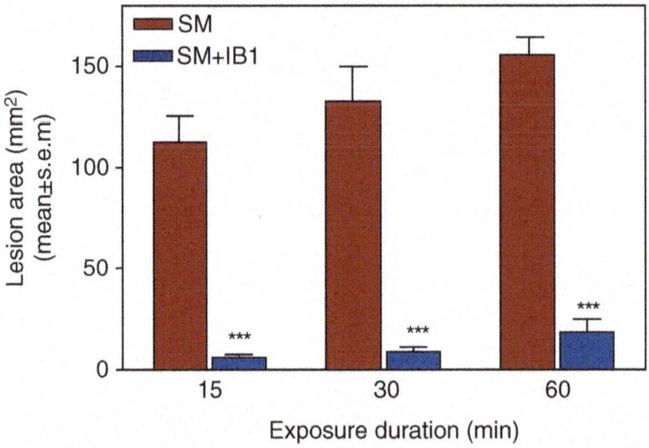

Fig. 11.2 Quantitative analysis of the area of the skin lesions 24 h following exposure to SM (1 μl droplets) for 15–60 min. IB1 afforded about 90% protection (0% protection assigned to SM controls, $***p < 0.001$ vs SM) when applied 1 h before exposure

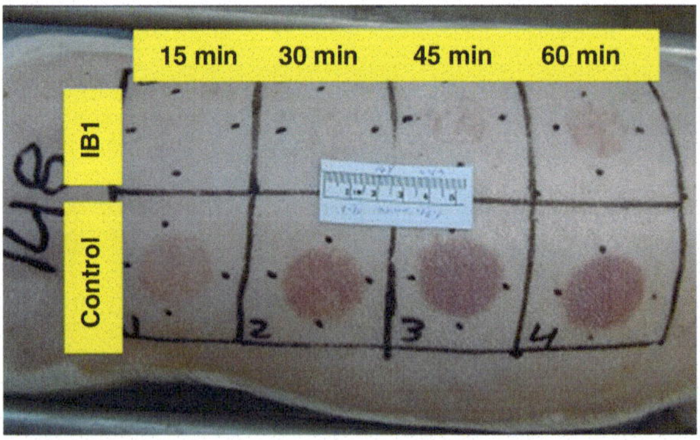

Fig. 11.3 The efficacy of IB1 against SM vapor exposure (15–60 min exposure durations) in pigs 24 h after exposure. Note the severe erythema in the untreated controls (lower panel) and the significant protection provided by IB1 (upper panel). IB1 was applied 1 h before exposure

Similar efficiency was obtained when tested against *SM vapor* (Fig. 11.3). Application of IB1 on the skin 1–6 h before exposure to SM vapor decreased significantly ($p < 0.05$ at 30 and 45 min) the extent of the damage as reflected in the erythema measurements (Fig. 11.4).

Histological evaluation of skin biopsies taken 1 week following exposure revealed severe damage in the untreated exposed controls compared to progressive

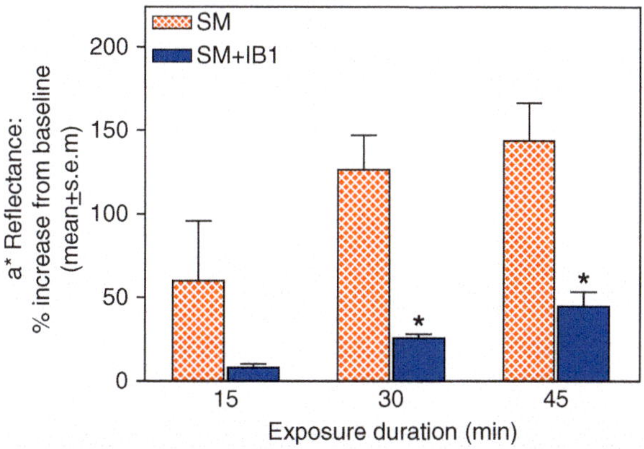

Fig. 11.4 Quantitative analysis of the extent of erythema, 24 h following exposure to SM vapor for exposure durations of 15–45 min. Note the substantial protection afforded by IB1 (*$p < 0.05$ vs SM)

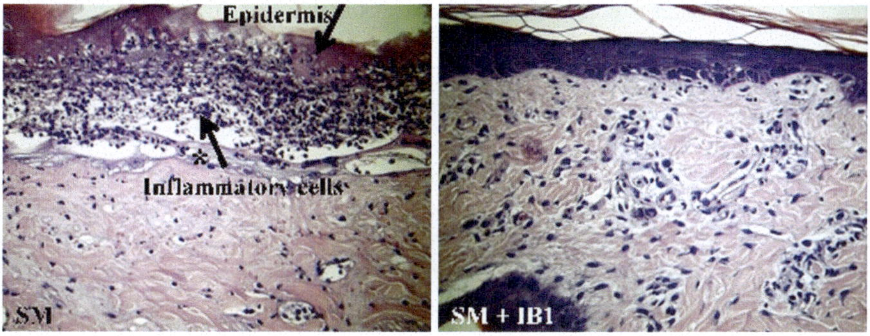

Fig. 11.5 Histological skin sections, taken 1 week following exposure to SM vapor (exposure duration of 1 h). Note the stratified regenerative epithelial coverage in the treated skin, compared to the inflammatory response and the very early healing stage of the epidermis in the untreated SM-exposed skin characterized by migration of vacuolated epidermal cells (asterisk in SM). H&E staining. Objective magnification ×40

healing in the IB1-treated areas (Fig. 11.5). While the IB1-treated skin was covered by stratified regenerative epidermal layer, only minor regeneration was observed in the untreated control, which was associated with massive infiltration of inflammatory cells.

Protection Efficacy Against VX

Pigs were exposed to a dose that was equivalent to $2LD_{50}$ of VX (in 1 μl droplets) and were decontaminated 1 or 4 h after agent's application.

Control unprotected animals displayed a time-dependent inhibition of blood ChE activity and exhibited clinical symptoms typical of organophosphate poisoning, including salivation, muscle fasciculation, respiratory distress, and death. When pigs were exposed for 1 h, the control unprotected animals exhibited typical moderate clinical symptoms, starting at 6 h after exposure. Inhibition of blood ChE activity reached its peak value (60%) 7 h after VX application (Fig. 11.6). All these animals survived the exposure. When IB1 was applied 12 h before exposure, under the same conditions, IB1 pretreated pigs did not exhibit any adverse clinical signs and ChE inhibition increased to a maximal value of 15% only (Fig. 11.6).

When exposed to a prolonged challenge of VX (4 h duration), most of the unprotected animals developed around 90% ChE inhibition within 4 h (Fig. 11.7) and died within 12–48 h. In contrast, all the pigs pretreated with IB1, despite the ChE inhibition, survived the 4 h challenge with $2LD_{50}$ (1.3 mg/kg) of VX and exhibited only minor short-term toxic symptoms, if any. The inhibition of ChE developed slowly and reached the peak of 80% inhibition only 8 h after VX application (Fig. 11.7).

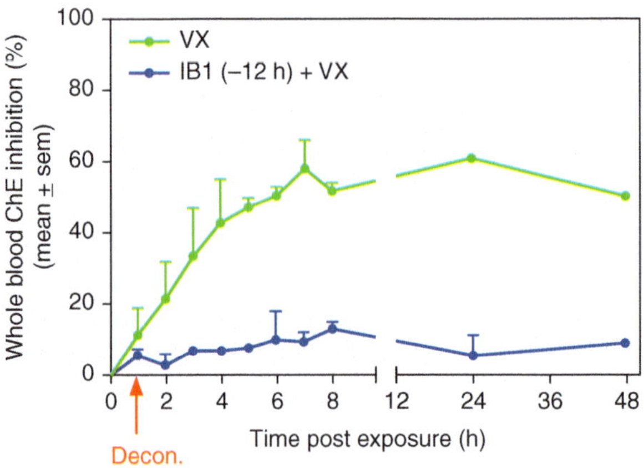

Fig. 11.6 The effect of IB1 against $2LD_{50}$ of VX (1.3 mg/kg, 1 h exposure) in pigs, expressed by the percent of inhibition in blood ChE activity. IB1 was applied 12 h before exposure. Note the lower inhibition of ChE activity in the IB1 pretreated animals

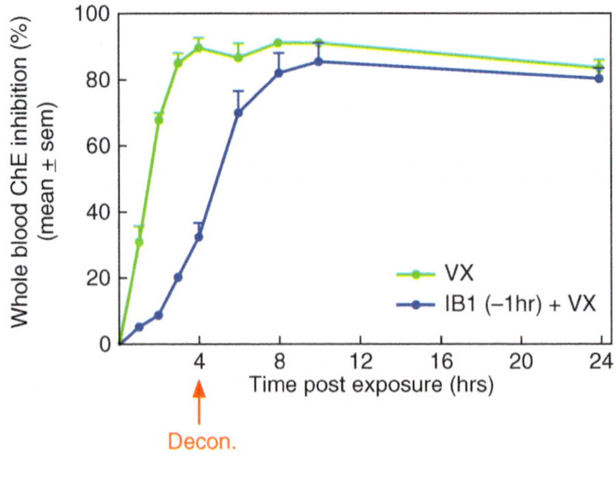

Fig. 11.7 The effect of IB1 against 2LD50 VX (1.3 mg/kg, 4 h exposure duration) in pigs, expressed by the percent of inhibition in blood ChE activity. IB1 was applied 1 h before exposure. Note the more moderate slope of ChE inhibition in IB1-treated animals, compared to the rapid increase in inhibition in the untreated group, which may have contributed to the better clinical outcome observed in these animals

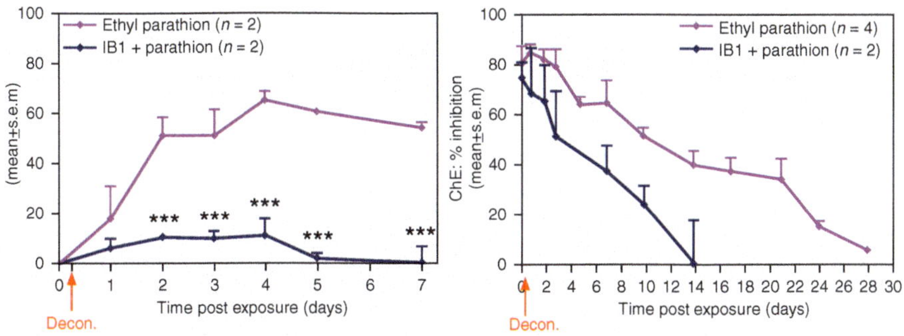

Fig. 11.8 The effect of IB1 against ethyl parathion intoxication (40 mg/kg for 6 h and 250 mg/kg, 2 h exposure) in pigs, expressed by the percent of inhibition in blood ChE activity. IB1 was applied 1 h before exposure. IB1 essentially eliminated inhibition of ChE after exposure to 40 mg/kg (∗∗∗$p < 0.001$ vs parathion). Following a higher dose, a faster return to normal enzyme activity in the IB1 pretreated animals is shown

Protection Efficacy Against Ethyl Parathion

Topical exposure of pigs to 40 mg/kg of ethyl parathion in a commercial formulation for 6 h resulted in a 60% inhibition of the ChE enzyme 4 days after exposure (Fig. 11.8A). The application of IB1 1 h before the exposure almost eliminated any inhibition of the enzyme ($p < 0.001$).

Exposure to 250 mg/kg of ethyl parathion for 2 h resulted in significant inhibition of whole blood ChE and typical clinical signs including salivation, fasciculation, and respiratory distress. The exposed pigs lost weight up to 10% of their body weight within 4 days of exposure and started to regain weight between days 5 and 7. The ChE inhibition reached a peak of about 85% at 24 h after exposure and then it subsided slowly until regaining almost full activity only 28 days postexposure (Fig. 11.8B).

Pigs that were exposed to ethyl parathion 1 h after application of IB1 exhibited high inhibition of ChE of almost 80% but it subsided faster and the enzyme regained its activity within 14 days (Fig. 11.8B). The pigs that were protected with IB1 had only very slight clinical symptoms such as minor salivation, fasciculation, and general weakness that lasted only 24 h.

Protection Efficacy Against Acrolein

Dermal exposure of pigs to acrolein liquid or vapor resulted in a dose- and time-dependent damage to the skin. Interestingly, the lesions developed first at the circumference of the exposed area, and with the increase in exposure duration and dose, a more significant damage was observed in the center as well (Figs. 11.9A, 11.10A).

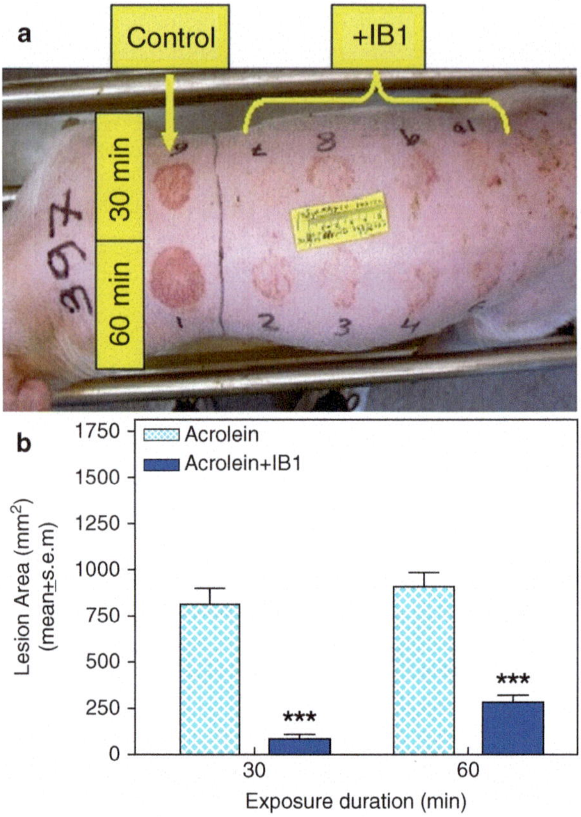

Fig. 11.9 The efficacy of IB1 in pigs, 24 h following exposure to acrolein vapor for exposure durations of 30 and 60 min. (**a**) Note the minor damage on the treated skin, compared to the severe lesions in the untreated control areas. IB1 was applied 1 h before exposure. (**b**) Quantitative analysis of skin lesions area 24 h following exposure to acrolein vapor for 30 and 60 min. IB1 afforded a significant protection of 70–90% (0% protection assigned to acrolein controls) when applied 1 h before exposure (***$p < 0.001$ vs acrolein). ($n = 4$ pigs: $n = 4$ for each 30 and 60 min control sites and $n = 16$ for each 30 and 60 min IB1 protected sites)

IB1 afforded a significant protection. Following exposure to acrolein vapor for 30 min almost full protection (90%) was observed ($p < 0.001$) and following a 60-min exposure only small lesions developed producing 70% protection (Fig. 11.9, $p < 0.001$).

Exposure to acrolein liquid after application of IB1 (Figs.11.10, 11.11) afforded slightly less protection exhibiting somewhat larger lesions, compared to those that developed after vapor exposure. Following exposure to acrolein liquid for 30 min and 60 min, 55–40% protection was observed, respectively, yet the difference between the nonprotected exposed areas and the protected areas was obvious (Fig. 11.10, $p < 0.005$).

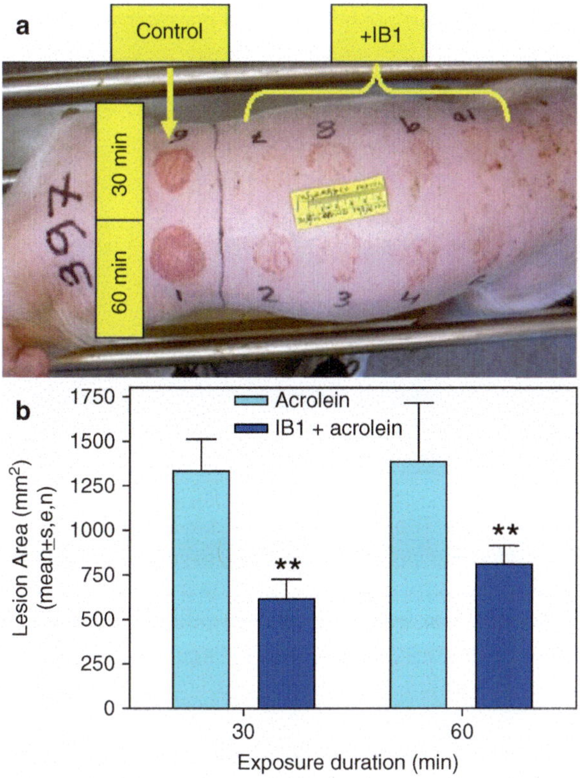

Fig. 11.10 The efficacy of IB1 in pigs, 24 h following exposure to acrolein (50 μl droplets) for exposure durations of 30 and 60 min. (**a**) Note the minor damage on the treated skin, compared to the severe lesions in the untreated control areas. IB1 was applied 1 h before exposure. (**b**) Quantitative analysis of skin lesions area 24 h following exposure to acrolein liquid (50 μl droplets) for 30 and 60 min. IB1 afforded 40–55% protection (0% protection assigned to acrolein controls) when applied 1 h before exposure ($**p < 0.005$ vs acrolein). ($n = 4$ pigs: $n = 4$ for each 30 and 60 min control sites and $n = 16$ for each 30 and 60 min IB1 protected sites)

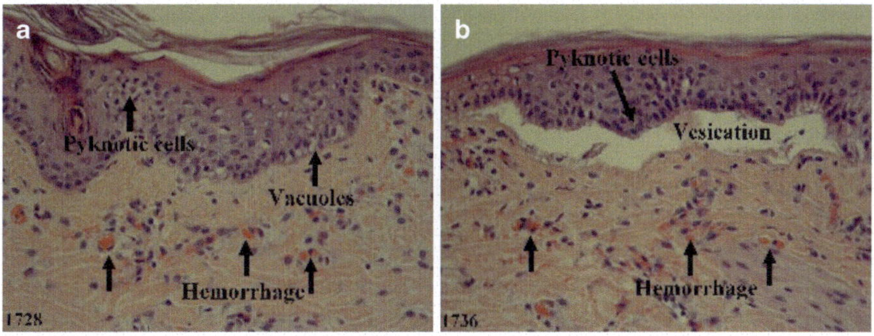

Fig. 11.11 Histological skin sections taken 6 h (**a**) and 24 h (**b**) after 1 h exposure to acrolein droplets (50 μl). Note the pyknotic cells and vacuoles in the epidermis and hemorrhage in the dermis (**a**, **b**) and the separation at the basement membrane (vesication) (**b**). H&E staining, objective magnification ×40

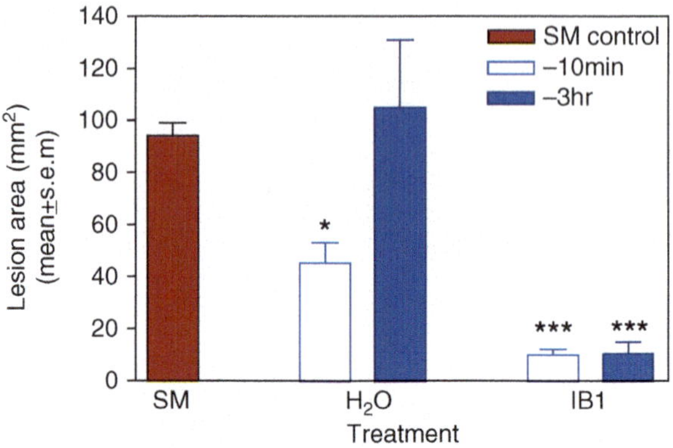

Fig. 11.12 Quantitative analysis of the area of the skin lesions 24 h following exposure to SM (1 μl droplets) for 60 min. Water afforded transient protection, while IB1 provided long-lasting hydration and therefore continuing significant protection ($*p < 0.05$, $***p < 0.001$ vs SM)

IB1: Mode of Protection

A. In vivo studies in pigs – Topically applied water 10 min before exposure to 1 μl droplets of SM provided some protection, that is, the damaged skin area was smaller than the untreated SM controls (Fig. 11.12). When water was applied 3 h before exposure, no protection was obtained, probably due to the rapid evaporation of water from the skin. In contrast, there was no change in the efficacy of IB1 that was applied under the same conditions (10 min vs 3 h) (Fig. 11.12).

B. Histochemistry of phospholipids in skin sections – The stratum corneum in the skin of naïve animals stains positively for phospholipids, demonstrating the lipophilic part of this layer. In contrast, when IB1-treated skin was stained, the reaction was slight and insignificant demonstrating the dynamic behavior of the stratum corneum (Fig. 11.13).

Discussion

The present study shows the high efficacy of the topical skin protectant, IB1 (Dermostyx), against percutaneous toxic agents in the pig model and its mode of protection by interaction with the stratum corneum.

There are two main ways of protecting the skin against chemical agents such as SM, VX, and TICs. The first method is a passive protection which involves covering the skin with protective clothes [1, 16]. This method has several drawbacks: first, the protective clothes are relatively heavy and uncomfortable to wear for a long period of time and therefore they cannot be used continuously as a protective measure. Second, the protective clothes do not cover completely the whole body, leaving areas unprotected such as the hands and neck and therefore they do not offer full protection. Furthermore, such protective measures are quite expensive, and that of course limits their usefulness. The second method of protection involves applying reactive materials to the skin, which react with the toxic agents and neutralize them

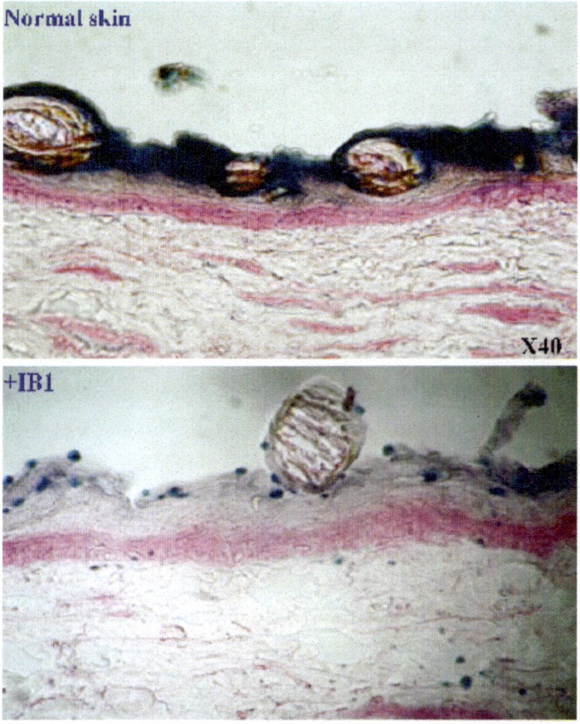

Fig. 11.13 Sudan Black B staining for phospholipids of the stratum corneum in naïve guinea pig skin (upper layer) (frozen sections) and following IB1 application. Note the intense staining in the normal skin and the decrease in positive staining for lipids after the application of the skin protectant. Objective magnification ×40

[16]. The drawback associated with this method is that it requires the application of active materials that are generally harmful by themselves and are as yet only limited in efficacy. Additionally, such reactive materials, generally, require the use of large quantities which are difficult to apply to the skin for a long time. IB1 overcomes these drawbacks. It provides a protective layer against a large variety of toxic agents for a long period of time. It is compatible with the skin and because it consists of ingredients widely used in cosmetics and medicine, it is safe for human use.

A single topical application of the protectant prior (10 min–12 h) to prolonged exposure (1–4 h) to the toxic agents reduced by over 85% the size and severity of skin lesions induced by high doses of SM (both liquid and vapor) and prevented the development of any clinical symptoms following extremely long exposure to lethal doses of VX. Highly effective protection was achieved also when IB1 was tested against TICs such as ethyl parathion and acrolein. It should be noted that although the protective values varied among the various agents yet the clinical signs of all the tested agents were substantially reduced by the pretreatment with IB1. Interestingly, high protection was afforded against both liquid and vapor CWAs. In comparison, the TSP used by the US military, Skin Exposure Reduction Paste Against Chemical

Warfare Agents (SERPACWA), was effective against liquid SM but not against SM vapor (personal communication) and provided significant but modest protection against VX [17].

The barrier properties of IB1 remain effective for at least 12 h after application (the maximum time tested), which is a relatively long period. The longest pretreatment duration that was tested for the efficacy of SERPACWA, the TSP used by the US military, was 5 h [17, 18]. IB1 is absorbed into the stratum corneum of the skin and remains there and we have shown that the ingredients are not absorbed into the circulation [3]. The protective mechanism of this preparation seemed to be primarily due to alterations in the physicochemical properties of the stratum corneum that turned hydrophilic by the glycerin. Thus, penetration of lipophilic compounds is prevented.

The stratum corneum is a layer of dead flattened keratin-filled cells (corneocytes) that is embedded in a matrix of stacked lipid lamellae in an array similar to "bricks and mortar" [19–21]. It is this unique structure that accounts for its selective permeability of topically applied lipophilic compounds such as CWAs and TICs and for its capacity to trap water in large quantities. Hydration of the skin is known to affect its barrier function and thereby exert a profound effect on the penetration of both lipophilic and hydrophilic molecules [22–24]. Glycerin is widely used in cosmetic formulations as a humectant and as a skin moisturizer, but compared to other humectants it has a long-lasting effect. In addition, glycerin is also highly hygroscopic and recognized by its ability to retain water in the skin. Thus, the role of glycerin in the protectant is to provide a hydrophilic stable barrier on the skin. Indeed, we have shown that topically applied water by itself provided some protection but only when applied close to the exposure (10 min), while no protection was achieved if applied 1–3 h before exposure, probably due to its rapid evaporation. When using glycerin, the hydration effect was long lasting and the lipophilic stratum corneum turned hydrophilic as demonstrated by the histochemical staining of phospholipids. Another advantage of glycerin is that it does not penetrate from the stratum corneum into the circulation as shown in preclinical [2] and Phase I clinical [3] studies.

The addition of magnesium sulfate into the glycerin solution decreased the solubility of the toxic agents in the stratum corneum water phase, a process known as "salting out." The added value of the salt in the protective mechanism was observed in vitro by the FINABEL test, which is a qualitative permeation test for chemical agents [17] (data not shown).

IB1 is a noncatalytic compound that does not contain reactive materials that may neutralize the toxic chemicals. Thus, although the penetration of the toxic chemicals is prevented they remain on the skin and decontamination should be performed when possible. Delay of decontamination is possible because of IB1 high safety and compatibility with the skin. IB1 is a mixture of widely used and safe ingredients and this prevents possible side effects. In contrast, SERPACWA consists of a mixture of perfluoroalkylpolyether and polytetrafluoroethylene (PRFE). The handling of smoking products, such as cigarettes, by personnel who have even small amounts of

SERPACWA on their hands may result in contamination that might lead to polymer fume fever [25].

The expected use of IB1 is by application on exposed and sensitive skin areas (armpits, groin, waist, wrists), when necessary for both military troops and civilian populations. It is easily applied on the skin and removed by rinsing with water and a quantity of 10–15 gr is sufficient for one application covering approximately 20% of the body surface.

In summary, IB1 (Dermostyx) has all the qualities required for efficient skin protectant: high efficacy against CWA agents (SM, VX) and TICs (ethyl parathion, acrolein), long-lasting protection (tested up to 12 h following single application), simple and readily available ingredients, and safe with no adverse effects or any toxicity.

References

1. Braue EH. Development of a reactive topical skin protectant. J Appl Toxicol. 1999;1:S47–53.
2. Kadar T, Fishbine E, Meshulam J, Sahar R, Amir A, Barness I. A topical skin protectant against chemical warfare agents. Isr Med Assoc J. 2003;5:1–3.
3. Eisenkraft A, Vidan A, Robenshtok E, Shochat T, Hourvitz A, Dushnitsky T. Phase I study of a protective cream against chemical warfare agents. Mil Med. 2009;174:47–55.
4. Duncan EJS, Brown A, Lundy P, et al. Site-specific percutaneous absorption of methyl salicylate and VX in domestic swine. J Appl Toxicol. 2002;22:141–8.
5. Kadar T, Fishbine E, Meshulam Y, Sahar R, Chapman S, Liani H, Barness I, Amir A. Treatment of skin injuries induced by sulfur mustard with calmodulin antagonists, using the pig model. J Appl Toxicol. 2000;20:S133–6.
6. Babin MC, Ricketts K, Skvorak JP, Gazaway M, Mitcheltree LW, Casillas RP. Systemic administration of candidate antivesicants to protect against topically applied sulfur mustard in the mouse ear vesicant model (MEVM). J Appl Toxicol. 2000;20:S141–4.
7. Dachir S, Fishbine E, Meshulam Y, Sahar R, Amir A, Kadar T. Screening of potential anti-inflammatory treatments against cutaneous sulfur mustard using the mouse ear vesicant model. Hum Exp Toxicol. 2002;21:197–203.
8. Dachir S, Fishbeine E, Meshulam Y, Sahar R, Chapman S, Amir A, Kadar T. Amelioration of sulfur mustard skin injury following a topical treatment with a mixture of a steroid and a NSAID. J Appl Toxicol. 2004;24:107–13.
9. Munro NB, Ambrose KR, Watson AP. Toxicity of the organophosphate chemical warfare agents GA, GB and VX. Implications for public protection. Environ Health Perspect. 1994;102:18–38.
10. Hayes GR, Funckes AJ Jr, Hartwell WV. Dermal exposure of human volunteers to parathion. Arch Environ Health. 1964;8:829–33.
11. Kramer RE, Wellman SE, Zhu H, Rockhold RW, Baker RC. A comparison of cholinesterase activity after intravenous, oral or dermal administration of methyl parathion. J Biomed Sci. 2002;9:140–8.
12. Ghilarducci DP, Tjeerdema RS. Fate and effects of acrolein. Environ Contam Toxicol. 1995;144:95–146.
13. Bein K, Leikauf GD. Acrolein – a pulmonary hazard. Mol Nutr Food Res. 2011;55:1342–60.
14. Dachir S, Cohen M, Cohen L, Buch H, Kadar T. Acute and long-term ocular effects of acrolein vapor on the eyes and potential therapies. Cutan Ocul Toxicol. 2015;34:286–93.

15. Johnson CD, Russell RL. A rapid simple radiometric assay for cholinesterase, suitable for multiple determinations. Anal Biochem. 1975;64:229–38.
16. Koper O, Lucas E, Klabunde KJ. Development of reactive topical skin protectants against sulfur mustard and nerve agents. J Appl Toxicol. 1999;19:S59–70.
17. Braue EH, Smith KH, Doxzon BF, Lumpkin HL, Clarkson ED. Efficacy studies of reactive skin decontamination lotion, M291 skin decontamination kit, 0.5% bleach, 1% soapy water, and skin exposure reduction paste against chemical warfare agents, part 1: guinea pigs challenged with VX. Cut Ocular Toxicol. 2011;30:15–28.
18. Braue EH, Smith KH, Doxzon BF, Lumpkin HL, Clarkson ED. Studies of reactive skin decontamination lotion, M291 skin decontamination kit, 0.5% bleach, 1% soapy water, and skin exposure reduction paste against chemical warfare agents, part 1: guinea pigs challenged with soman. Cutan Ocul Toxicol. 2011;30:29–37.
19. Elias PM. Dynamics of the epidermal barrier: new implications for percutaneous drug delivery, topical therapeutics and disease pathogenesis. Prog Dermatol. 1992;26:1–8.
20. Liu DK, Wannemacher RW, Snider TH, Hayes TL. Efficacy of the topical skin protectant in advanced development. In Proceedings of the 1998 Medical Defense Bioscience Review. US Army Medical Research and Materiel Command, MD, USA, pp. 1–8.
21. Silva CL, Topgaard D, Kocherbitov V, Sousa JJS, Pais AACC, Sparr E. Stratum corneum hydration: phase transformations and mobility in stratum corneum, extracted lipids and isolated corneocytes. Biochim Biophys Acta. 2007;1768:2647–59.
22. Reiger MM, Deem DE. Skin moisturizers. The effects of cosmetic ingredients on human stratum corneum. J Soc Cosmet Chem. 1974;25:253–62.
23. Batt MD, Fairhurst E. Hydration of the stratum corneum. Int J Cosmet Sci. 1986;8:253–64.
24. Fluhr JW, Gloor M, Lehmann L, Lazzerini S, Distante F, Berardesca E. Glycerol accelerates recovery of barrier function in vivo. Acta Derm Venereol. 1999;79:418–21.
25. Skin exposure reduction paste against chemical warfare agents (SERPACWA). www.accessdata.fda.gov/drugsatfda_docs/label/2000/21084lbl.pdf.

Chapter 12
Understanding the Impact of Responder Management Strategies on Public Experiences and Behaviour During Mass Casualty Decontamination

Holly Carter, John Drury, and Richard Amlôt

As demonstrated by the extensive research presented within this volume, there is now a wealth of evidence relating to best practices in terms of optimising physical and technical aspects of skin decontamination in response to chemical, biological, radiological, and nuclear (CBRN) incidents. There is another factor that must also be considered when ensuring that skin decontamination is as effective as possible: will those affected be prepared to undertake recommended decontamination actions? Traditionally, the answer to this question has relied on two (contradictory) assumptions. The first is that people will automatically take actions recommended to them in these situations; they will be frightened and will rely on emergency responders to help them [5, 8]. The second is that people will not take recommended decontamination actions; they will behave in an irrational and disorderly way, and emergency responders will need to control this disorderly and irrational behaviour [5, 12].

However, recent research has demonstrated that public behaviour is much more nuanced in these situations, and that the way in which members of the public behave will be determined in large part by the way in which the incident is managed. This is particularly the case during incidents involving *mass* decontamination, in which there will be a relatively small number of emergency responders compared to members of the public. When decontamination is required, people will respond both to the perceived threat (the possibility of being contaminated) and the way the threat is managed (actions taken by emergency responders). The way an incident is managed will therefore affect the way members of the public respond. Understanding how responder management strategies can affect public behaviour, and hence the efficacy of decontamination, is crucial to ensuring the success of the decontamination process.

H. Carter · R. Amlôt (✉)
Emergency Response Department Science and Technology, Public Health England, Salisbury, UK
e-mail: Richard.Amlot@phe.gov.uk

J. Drury
School of Psychology, University of Sussex, Brighton, UK

H. Zhu, H. I. Maibach (eds.), *Skin Decontamination*,
https://doi.org/10.1007/978-3-030-24009-7_12

Incidents involving mass decontamination involve intergroup encounters between a crowd and emergency responders, and it is therefore helpful to consider principles from crowd behaviour theories when examining public behaviour during mass decontamination. In particular, the social identity approach [48, 49] has been beneficial in facilitating an understanding of public behaviour in this context. The social identity approach suggests that people have both personal and social identities, and that social identities are based on group memberships. When people come to share a social identity, it affects the way in which they interact with members of their own social group, and also with members of other social groups. In particular, when people share a social identity, they are more likely to cooperate with other group members, and act in accordance with group norms. People come to share a social identity when they perceive themselves as similar to other group members at some level of comparison. Some of the factors that enhance the likelihood of categorising oneself as similar to others include proximity to others, a sense of shared fate with other group members, and the perception of a shared threat; these are all factors that are associated with incidents involving mass decontamination, and hence application of the social identity approach can facilitate an improved understanding of public behaviour in this context.

This chapter has three key aims. First, we will describe research into likely public behaviour during mass emergencies, and demonstrate how the way in which an incident is managed will affect the way in which members of the public respond. Second, we will highlight how an effective responder management strategy can promote positive public behaviours during mass decontamination. Third, to outline some specific recommendations for optimising the way in which incidents involving mass decontamination are managed.

Why It Is Important to Understand Public Behaviour

Incidents involving CBRN agents are likely to be very frightening for members of the public, because they are unfamiliar and ambiguous (e.g. [15, 18, 41]). People will also probably be unfamiliar with the decontamination process, and it is possible that decontamination could be more stressful for the people affected than the CBRN incident itself [34]. This is especially likely in incidents where decontamination is not managed effectively [5].

Until recently, planning for incidents involving mass decontamination has focused on technical aspects, such as developing and testing decontamination equipment, and there hasn't been much consideration of likely public experiences and behaviour during the decontamination process (e.g. [5, 12]). Where likely public behaviour has been considered, there is often a reliance on common myths about disasters, such as public disorder or mass panic. However, over 50 years of research has shown that panic occurs very rarely (if at all) during mass emergencies and disasters, and that people are much more likely to behave in a helpful and cooperative way (e.g. [1, 2, 16, 17, 20–24, 35, 36, 40]).

The reliance on common myths about disasters can lead to a focus on the need to impose control on the actions of members of the public, with a perception that imposing such control will prevent people from 'panicking' and behaving in a disorderly way (e.g. [3, 25]). These types of control management strategies can involve withholding information from members of the public (e.g. [27, 30, 31]), and failure to respect the needs of the public (e.g. [5, 32]). This reliance on control management strategies is concerning, because research shows that these types of control management strategies may create public disorder, rather than preventing it (e.g. [26, 42, 44, 47]). The reason for this is that members of the public may see attempts to control or coerce them as illegitimate action on the part of emergency responders. This perception that responders are behaving in an illegitimate way may result in members of the public uniting to challenge the authority of emergency responders, thus creating the very disorder that emergency responders were hoping to prevent (e.g. [43, 45, 47]).

In addition to having the potential to create public disorder, withholding information from members of the public will make it difficult for them to undergo decontamination (even if they are willing to). As noted above, during incidents involving decontamination, there will likely be a relatively small number of responders, compared to members of the public. Because of this, members of the public will need to take action to help themselves: this will not be possible if they are not given information about the actions they need to take [9].

There is therefore a need to update planning and guidance for mass decontamination, to make sure that these are based on relevant theory and research about public behaviour, and not on outdated assumptions about mass panic. We have carried out extensive research to understand how members of the public are likely to experience mass decontamination, and how the way in which responders manage an incident involving mass decontamination will affect the way in which members of the public respond. Our research has been used to inform guidance and training for emergency responders and policy makers in planning for and managing mass decontamination, and the key findings are described below.

How Effective Management Can Promote Improved Decontamination Outcomes

In terms of promoting positive public behaviours in mass casualty decontamination, an effective management strategy will achieve five key things: (1) it will get people to agree to undergo decontamination; (2) it will help people to undergo decontamination quickly and efficiently; (3) it will encourage people to cooperate with each other during decontamination; (4) it will make people feel less anxious; and (5) it will ensure that those with greater functional needs are able to undergo decontamination. In order to understand how effective management can improve decontamination outcomes, a number of research studies have been carried out. These include a review of real-life small-scale incidents involving decontamination [5], a review of the literature relating to decontamination of members of vulnerable groups [12], focus groups with members of the public [13, 14], analysis of data from mass decontamination field exercises [6, 7], and mass decontamination online and field experiments [9, 10]. Each of these outcomes is described in further detail below, alongside relevant research.

Getting People to Agree to Undergo Decontamination

Getting people to agree to undergo decontamination will be crucial to the success of the decontamination process. For decontamination to be successful, people will need to agree to undertake any actions recommended by emergency responders. These actions may include disrobing, undergoing improvised and/or interim decontamination, and undergoing a decontamination shower in a specialist mass decontamination unit.

As mentioned above, decontamination may be frightening and embarrassing for members of the public, and this may make them reluctant to agree to undergo decontamination (e.g. [32, 50, 51]). A review of small-scale decontamination incidents showed that refusal to undergo decontamination was common [5]. This was especially the case during incidents in which people felt that they had not received sufficient information from emergency responders about the decontamination process, and when they felt that their needs for privacy and modesty had not been respected. Any reluctance of people to undergo decontamination will delay decontamination, and could potentially cost lives (e.g. [28]). It is therefore essential that people agree to undergo decontamination, and that they do so in a quick and efficient way.

Emergency responders can encourage people to agree to undergo decontamination by doing two key things. First, emergency responders should explain to members of the public why it is necessary for them to undergo decontamination. If people don't understand why decontamination is important they are unlikely to agree to do it. Explanations should be health-focused where possible, should explain how undergoing decontamination will reduce the risk of further harm from the contaminant and will also potentially prevent secondary contamination of other people and places [9, 11]. Second, by showing respect for public needs for privacy. If people don't feel that their needs for privacy and modesty have been met, they are unlikely to agree to undergo decontamination. While it may not always be possible to provide people with the level of privacy they would like, it is important to communicate why this is the case, and therefore demonstrate an understanding of and respect for public needs [11].

Doing these two things will demonstrate that responders are managing the incident in a legitimate way and will promote trust in emergency responders and the information that they provide. A key finding from our research into public behaviour during mass decontamination is that a perception that responders are managing an incident in a legitimate way is crucial for getting people to agree to undergo decontamination. When people feel that they have received effective communication, and that their needs for privacy have been met, this results in increased perceived legitimacy of emergency responders and the actions that they are taking. This is crucial, because this perception of responder legitimacy facilitates the formation of shared identity between members of the public and emergency responders which, as noted above, enhances cooperation with other group members and encourages people to act in accordance with group norms (e.g. the norm of undergoing decontamination). Shared identity between members of the public and emergency responders therefore encourages people to agree to undergo decontamination [11].

Helping People to Undergo Decontamination Quickly and Efficiently

As the section above demonstrates, getting people to agree to undergo decontamination is a crucial first step in ensuring that decontamination is successful. The next step is to make sure that people know what they need to do, to help them to undergo decontamination quickly and efficiently. The key to quick and efficient decontamination is to provide people with sufficient practical information about the actions that they need to take. Findings from decontamination field exercises show that people consistently report that they have not received practical information about what to do during the decontamination process, and consequently, that they are confused and don't know what actions to take [6, 7].

To understand more about the effect of different levels of information on public behaviour during mass decontamination, we carried out a mass decontamination field experiment. During this experiment, three different groups of participants were provided with different levels of information before they underwent decontamination. Information included explanations about the importance of decontamination, updates about actions responders were taking, and practical information about the actions that participants needed to take during the decontamination process [9]. Participants were timed going through decontamination to enable a comparison of decontamination efficiency between groups. The optimum time for participants to complete the entire decontamination process was 9 minutes and 30 seconds. Findings showed that those who were provided with the most detailed information went through the decontamination process more quickly and efficiently than those who were provided with less detailed information, and in closest to the optimum time. In fact, of those who received the less detailed information, the slowest participants took 19 minutes and 48 seconds to undergo the full decontamination process; this is almost twice as long as the process should have taken.

This therefore illustrates how important it is for emergency responders to provide people with detailed information about the actions people need to take during decontamination, and not to assume that people will know what actions they need to take. It has sometimes been suggested by emergency responders and policy makers that during decontamination there will not be time to provide people with information, and that doing so will delay the decontamination process. The findings presented here show that the opposite is true: the more information that people can be provided with about what to do during decontamination, the more quick and efficient the process is likely to be.

Encouraging People to Cooperate with Each Other During Decontamination

As well as being willing and able to undergo decontamination quickly and efficiently, those involved will also need to cooperate with each other to make sure that the decontamination process runs smoothly. Cooperating with each other in the context of decontamination involves two different aspects:

1. Behaving in an orderly and cooperative way during decontamination (e.g. forming an orderly queue to go through the decontamination process). As noted at the start of this chapter, this type of orderly and cooperative behaviour is common during mass emergencies, and disorderly behaviour tends to be rare (e.g. [2, 16, 17, 19, 29, 35, 36]).
2. Actively helping others (e.g. helping to assist someone who has difficulty walking to go through the decontamination process). This type of active helping has also been shown to be common during mass emergencies and disasters, particularly where people experience a sense of shared social identity with each other (e.g. [22–24]).

Given the low number of responders to members of the public during incidents requiring decontamination, the more that members of the public are willing to cooperate with and assist each other during decontamination, the more smoothly the decontamination process is likely to run. It is therefore important to understand what makes people more or less likely to behave helpfully and cooperatively during decontamination, so that such behaviour can be encouraged.

The social identity approach [48, 49] suggests that people are more likely to cooperate with each other if they identify with each other. In mass emergencies, people often experience a sense of shared fate (in relation to the emergency) that leads them to identify with others 'in the same boat' (e.g. [22–24]). When there is a shared identity amongst a group of people, this results in:

1. The internalisation of shared goals and motivation to contribute to the achievement of such goals (in this case, the goal of undergoing decontamination) [33].
2. A sense of collective efficacy, which is a belief that those involved in the incident can work together to achieve shared goals, and to overcome any challenges that they face [23].
3. Motivation to help and cooperate with other group members [37–39].

A sense of shared identity will therefore be crucial for encouraging those affected to cooperate with each other when undergoing decontamination. As described above, those involved in a mass emergency are likely to experience a sense of shared identity, as a result of the sense of shared fate that they all face. In the case of incidents involving mass decontamination, it is important that people also identify with the emergency responders managing the incident. If members of the public experience shared identity with each other, and not with emergency responders, they may work together to challenge responder authority, rather than to go through decontamination [11, 26, 46, 47].

To ensure that identification is also shared between members of the public and emergency responders, it is again crucial that emergency responders communicate effectively with members of the public. As described above, effective communication results in perceptions that responders are managing the incident in a legitimate way. Perceptions of responder legitimacy have been shown to be key in promoting shared identity between members of the public and emergency responders during mass decontamination [7, 9, 10]. Effective communication therefore encourages people to cooperate with each other in two ways (e.g. [7, 9, 10]):

1. It promotes *willingness* to cooperate with each other, by establishing trust, which in turn enhances identification with emergency responders and ensures that undergoing decontamination is accepted as a shared goal.
2. It promotes *ability* to cooperate with each other – by providing people with the information that they need in order to know what to do during decontamination, and therefore to be able to work together. Ensuring that people know what to do during decontamination promotes a sense of collective agency, enabling people to work together to achieve shared goals (i.e. decontamination).

Making People Feel Less Anxious

As described at the beginning of this chapter, CBRN incidents have the potential to be very frightening for those involved, because they are unfamiliar and ambiguous (e.g. [15, 18, 41]). The decontamination process is also likely to be unfamiliar and frightening for those involved [34]. Decontamination involves the need to remove clothes and undergo a shower in front of others. It is therefore likely to be embarrassing, which may result in high levels of public anxiety.

It is important that emergency responders understand that while panic will be rare, and people are likely to behave rationally, they are still likely to be anxious. While a certain level of anxiety is to be expected during incidents involving CBRN agents, it is important that this concern is in proportion to the potential effects of any contaminant, rather than in relation to the decontamination process itself. Understanding what factors may increase public anxiety about the decontamination process will help emergency responders to manage this when carrying out decontamination.

Our review of findings from small-scale incidents involving decontamination revealed the potential for high levels of anxiety amongst members of the public about the decontamination process. This was especially the case during incidents in which those affected felt they had not received adequate information about the decontamination process, and when they felt that their concerns about dignity and modesty had not been addressed [5, 32, 50, 51].

To reduce public anxiety about the decontamination process, it is therefore important that emergency responders communicate with those affected about why it is important for them to undergo decontamination, and how decontamination will help to protect them (and others) from the effects of any contaminant. It is also important that those affected feel that their needs for privacy and modesty are being considered during the decontamination process. Failure to respect public needs for privacy has been shown to be a key factor in increasing public anxiety, and reducing public compliance, during decontamination [4–7, 9, 11].

Understanding the Needs of Vulnerable Groups

As well as the review of small-scale incidents, we also carried out a review to examine the literature relating to decontamination of members of vulnerable groups [12]. This revealed that there are a large number of different factors that may make someone vulnerable during decontamination, and there is often considerable overlap between the needs of different vulnerable groups. Because of this, it is helpful to take a 'functional needs' approach. This type of approach involves considering the greater needs that some people may have during decontamination [12]. There are four main functional needs that should be considered when planning for mass decontamination: (1) impaired ability to physically undergo decontamination (e.g. anyone who may struggle to undergo decontamination unassisted); (2) impaired ability to communicate during the decontamination process (e.g. difficulty in seeing, hearing, or understanding instructions); (3) different social or cultural needs (e.g. cultural or religious norms); and (4) pre-existing health factors or medical conditions (e.g. any factors that may make someone more susceptible to the effects of contamination or may make it more difficult for them to successfully undergo the decontamination process).

The review of literature relating to the needs of vulnerable groups during decontamination highlighted several potential recommendations for those with different functional needs. From the findings of this review, we suggest that emergency responders should: treat each individual as an expert in his or her own needs during decontamination; implement a buddy system, whereby a person with additional functional needs is paired with another member of the public during decontamination; provide simple pictorial instructions; consider allowing individuals to retain any functional aids that they may have (e.g. prosthetic limbs, walking aids, hearing aids) during the decontamination process; and consider potential ethical, religious, and cultural needs when asking people to disrobe.

Recommendations for Optimising Management of Mass Decontamination

1. *Responders should communicate openly and honestly with members of the public, and should provide regular updates about any actions that they are taking.* This will help to establish trust and a perception that responders are managing the incident in a legitimate way, which will promote compliance with responder instructions.
2. *Emergency responders should communicate in a health-focused way about the importance of decontamination.* Specifically, responders should communicate: (1) *why* decontamination is necessary, in terms of removing any potential contaminant from the skin and preventing any further risks to health; (2) *how* decontamination will protect someone, and their loved ones. Failure to remove contaminant from someone's skin could result in secondary contamination of other people and places, including potentially a person's home and family; and (3) *what* the process will involve. It is important that members of the public understand exactly what the decontamination process will involve before they undergo it, since this is likely to reduce public anxiety, and increase public compliance.
3. *Emergency responders should provide members of the public with sufficient practical information during the decontamination process.* Provision of sufficient practical information during the decontamination process improves the speed and efficiency of decontamination, reduces confusion, and could therefore save lives during a real incident involving mass decontamination.
4. *Emergency responders should respect public needs for privacy and modesty.* Failure to respect public needs for privacy can reduce public compliance, and therefore result in delays to decontamination.
5. *Emergency responders should treat everyone as an expert in his or her own needs during decontamination.* Treating each person as an individual will demonstrate respect for their needs, which should result in increased perceptions of legitimacy, and increased compliance. Training and exercising should be carried out with those with different functional needs, to ensure that plans are in place should a real incident occur.

The evidence presented within this chapter demonstrates that if an incident involving mass decontamination is managed effectively (in line with the recommendations presented), this will increase the perceived legitimacy of responders and the actions they are taking, and will therefore promote compliance with responder instructions. The five recommendations presented here could therefore improve behavioural and psychological outcomes during mass decontamination, which could result in lives being saved during a real incident.

However, if an incident is not managed effectively, members of the public may unite to challenge the authority of emergency responders, resulting in non-compliance with decontamination procedures. A particular problem can be when 'control' management strategies are used. Such control strategies can lead to a belief that emergency responders are behaving in an unfair or illegitimate way, which can lead to reduced public compliance, and even attempts to challenge responders' authority. A key finding from this research is that the way in which emergency responders manage an incident will affect the nature of the relationship between emergency responders and members of the public. This will in turn affect the way in which members of the public behave and will ultimately affect the outcomes of the incident.

Acknowledgement Richard Amlôt and Holly Carter are affiliated to the National Institute for Health Research Health Protection Research Unit (NIHR HPRU) in Emergency Preparedness and Response at King's College London in partnership with Public Health England (PHE), in collaboration with the University of East Anglia and Newcastle University. The views expressed are those of the authors and not necessarily those of the NHS, the NIHR, the Department of Health or Public Health England.

References

1. Aguirre BE. Commentary on "Understanding mass panic and other collective responses to threat and disaster". Emergency evacuations, panic, and social psychology. Psychiatry. 2005;68(2):121–9.
2. Aguirre BE, Torres MR, Gill KB, Hotchkiss HL. Normative collective behaviour in the station building fire. Soc Sci Q. 2011;92(1):100–18.
3. Auf der Heide E. Common misconceptions about disasters: panic, the 'disaster syndrome', and looting. In: O'Leary M, editor. The first 72 hours: a community approach to disaster preparedness. Lincoln, Nebraska: iUniverse Publishing; 2004. p. 340–80.
4. Carter H, Drury J, Rubin GJ, Williams R, Amlôt R. Public experiences of mass casualty decontamination. Biosecur Bioterror. 2012;10(3):280–9.
5. Carter H, Drury J, Rubin GJ, Williams R, Amlôt R. Communication during mass casualty decontamination: highlighting the gaps. Int J Emerg Serv. 2013a;2(1):29–48.
6. Carter H, Drury J, Rubin GJ, Williams R, Amlôt R. The effect of communication on anxiety and compliance during mass decontamination. Disaster Prev Manag. 2013b;22(2):132–47.
7. Carter H, Drury J, Amlôt R, Rubin GJ, Williams R. Perceived responder legitimacy and group identification predict cooperation and compliance in a mass decontamination field exercise. Basic Appl Soc Psychol. 2013c;35(6):575–85.
8. Carter H, Drury J, Rubin GJ, Williams R, Amlôt R. Emergency responders' experiences of and expectations regarding decontamination. Int J Emerg Serv. 2014a;3(2):179–92.
9. Carter H, Drury J, Rubin GJ, Williams R, Amlôt R. Effective responder communication improves efficiency and psychological outcomes in a mass decontamination field experiment: implications for public behaviour in the event of a chemical incident. PLoS One. 2014b;9(3):e89846.
10. Carter H, Drury J, Amlôt R, Rubin GJ, Williams R. Effective responder communication, perceived responder legitimacy and group identification predict public cooperation and compliance in a mass decontamination visualisation experiment. J Appl Soc Psychol. 2015a;45(3):173–89.

11. Carter H, Drury J, Amlôt R, Rubin GJ, Williams R. Applying crowd psychology to develop recommendations for the management of mass decontamination. Health Secur. 2015b;13(1):45–53.
12. Carter H, Amlôt R. Mass casualty decontamination guidance and psychosocial aspects of CBRN incident management: a review and synthesis. PLoS Curr. 2016;27(1). https://doi.org/10.1371/currents.dis.c2d3d652d9d07a2a620ed5429e017ef5.
13. Carter H, Weston D, Betts N, Wilkinson S, Amlôt R. Public perceptions of emergency decontamination: effects of intervention type and responder management strategy during a focus group study. PLoS One. 2018;13(4):e0195922.
14. Carter H, Weston D, Symons C, Amlôt R. Public perceptions of pre-incident information campaign materials for the initial response to a chemical incident: the 'Remove, Remove, Remove' campaign. Disaster Prev Manag. (In press).
15. Cornish P. The CBRN system: assessing the threat of terrorist use of chemical, biological, radiological and nuclear weapons in the United Kingdom. London: Chatham House; 2007.
16. Cornwell B. Panic or situational constraints? The case of the M/V Estonia. Int J Mass Emerg Disasters. 2001;19(1):5–25.
17. Cornwell B. Bonded fatalities: relational and ecological dimensions of a fire evacuation. Sociol Q. 2003;44(4):617–38.
18. DiGiovanni C. Domestic terrorism with chemical or biological agents: psychiatric aspects. Am J Psychiatr. 1999;156(10):1500–5.
19. Donald I, Canter D. Behavioural aspects of the King's cross disaster. In: Canter D, editor. Fires and human behaviour. 2nd ed. David Fulton Publishers: London; 1990. p. 15–30.
20. Drury J. The role of social identity processes in mass emergency behaviour: an integrative review. Eur Rev Soc Psychol. 2018;29(1):38–81. https://doi.org/10.1080/10463283.2018.1471948.
21. Drury J, Carter H, Cocking C, Ntontis E, Tekin Guven S, Amlôt R. Facilitating collective psychosocial resilience in the public in emergencies: twelve recommendations based on the social identity approach. Front Public Health. (submitted).
22. Drury J, Cocking C, Reicher S. Everyone for themselves? A comparative study of crowd solidarity among emergency survivors. Br J Soc Psychol. 2009b;48:487–506.
23. Drury J, Cocking C, Reicher S. The nature of collective resilience: survivor reactions to the 2005 London bombings. Int J Mass Emerg Disasters. 2009a;27(1):66–95.
24. Drury J, Cocking C, Reicher S, Burton A, Schofield D, Hardwick A, Graham D, Langston P. Cooperation versus competition in a mass emergency evacuation: a new laboratory simulation and a new theoretical model. Behav Res Methods. 2009c;41(3):957–70.
25. Drury J, Novelli D, Stott C. Psychological disaster myths in the perception and management of mass emergencies. J Appl Soc Psychol. 2013;43(11):2259–70.
26. Drury J, Reicher S. Collective action and psychological change: the emergence of new social identities. Br J Soc Psychol. 2000;39:579–604.
27. Dynes RR. Community emergency planning: false assumptions and inappropriate analogies. Int J Mass Emerg Disasters. 1994;12(2):141–58.
28. Edwards NA, Caldicott DGE, Eliseo T, Pearce A. Truth hurts – hard lessons from Australia's largest mass casualty exercise with contaminated patients. Emerg Med Australas. 2006;18(2):185–95.
29. Feinberg WE, Johnson NR. The ties that bind: a macro-level approach to panic. Int J Mass Emerg Disasters, 2001;19(3).
30. Furedi F. Fear and security: a vulnerability-led policy response. Soc Policy Adm. 2008;42(6):645–61.
31. Gannt P, Gannt R. Disaster psychology: dispelling the myths of panic. Prof Saf. 2012;2012:42–9.
32. Hanley C. Residents sickened by pesticide cloud; ag officials insider changing rules. Latino News; 1999. Retrieved 7 October, 2010, from http://wearcam.org/decon/decon_like_rape_dec99.html
33. Haslam SA, Jetten J, Waghorn C. Social identification, stress and citizenship in teams: a five-phase longitudinal study. Stress Health. 2009;25:21–30.

34. Holloway HC, Norwood AE, Fullerton CS, Engel CC, Ursano RJ. The threat of biological weapons: prophylaxis and mitigation of psychological and social consequences. J Am Med Assoc. 1997;278(5):425–7.
35. Johnson NR. Panic at "the who concert stampede": an empirical assessment. Soc Probl. 1987;34(4):362–73.
36. Johnson NR. Fire in a crowded theatre: a descriptive investigation of the emergence of panic. Int J Mass Emerg Disasters. 1988;6(1):7–26.
37. Levine M, Cassidy C, Brazier G, Reicher S. Self-categorization and bystander non-intervention: two experimental studies. J Appl Soc Psychol. 2002;32(7):1452–63.
38. Levine M, Prosser A, Evans D, Reicher S. Identity and emergency intervention: how social group membership and inclusiveness of group boundaries shape helping behaviour. Personal Soc Psychol Bull. 2005;31:443.
39. Levine M, Thompson K. Identity, place, and bystander intervention: social categories and helping after natural disasters. J Soc Psychol. 2004;144(3):229–45.
40. Quarantelli EL. The nature and conditions of panic. Am J Sociol. 1954;60(3):267–75.
41. Regis E. Evaluating the threat: does mass biopanic portend mass destruction? Sci Am. 2001;285(6):21–3.
42. Reicher S. 'The Battle of Westminster': developing the social identity model of crowd behaviour in order to explain the initiation and development of collective conflict. Eur J Soc Psychol. 1996;26:115–34.
43. Reicher S. The psychology of crowd dynamics. In: Hogg MA, Tindale RS, editors. Blackwell handbook of social psychology: group processes. Oxford: Blackwell; 2001.
44. Stott C, Drury J. Crowds, context and identity: dynamic categorisation processes in the 'poll tax riot'. Hum Relat. 2000;53:247–73.
45. Stott C, Hoggett J, Pearson G. 'Keeping the peace': social identity, procedural justice and the policing of football crowds. Br J Criminol. 2012;52:381–99.
46. Stott C, Hutchison P, Drury J. 'Hooligans' abroad? Inter-group dynamics, social identity and participation in collective 'disorder' at the 1998 World Cup Finals. Br J Soc Psychol. 2001;40:359–84.
47. Stott C, Reicher S. How conflict escalates: the inter-group dynamics of collective football crowd 'violence'. Sociology. 1998;32:353–77.
48. Tajfel H, Turner J. An integrative theory of intergroup conflict. In: Austin WG, Worchel S, editors. The social psychology of intergroup relations. Monterey, CA: Wadsworth; 1979.
49. Turner JC, Hogg MA, Oakes PJ, Reicher SD, Wetherell MS. Rediscovering the social group: a self-categorization theory. Oxford, UK: Blackwell; 1987.
50. United States Fire Administration. Fire Department response to biological threat at B'nai B'rith headquarters. Washington, DC: United States Fire Administration; 1997.
51. Vogt BM, Sorensen JH. How clean is safe? Improving the effectiveness of decontamination of structures and people following chemical and biological incidents. Tennessee: Oak Ridge National Laboratory; 2002.

Appendix: Skin, Hair, and Nail – Abbreviated Decontamination Bibliography[1]

Radiation (Radioisotopes)[2]

Nishad, D. K., et al. (2018). "Decontamination of rat and human skin experimentally contaminated with 99mTc, 201Tl and 131I radionuclides using "Dermadecon"–a skin decontamination kit: an efficacy study." Cutaneous and Ocular Toxicology 37(1): 1–8.

Abstract: Radioactive skin contamination is one of the most likely risks which occurs after accidental or occupational radiological accidents apart from internal contamination. In such cases where the radioactive contamination has occurred, the person who is contaminated should be decontaminated as early as possible to reduce the damaging health effects of radiation. In the present study, the decontamination efficiency of a developed skin decontamination kit "dermadecon" has been evaluated in animal models and human subjects using gamma scintigraphy. Decontamination efficiency (percentage of the radioactive contaminant removed) was calculated for each radioactive isotope of the study and compared with control where general washing procedure was followed using liquid and soap. The effectiveness of the kit was calculated in animal model with respect to ^{99m}Tc-sodium-pertechnetate ($^{99m}TcO^{4-}$), ^{201}TlCl and ^{131}I and was found 92.84 ± 4.9%, 91.18 ± 3.23% and 94.67 ± 2.92%, respectively. Whereas, in case of human skin, the decontamination efficiency for $^{99m}TcO^{4-}$ was observed to be 95.00 ± 3.21%. On the basis of findings from the study, it can be concluded that the decontamination agents of the used skin decontamination kit are effective for removal of localized radioactive contaminants from skin, as compared with normal decontamination using soap and water.

[1] The editors welcome additional references...

[2] Newest-Oldest.

H. Zhu, H. I. Maibach (eds.), *Skin Decontamination*,
https://doi.org/10.1007/978-3-030-24009-7

Tazrart, A., et al. (2017). "Penetration and decontamination of americium-241 ex vivo using fresh and frozen pig skin." Chemico-Biological Interactions 267: 40–47.

Abstract: Skin contamination is one of the most probable risks following major nuclear or radiological incidents. However, accidents involving skin contamination with radionuclides may occur in the nuclear industry, in research laboratories and in nuclear medicine departments. This work aims to measure the penetration of the radiological contaminant Americium (^{241}Am) in fresh and frozen skin and to evaluate the distribution of the contamination in the skin. Decontamination tests were performed using water, Fuller's earth and diethylene triamine pentaacetic acid (DTPA), which is the recommended treatment in case of skin contamination with actinides such as plutonium or americium. To assess these parameters, we used the Franz cell diffusion system with full-thickness skin obtained from pigs' ears, representative of human skin. Solutions of ^{241}Am were deposited on the skin samples. The radioactivity content in each compartment and skin layers was measured after 24 h by liquid scintillation counting and alpha spectrophotometry. The Am cutaneous penetration to the receiver compartment is almost negligible in fresh and frozen skin. Multiple washings with water and DTPA recovered about 90% of the initial activity. The rest remains fixed mainly in the *stratum corneum*. Traces of activity were detected within the epidermis and dermis which is fixed and not accessible to the decontamination.

An, D. D., et al. (2017). "From early prophylaxis to delayed treatment: Establishing the plutonium decorporation activity window of hydroxypyridinonate chelating agents." Chemico-Biological Interactions 267: 80–88.

Abstract: The potential consequences of a major radiological event are not only large-scale external radiation exposure of the population, but also uncontrolled dissemination of, and internal contamination with, radionuclides. When planning an emergency response to radiological and nuclear incidents, one must consider the need for not only post-exposure treatment for contaminated individuals, but also prophylactic measures to protect the workforce facing contaminated areas and patients in the aftermath of such events. In addition to meeting the desired criteria for post-exposure treatments such as safety, ease of administration, and broad-spectrum efficacy against multiple radionuclides and levels of challenge, ideal prophylactic countermeasures must include rapid onset; induce minimal to no performance-decrementing side effects; be compatible with current military Chemical, Biological, Radiological, Nuclear, and Explosive countermeasures; and require minimal logistical burdens. Hydroxypyridinone-based actinide decorporation agents have shown the most promise as decorporation strategies for various radionuclides of concern, including the actinides plutonium and americium. The studies presented here probe the extent of plutonium decorporation efficacy for two chelating agents, 3,4,3-LI(1,2-HOPO) and 5-LIO(Me-3,2-HOPO), from early pre-exposure time points to a delay of up to 7 days in parenteral or oral treatment administration, i.e., well beyond the initial hours of emergency response. Despite delayed treatment after a contamination event, both ligands clearly enhanced plutonium elimination through the investigated 7-day post-treatment period. In addition, a remarkable prophylactic efficacy was revealed for 3,4,3-LI(1,2-HOPO) with treatment as early as 48 h before the plutonium challenge. This work provides new perspectives in the indication and use of experimental actinide decorporation treatments.

Sharma, N., et al. (2017). "Ex-vivo complexation, skin permeation, interaction and cytodermal toxicity studies of p-tertbutylcalix [4] arene nanoemulsion for radiation decontamination." Life Sciences 168: 65–76.

Abstract: *p-tertbutylcalix*[4]*arene* loaded nanoemulsion has been designed, characterized and evaluated for skin decontamination of radionuclides of interest in nuclear and radiological emergencies. Further, nanoemulsion was evaluated for Ex-vivo complexation, skin permeation, interaction and cytodermal toxicity.

- **Reference Type**: Journal Article
- **Record Number**: 5
- **Author**: Patyar, Rakesh Raman and Patyar, Sazal
- **Year**: 2017
- **Title**: Role of drugs in the prevention and amelioration of radiation induced toxic effects
- **Journal**: European Journal of Pharmacology
- **Short Title**: Role of drugs in the prevention and amelioration of radiation induced toxic effects
- **ISSN**: 0014-2999

Abstract: As the use of radiation technology for nuclear warfare or for the benefits of mankind (e.g. in radiotherapy or radio-diagnosis) is increasing tremendously, the risk of associated side effects is becoming a cause of concern. These effects, ranging from nausea/vomiting to death, may result from accidental or deliberate exposure and begin in seconds. Through this review paper, efforts have been done to critically review different compounds which have been investigated as radioprotectors and radiation mitigators. Radioprotectors are compounds which are administered just before or at the time of irradiation so as to minimize the radiation induced damage to normal tissues. And radiation mitigators are the compounds which can even minimize or ameliorate post irradiation-toxicity provided they are administered before the onset of toxic symptoms. A variety of agents have been investigated for their preventive and ameliorative potential against radiation induced toxic effects. This review article has focused on various aspects of the promising representative agents belonging to different classes of radioprotectors and mitigators. Many compounds have shown promising results, but till date only *amifostine* and *palifermin* are clinically approved by FDA. To fill this void in pharmacological armamentarium, focus should be shifted towards novel approaches.

Grives, S., et al. (2015). "Ex vivo uranium decontamination efficiency on wounded skin and *in vitro* skin toxicity of a calixarene-loaded nanoemulsion." Journal of Pharmaceutical Sciences 104(6): 2008–2017.
Abstract: The present work aims at studying the decontamination efficacy of a calixarene-loaded nanoemulsion on two *ex vivo* wounded skin models mimicking superficial stings or cuts contaminated with uranium, and on a third model using excoriation. The decontaminating formulation was compared with the currently used radio-decontaminating soapy water (Trait rouge®) treatment. Moreover, to assess skin damage potentially induced by the undiluted nanoemulsion, *in vitro* toxicity studies were conducted on an *in vitro* reconstructed human epidermis, coupled with three different toxicity tests [3-(4,5-dimethylthiazol-2-yl)-2,5 diphenyl tetrazolium bromide, lactate dehydrogenase, and interleukin-1-α]. This work demonstrated not only a significant decontamination activity of the calixarene nanoemulsion on wounded skin, ranging from 92% to 94% of the applied uranium solution according to the *ex vivo* model used, but also the absence of side effects of this promising treatment. (© 2015 Wiley Periodicals, Inc. and the American Pharmacists Association J Pharm Sci 104:2008–2017, 2015)

Rana, S., et al. (2014). "Scintigraphic evaluation of decontamination lotion for removal of radioactive contamination from skin." Disaster Medicine and Public Health Preparedness 8(2): 130–135.
Abstract: Skin contamination is one of the most likely risks after accidental or occupational radiological accidents. Using scintigraphy, we assessed a topical lotion for its decontamination efficacy (DE) after exposure with short-lived medical radioisotopes technetium Tc 99m (99mTc) and thallium 201Tl (201Tl).

Rana, S., et al. (2014). "p-Tertbutylcalix [4] arene nanoemulsion: Preparation, characterization and comparative evaluation of its decontamination efficacy against Technetium-99m, Iodine-131 and Thallium-201." Colloids and Surfaces B: Biointerfaces 117: 114–121.
Abstract: This study aimed to develop *p*-tertbutylcalix[4]arene o/w nanoemulsion for decontamination of radioisotopes from skin. Formulation was characterized using dynamic light scattering (DLS), transmission electron microscopy (TEM), multi-photon confocal microscopy techniques and *in vitro* dissolution studies. *In vivo* evaluation of nano-emulsion was done using nuclear medicine technique. Stability studies and dermal toxicity studies were also carried out. Comparative decontamination efficacy (DE) studies were performed on synthetic human tissue equivalent material and Sprague Dawley rat against three commonly used medical radioisotopes, i.e., Technetium-99m (^{99m}Tc), Iodine-131 (^{131}I) and Thallium-201 (^{201}Tl). Decontamination was performed using cotton swabs soaked in nanoemulsion at different time intervals of contaminants exposure. Whole body imaging and static counts were recorded using gamma camera before and after each decontamination attempt data was analyzed using one way analysis of variance (ANOVA) and found to be statistically significant ($p < 0.05$). DE of the nanoemulsion loaded with *p*-tertbutylcalix[4]arene was observed to be 88 ± 5%, 90 ± 3% and 89 ± 3% for

^{99m}Tc, ^{131}I and ^{201}Tl respectively. Dermal toxicity studies revealed no significant differences between treated and control animals. Skin histopathology slides with and without API (Active pharmaceutical ingredients) also found to be comparable. *p*-Tertbutylcalix[4]arene loaded nanoemulsion shows great promise for skin decontamination against broad ranges of radiological contaminants besides being stable and safe.

- **Reference Type**: Journal Article
- **Record Number**: 42
- **Author**: Phan, Guillaume, Semili, Naïma, Bouvier-Capely, Céline, Landon, Géraldine, Mekhloufi, Ghozlene, Huang, Nicolas, Rebière, François, Agarande, Michelle and Fattal, Elias
- **Year**: 2013
- **Title**: Calixarene cleansing formulation for uranium skin contamination
- **Journal**: Health Physics
- **Volume**: 105
- **Issue**: 4
- **Pages**: 382–389
- **Short Title**: Calixarene cleansing formulation for uranium skin contamination
- **ISSN**: 0017-9078
- **DOI**: https://doi.org/10.1097/HP.0b013e318298e8d3
- **Accession Number**: 00004032-201310000-00011

Keywords: Chelation; Contamination; Occupational safety; Uranium

Abstract: Abstract An oil-in-water cleansing emulsion containing calixarene molecule, an actinide specific chelating agent, was formulated in order to improve the decontamination of uranium from the skin. Commonly commercialized cosmetic ingredients such as surfactants, mineral oil, or viscosifying agents were used in preparing the calixarene emulsion. The formulation was characterized in terms of size and apparent viscosity measurements and then was tested for its ability to limit uranyl ion permeation through excoriated pig-ear skin explants in 24-h penetration studies. Calixarene emulsion effectiveness was compared with two other reference treatments consisting of DTPA and EHBP solutions. Application of calixarene emulsion induced the highest decontamination effect with an 87% decrease in uranium diffusion flux. By contrast, EHBP and DTPA solutions only allowed a 50% and 55% reduction of uranium permeation, respectively, and had the same effect as a simple dilution of the contamination by pure water. Uranium diffusion decrease was attributed to uranyl ion-specific chelation by calixarene within the formulation, since no significant effect was obtained after application of the same emulsion without calixarene. Thus, calixarene cleansing emulsion could be considered as a promising treatment in case of accidental contamination of the skin by highly diffusible uranium compounds. Health Phys. 105(4):000-000; 2013

URL: https://journals.lww.com/health-physics/Fulltext/2013/10000/Calixarene_Cleansing_Formulation_for_Uranium_Skin.11.aspx

- **Reference Type**: Journal Article
- **Record Number**: 86
- **Author**: Rana, Sudha, Dutta, Mita, Soni, Nakshe L, Chopra, Mahendra K, Kumar, Vinod, Goel, Rajeev, Bhatnagar, Aseem, Sultana, Sarwat and Sharma, Rakesh Kumar
- **Year**: 2012
- **Title**: Decontamination of human and rabbit skin experimentally contaminated with 99m Tc radionuclide using the active components of "Shudhika"—a skin decontamination kit
- **Journal**: Prehospital and Disaster Medicine
- **Volume**: 27
- **Issue**: 2
- **Pages**: 162–166
- **Short Title**: Decontamination of human and rabbit skin experimentally contaminated with 99m Tc radionuclide using the active components of "Shudhika"—a skin decontamination kit
- **ISSN**: 1945-1938

Abstract: INTRODUCTION: Radioactive contamination can occur as a result of accidental or intentional release of radioactive materials (RM) into the environment. RM may deposit on clothing, skin, or hair. Decontamination of contaminated persons should be done as soon as possible to minimize the deleterious health effects of radiation. The goal of this study was to evaluate the decontamination efficiency (for residual contaminant) of the active components of "Shudhika," an indigenously developed skin decontamination kit. The study kit is for external radioactive decontamination of intact skin.

METHODS: Decontamination efficiency was evaluated on the skin surface of rabbit (n = 6) and human volunteers (n = 13). 99mTc sodium pertechnetate (200-250 μCi) was used as the radio-contaminant. Skin surface area (5 × 5 cm^2) of thoracic abdominal region of the rabbit and the forearm and the palm of human volunteers were used for the study. Decontamination was performed by using cotton swabs soaked with chemical decontamination agents of the kit.

RESULTS: Decontamination efficiency (% of the contaminant removed) was calculated for each component of the study. Overall effectiveness of the kit was calculated to be 85% ± 5% in animal and 92% ± 3% in human skin surfaces. Running water and liquid soap with water was able to decontaminate volunteers' hand and animal skin up to 70% ± 5%. Chemical decontamination agents were applied only for trace residues (30% ± 5%). Efficiency of all the kit components was found up to be 20% ± 3% (animal) and 28% ± 2 (human), respectively. Residual contamination after final decontamination attempt for both the models was observed to be 12% ± 3% and 5% ± 2%. After 24 and 48 hours of the decontamination procedure, skin was found to be normal (no redness, erythema and edema were observed).

CONCLUSION: Decontaminants of the study kit were effective in removal of localized radioactive skin contamination when water is ineffective for further decontamination. By using the chemical decontaminants of the study kit, the use of water and radioactive waste generation could be reduced. Cross-contamination could also be avoided. During radiologic emergencies where water may be radioactively contaminated, the study kit could be used.

Schulze, P. and W. Lake (2008). Guidelines for mass casualty decontamination during a HAZMAT/weapon of mass destruction incident. Volumes 1 and 2, US Army Chemical Biological, Radiological and Nuclear School and US Army Edgewood Chemical Biological Center.
Abstract: N/A

Bernaola, O. and A. Filevich (1970). "Fast drying strippable protective cover for radioactive decontamination." Health Physics 19(5): 685–687.
Abstract: N/A

- **Reference Type**: Journal Article
- **Record Number**: 55
- **Author**: Vorob'ev, AM
- **Year**: 1967
- **Title**: Selection of mixtures of wetting agents for cleansing the skin of radioactive contamination
- **Journal**: Gigiena i sanitariia
- **Volume**: 32
- **Issue**: 7
- **Pages**: 45
- **Short Title**: Selection of mixtures of wetting agents for cleansing the skin of radioactive contamination
- **ISSN**: 0016-9900

Chemical Warfare Agents (CWAs)

Cao, Y., et al. (2018). "Binding affinity and decontamination of dermal decontamination gel to model chemical warfare agent simulants." Journal of Applied Toxicology 38(5): 724–733.
Abstract: Six chemical warfare agent simulants (trimethyl phosphate, dimethyl adipate, 2-chloroethyl methyl sulfide, diethyl adipate, chloroethyl phenyl sulfide and diethyl sebacate) were studied in *in vitro* human skin to explore relationship between dermal penetration/absorption and the mechanisms of simulant partitioning between stratum corneum (SC) and water as well as between dermal decontamination gel (DDGel) and water. Both binding affinity to and decontamination of simulants using DDGel were studied. Partition coefficients of six simulants between SC and water (Log $P_{SC/w}$) and between DDGel and water (Log $P_{DDGel/w}$) were determined. Results showed that DDGel has a similar or higher binding affinity to each simulant compared to SC. The relationship between Log P octanol/water and Log $P_{SC/w}$ as well as between Log P octanol/water and Log $P_{DDGel/w}$ demonstrated that partition coefficient of simulants correlated to their lipophilicity or hydrophilicity. Decontamination efficiency results with DDGel for these simulants were consistent with binding affinity results. Amounts of percentage dose of chemicals in DDGel of trimethyl phosphate, dimethyl adipate,

2-chloroethyl methyl sulfide, diethyl adipate, chloroethyl phenyl sulfide and diethyl sebacate were determined to be 61.15, 85.67, 75.91, 53.53, 89.89 and 76.58, with corresponding amounts absorbed in skin of 0.96, 0.65, 1.68, 0.72, 0.57 and 1.38, respectively. *In vitro* skin decontamination experiments coupled with a dermal absorption study demonstrated that DDGel can efficiently remove chemicals from skin surface, back-extract from the SC, and significantly reduced chemical penetration into skin or systemic absorption for all six simulants tested. Therefore, DDGel offers a great potential as a NextGen skin Decon platform technology for both military and civilian use.

- **Reference Type**: Journal Article
- **Record Number**: 1
- **Author**: Carniato, F., Bisio, C., Evangelisti, C., Psaro, R., Dal Santo, V., Costenaro, D., Marchese, L. and Guidotti, M.
- **Year**: 2018
- **Title**: Iron-montmorillonite clays as active sorbents for the decontamination of hazardous chemical warfare agents
- **Journal**: Dalton Transactions (Cambridge, England: 2003)
- **Volume**: 47
- **Issue**: 9
- **Pages**: 2939-2948
- **Date**: 2018/02/27
- **Short Title**: Iron-montmorillonite clays as active sorbents for the decontamination of hazardous chemical warfare agents
- **Alternate Journal**: Dalton Trans
- **ISSN**: 1477-9226
- **DOI**: https://doi.org/10.1039/c7dt03859c
- **Accession Number**: 29441378
- **URL**: http://europepmc.org/abstract/MED/29441378; https://doi.org/10.1039/c7dt03859c; http://pubs.rsc.org/en/content/articlepdf/2018/dt/c7dt03859c
- **'File' Attachments**: internal-pdf://3829176425/Carniato-2018-Iron-montmorillonite clays as ac.pdf
- **Author Address**: Department of Sciences and Technological Innovation, University of Eastern Piedmont, viale T. Michel 11, 15121 Alessandria, Italy. chiara.bisio@uniupo.it.
- **Name of Database**: PubMed
- **Language**: English

Abstract: A class of heterogeneous catalysts based on commercial bentonite from natural origin, containing at least 80 wt% of montmorillonite clay, was designed to transform selectively and under mild conditions toxic organosulfur and organophosphorus chemical warfare agents into non-noxious products with a reduced impact on health and environment. The bentonite from the natural origin was modified by introducing iron species and acid sites in the interlayer space, aiming to obtain a sorbent with strong catalytic oxidising and hydrolytic properties. The catalytic performance of these materials was evaluated in the oxidative abatement of (2-chloroethyl)ethyl sulfide (CEES), a simulant of sulfur mustard, in the presence of aqueous hydrogen peroxide as an oxidant. A new decontamination formulation was, moreover, proposed and obtained by mixing sodium perborate, as a solid oxidant, to iron-bentonite catalysts. Solid-phase decontamination tests, performed on a cotton textile support contaminated with organosulfide and organophosphonate simulant agents revealed the good activity of the solid formulation, especially in the *in situ* detoxification of blistering agents. Tests carried out on the real blistering warfare agent, sulfur mustard (HD agent), showed that, thanks to the co-presence of the iron-based clay together with the solid oxidant component, a good decontamination of the test surface from the real warfare agent could be achieved (80% contaminant degradation, under ambient conditions, in 24 h).

Spiandore, M., et al. (2017). "Efficacy of scalp hair decontamination following exposure to vapours of sulphur mustard simulants 2-chloroethyl ethyl sulphide and methyl salicylate." Chemico-Biological Interactions 267: 74–79.
Abstract: Chemical warfare agents are an actual threat and victims' decontamination is a main concern when mass exposure occurs. Skin decontamination with current protocols has been widely documented, as well as surface decontamination. However, considering hair ability to trap chemicals in vapour phase, we investigated hair decontamination after exposure to sulphur mustard simulants methyl salicylate and 2-chloroethyl ethyl sulphide. Four decontamination protocols were tested on hair, combining showering and emergency decontamination (use of Fuller's earth or Reactive Skin Decontamination Lotion RSDL®). Both simulants were recovered from hair after treatment, but contents were significantly reduced (42–85% content allowance). Showering alone was the least efficient protocol. Concerning 2-chloroethyl ethyl sulphide, protocols did not display significant differences in decontamination efficacy. For MeS, use of emergency decontaminants significantly increased showering efficacy (10–20% rise), underlining their usefulness before thorough decontamination. Our results highlighted the need to extensively decontaminate hair after chemical exposure. Residual amounts after decontamination are challenging, as their release from hair could lead to health issues.

Lydon, H. L., et al. (2017). "Development of haemostatic decontaminants for treatment of wounds contaminated with chemical warfare agents. 3: Evaluation of *in vitro* topical decontamination efficacy using damaged skin." Journal of Applied Toxicology 37(8): 976–984.
Abstract: Previous studies have demonstrated that haemostatic products with an absorptive mechanism of action retain their clotting efficiency in the presence of toxic materials and are effective in decontaminating chemical warfare (CW) agents when applied to normal, intact skin. The purpose of this *in vitro* study was to assess three candidate haemostatic products for effectiveness in the decontamination of superficially damaged porcine skin exposed to the radiolabelled CW agents, soman (GD), VX and sulphur mustard (HD). Controlled physical damage (removal of the upper 100 μm skin layer) resulted in a significant enhancement of the dermal absorption of all three CW agents. Of the haemostatic products assessed,

WoundStat™ was consistently the most effective, being equivalent in performance to a standard military decontaminant (fuller's earth). These data suggest that judicious application of haemostatic products to wounds contaminated with CW agents may be a viable option for the clinical management of casualties presenting with contaminated, haemorrhaging injuries. Further studies using a relevant animal model are required to confirm the potential clinical efficacy of WoundStat™ for treating wounds contaminated with CW agents. (Copyright © 2017 John Wiley & Sons, Ltd.)

Das, L. M., et al. (2016). "Early indicators of survival following exposure to mustard gas: Protective role of 25 (OH) D." Toxicology Letters 248: 9–15.
Abstract: The use of sulfur mustard (SM) as a chemical weapon for warfare has once again assumed center stage, endangering civilian and the military safety. SM causes rapid local skin vesication and late-onset systemic toxicity. Most studies on SM rely on obtaining tissue and blood for characterizing burn pathogenesis and assessment of systemic pathology, respectively. However the present study focuses on developing a non-invasive method to predict mortality from high dose skin SM exposure. We demonstrate that exposure to SM leads to a dose dependent increase in wound area size on the dorsal surface of mice that is accompanied by a progressive loss in body weight loss, blood cytopenia, bone marrow destruction, and death. Thus our model utilizes local skin destruction and systemic outcome measures as variables to predict mortality in a novel skin-based model of tissue injury. Based on our recent work using vitamin D (25(OH)D) as an intervention to treat toxicity from SM-related compounds, we explored the use of 25(OH)D in mitigating the toxic effects of SM. Here we show that 25(OH)D offers protection against SM and is the first known demonstration of an intervention that prevents SM-induced mortality. Furthermore, 25(OH)D represents a safe, novel, and readily translatable potential countermeasure following mass toxic exposure.

- **Reference Type**: Journal Article
- **Record Number**: 21
- **Author**: Zhao, Junjie, Lee, Dennis T, Yaga, Robert W, Hall, Morgan G, Barton, Heather F, Woodward, Ian R, Oldham, Christopher J, Walls, Howard J, Peterson, Gregory W and Parsons, Gregory N
- **Year**: 2016
- **Title**: Ultra-fast degradation of chemical warfare agents using MOF–nanofiber kebabs
- **Journal**: Angewandte Chemie International Edition
- **Volume**: 55
- **Issue**: 42
- **Pages**: 13224–13228
- **Short Title**: Ultra-fast degradation of chemical warfare agents using MOF–nanofiber kebabs
- **ISSN**: 1521-3773
- **URL**: https://onlinelibrary.wiley.com/doi/abs/10.1002/anie.201606656

Abstract: The threat associated with chemical warfare agents (CWAs) motivates the development of new materials to provide enhanced protection with a reduced burden. Metal–organic frame-works (MOFs) have recently been shown as highly effective catalysts for detoxifying CWAs, but challenges still remain for integrating MOFs into functional filter media and/or protective garments. Herein, we report a series of MOF–nanofiber kebab structures for fast degradation of CWAs. We found TiO_2 coatings deposited via atomic layer deposition (ALD) onto polyamide-6 nanofibers enable the formation of conformal Zr-based MOF thin films including UiO-66, UiO-66-NH_2, and UiO-67. Cross-sectional TEM images show that these MOF crystals nucleate and grow directly on and around the nanofibers, with strong attachment to the substrates. These MOF-functionalized nanofibers exhibit excellent reactivity for detoxifying CWAs. The half-lives of a CWA simulant compound and nerve agent soman (GD) are as short as 7.3 min and 2.3 min, respectively. These results therefore provide the earliest report of MOF–nanofiber textile composites capable of ultra-fast degradation of CWAs.

- **Reference Type**: Journal Article
- **Record Number**: 85
- **Author**: Matar, Hazem, Guerreiro, Antonio, Piletsky, Sergey A, Price, Shirley C and Chilcott, Robert P
- **Year**: 2016
- **Title**: Preliminary evaluation of military, commercial and novel skin decontamination products against a chemical warfare agent simulant (methyl salicylate)
- **Journal**: Cutaneous and Ocular Toxicology
- **Volume**: 35
- **Issue**: 2
- **Pages**: 137–144
- **Short Title**: Preliminary evaluation of military, commercial and novel skin decontamination products against a chemical warfare agent simulant (methyl salicylate)
- **ISSN**: 1556-9527

Abstract: Rapid decontamination is vital to alleviate adverse health effects following dermal exposure to hazardous materials. There is an abundance of materials and products which can be utilised to remove hazardous materials from the skin. In this study, a total of 15 products were evaluated, 10 of which were commercial or military products and five were novel (molecular imprinted) polymers. The efficacies of these products were evaluated against a 10 µl droplet of 14C-methyl salicylate applied to the surface of porcine skin mounted on static diffusion cells. The current UK military decontaminant (Fuller's earth) performed well, retaining 83% of the dose over 24 h and served as a benchmark to compare with the other test products. The five most effective test products were Fuller's earth (the current UK military decontaminant), Fast-Act® and three novel polymers [based on itaconic acid, 2-trifluoromethylacrylic acid and N,N-methylenebis(acrylamide)]. Five products (medical moist-free wipes, 5% FloraFree™ solution, normal baby wipes, baby wipes for sensitive skin and Diphotérine™) enhanced the dermal absorption of 14C-methyl salicylate. Further work is required to establish the performance of the most effective products identified in this study against chemical warfare agents.

McElroy, C. S. and B. J. Day (2016). "Antioxidants as potential medical countermeasures for chemical warfare agents and toxic industrial chemicals." Biochemical Pharmacology 100: 1–11.

Abstract: The continuing horrors of military conflicts and terrorism often involve the use of chemical warfare agents (CWAs) and toxic industrial chemicals (TICs). Many CWA and TIC exposures are difficult to treat due to the danger they pose to first responders and their rapid onset that can produce death shortly after exposure. While the specific mechanism(s) of toxicity of these agents are diverse, many are associated either directly or indirectly with increased oxidative stress in affected tissues. This has led to the exploration of various antioxidants as potential medical countermeasures for CWA/TIC exposures. Studies have been performed across a wide array of agents, model organisms, exposure systems, and antioxidants, looking at an almost equally diverse set of endpoints. Attempts at treating CWAs/TICs with antioxidants have met with mixed results, ranging from no effect to nearly complete protection. The aim of this commentary is to summarize the literature in each category for evidence of oxidative stress and antioxidant efficacy against CWAs and TICs. While there is great disparity in the data concerning methods, models, and remedies, the outlook on antioxidants as medical countermeasures for CWA/TIC management appears promising.

- **Reference Type**: Journal Article
- **Record Number**: 7
- **Author**: Matar, Hazem, Guerreiro, Antonio, Piletsky, Sergey A, Price, Shirley C and Chilcott, Robert P
- **Year**: 2016
- **Title**: Preliminary evaluation of military, commercial and novel skin decontamination products against a chemical warfare agent simulant (methyl salicylate)
- **Journal**: Cutaneous and Ocular Toxicology
- Volume: 35
- **Issue**: 2
- **Pages**: 137–144
- **Short Title**: Preliminary evaluation of military, commercial and novel skin decontamination products against a chemical warfare agent simulant (methyl salicylate)
- **ISSN**: 1556-9527

Abstract: Rapid decontamination is vital to alleviate adverse health effects following dermal exposure to hazardous materials. There is an abundance of materials and products which can be utilised to remove hazardous materials from the skin. In this study, a total of 15 products were evaluated, 10 of which were commercial or military products and five were novel (molecular imprinted) polymers. The efficacies of these products were evaluated against a 10 µl droplet of 14C-methyl salicylate applied to the surface of porcine skin mounted on static diffusion cells. The current UK military decontaminant (Fuller's earth) performed well, retaining 83% of the dose over 24 h and served as a benchmark to compare with the other test products. The five most effective test products were Fuller's earth (the current UK military decontaminant), Fast-Act® and three novel polymers [based on itaconic acid, 2-trifluoromethylacrylic acid and N,N-methylenebis(acrylamide)]. Five products (medical moist-free wipes, 5% FloraFree™ solution, normal baby wipes, baby wipes for sensitive skin and Diphotérine™) enhanced the dermal absorption of 14C-methyl salicylate. Further work is required to establish the performance of the most effective products identified in this study against chemical warfare agents.

Dalton, C. H., et al. (2015). "Development of haemostatic decontaminants for the treatment of wounds contaminated with chemical warfare agents. 2: Evaluation of *in vitro* topical decontamination efficacy using undamaged skin." Journal of Applied Toxicology 35(5): 543–550.

Abstract: The risk of penetrating, traumatic injury occurring in a chemically contaminated environment cannot be discounted. Should a traumatic injury be contaminated with a chemical warfare (CW) agent, it is likely that standard haemostatic treatment options would be complicated by the need to decontaminate the wound milieu. Thus, there is a need to develop haemostatic products that can simultaneously arrest haemorrhage and decontaminate CW agents. The purpose of this study was to evaluate a number of candidate haemostats for efficacy as skin decontaminants against three CW agents (soman, VX and sulphur mustard) using an *in vitro* diffusion cell containing undamaged pig skin. One haemostatic product (WoundStat™) was shown to be as effective as the standard military decontaminants Fuller's earth and M291 for the decontamination of all three CW agents. The most effective haemostatic agents were powder-based and use fluid absorption as a mechanism of action to sequester CW agent (akin to the decontaminant Fuller's earth). The envisaged use of haemostatic decontaminants would be to decontaminate from within wounds and from damaged skin. Therefore, WoundStat™ should be subject to further evaluation using an *in vitro* model of damaged skin. (Copyright © 2014 Crown copyright. *Journal of Applied Toxicology* © 2014 John Wiley & Sons, Ltd.)

Capoun, T. and J. Krykorkova (2014). "Comparison of selected methods for individual decontamination of chemical warfare agents." Toxics 2(2): 307–326.

Abstract: This study addresses the individual decontamination of chemical warfare agents (CWA) and other hazardous substances. The individual decontamination applies to contaminated body surfaces, protective clothing and objects immediately after contamination, performed individually or by mutual assistance using prescribed or improvised devices. The article evaluates the importance of individual decontamination, security level for Fire and Rescue Service Units of the Czech Republic (FRS CR) and demonstrates some of the devices. The decontamination efficiency of selected methods (sorbent, glove and sponge, two-chamber foam device and wiping with alcohol) was evaluated for protective clothing and painted steel plate contaminated with O-ethyl-S-(diisopropylaminoethyl)-methylthiophosphonate (VX), sulfur mustard, o-cresol and acrylonitrile. The methods were assessed from an economic point of view and with regard to specific user parameters, such as the decontamination of surfaces or materials with poor accessibility and vertical surfaces, the need for a water rinse as well as toxic waste and its disposal.

- **Reference Type**: Journal Article
- **Record Number**: 17
- **Author**: Osovsky, Ruth, Kaplan, Doron, Nir, Ido, Rotter, Hadar, Elisha, Shmuel and Columbus, Ishay
- **Year**: 2014
- **Title**: Decontamination of adsorbed chemical warfare agents on activated carbon using hydrogen peroxide solutions
- **Journal**: Environmental Science & Technology
- **Volume**: 48
- **Issue**: 18
- **Pages**: 10912–10918
- **Short Title**: Decontamination of adsorbed chemical warfare agents on activated carbon using hydrogen peroxide solutions
- **ISSN**: 0013-936X

Abstract: Mild treatment with hydrogen peroxide solutions (3–30%) efficiently decomposes adsorbed chemical warfare agents (CWAs) on microporous activated carbons used in protective garments and air filters. Better than 95% decomposition of adsorbed sulfur mustard (HD), sarin, and VX was achieved at ambient temperatures within 1–24 h, depending on the H_2O_2 concentration. HD was oxidized to the nontoxic HD-sulfoxide. The nerve agents were perhydrolyzed to the respective nontoxic methylphosphonic acids. The relative rapidity of the oxidation and perhydrolysis under these conditions is attributed to the microenvironment of the micropores. Apparently, the reactions are favored due to basic sites on the carbon surface. Our findings suggest a potential environmentally friendly route for decontamination of adsorbed CWAs, using H_2O_2 without the need of cosolvents or activators.

Rolland, P., et al. (2013). "Hairy skin exposure to VX *in vitro*: Effectiveness of delayed decontamination." Toxicology *In Vitro* 27(1): 358–366.

Abstract: The chemical warfare agents such as VX represent a threat for both military and civilians, which involves an immediate need of effective decontamination systems. Since human scalp is usually unprotected compared to other body regions covered with clothes, it could be a preferential site of exposure in case of terrorist acts. The purpose of this study was to determine if skin decontamination could be efficient when performed more than 1 h after exposure. In addition, the impact of hairs in skin contamination was investigated. By using *in vitro* skin models, we demonstrated that about 75% of the applied quantity of VX was recovered on the skin surface 2 h after skin exposition, which means that it is worth decontaminating even if contamination occurred 2 h before. The stratum corneum reservoir for VX was quickly established and persistent. In addition, the presence of hairs modified the percutaneous penetration of the nerve agent by binding of VX to hairs. Hair shaft has thus to be taken into account in the decontamination process. Reactive Skin Decontamination Lotion (RSDL) and Fuller's Earth (FE) were active in the skin decontamination 45 min post-exposure, but RSDL was more efficient in reducing the amount of VX either in the skin or in the hair.

- **Reference Type**: Journal Article
- **Record Number**: 9
- **Author**: Misik, Jan, Pavlikova, Ruzena, Josse, Denis, Cabal, Jiri and Kuca, Kamil
- **Year**: 2012
- **Title**: *In vitro* skin permeation and decontamination of the organophosphorus pesticide paraoxon under various physical conditions – evidence for a wash-in effect
- **Journal**: Toxicology Mechanisms and Methods
- **Volume**: 22
- **Issue**: 7
- **Pages**: 520–525
- **Short Title**: *In vitro* skin permeation and decontamination of the organophosphorus pesticide paraoxon under various physical conditions – evidence for a wash-in effect
- **ISSN**: 1537-6516

Abstract: Misuse of various chemicals, such as chemical warfare agents, industrial chemicals or pesticides during warfare or terrorists attacks requires adequate protection. Thus, development and evaluation of novel decontamination dispositives and techniques are needed. In this study, *in vitro* permeation and decontamination of a potentially hazardous compound paraoxon, an active metabolite of organophosphorus pesticide parathion, was investigated. Skin permeation and decontamination experiments were carried out in modified Franz diffusion cells. Pig skin was used as a human skin model. Commercially produced detergent-based washing solutions FloraFree™ and Argos™ were used as decontamination means. The experiments were done under "warm", "cold", "dry" and "wet" skin conditions in order to determine an effect of various physical conditions on skin permeation of paraoxon and on a subsequent decontamination process. There was no significant difference in skin permeation of paraoxon under warm, cold and dry conditions, whereas wet conditions provided significantly higher permeation rates. In the selected conditions, decontamination treatments performed 1 h after a skin exposure did not decrease the agent volume that permeated through the skin. An exception were wet skin conditions with non-significant decontamination efficacy 18 and 28% for the FloraFree™ and Argos™ treatment, respectively. In contrast, the skin permeation of paraoxon under warm, cold and dry conditions increased up to 60–290% following decontamination compared to non-decontaminated controls. This has previously been described as a skin wash-in effect.

Misik, J., et al. (2012). "*In vivo* decontamination of the nerve agent VX using the domestic swine model." Clinical Toxicology 50(9): 807–811.

Abstract: The purpose of this *in vivo* study was to assess a new, putatively optimised method for mass casualty decontamination ("ORCHIDS protocol") for effectiveness in removing the chemical warfare agent VX from the skin of anaesthetised, domestic white pigs. ORCHIDS protocol consists of a 1.5-minute shower with a mild detergent (Argos™) supplemented by physical removal. A standard method of wet decontamination was used for comparison. Experimental animals were divided into four groups (A–D). Two groups were exposed to a supra-lethal percutaneous dose ($5 \times LD_{50}$; 300 μg kg^{-1}) of VX for 1 h prior to decontamination with either the ORCHIDS (C) or standard protocol (D). A third (B, positive control) group was exposed but not subject to decontamination. Blank controls (A) received anaesthesia and the corresponding dose of normal saline instead of VX. Observations of the clinical signs of intoxication were supplemented by measurements of whole blood cholinesterase (ChE) performed on samples of arterial blood acquired at 30-minute intervals for the duration of the study (up to 6 h). Untreated (B) animals displayed typical cholinergic signs consistent with VX intoxication (local fasciculation, mastication, salivation, pilo-erection and motor convulsions) and died 165–240 min post exposure. All animals in both decontamination treatment groups (C, D) survived the duration of the study and exhibited less severe signs of cholinergic poisoning. Thus, both the standard and ORCHIDS protocol were demonstrably effective against exposure to the potent nerve agent VX, even after a delay of 1 h. A critical advantage of the ORCHIDS protocol is the relatively short shower duration (1½ min compared to 3 min). In practice, this could substantially improve the rate at which individuals could be decontaminated by emergency responders following exposure to toxic materials such as chemical warfare agents.

- **Reference Type**: Journal Article
- **Record Number**: 15
- **Author**: Clarkson, Edward D, Schulz, Susan M, Railer, Roy F and Smith, Kelly H
- **Year**: 2012
- **Title**: Median lethal dose determination for percutaneous exposure to soman and VX in guinea pigs and the effectiveness of decontamination with M291 SDK or SANDIA foam
- **Journal**: Toxicology Letters
- **Volume**: 212
- **Issue**: 3
- **Pages**: 282–287
- **Short Title**: Median lethal dose determination for percutaneous exposure to soman and VX in guinea pigs and the effectiveness of decontamination with M291 SDK or SANDIA foam
- **ISSN**: 0378-4274
- **URL**: https://www.sciencedirect.com/science/article/pii/S0378427412011642?via%3Dihub

Abstract: Soman (GD) and VX are chemical warfare agents that can be absorbed through the skin. We determined the median lethal dose (MLD) for the cutaneous application of GD and VX in anesthetized haired guinea pigs and then tested the ability of a currently fielded decontamination kit, the M291 Skin Decontamination

Kit (SDK), and decontaminating foam made by SANDIA Labs to decontaminate areas that have been exposed to cutaneous applications of GD and VX. The fur of guinea pigs was clipped on the left flank 24 h prior to exposure. Animals were anesthetized and 5 min later neat GD or neat VX was applied. The MLD for percutaneous exposure to GD was 11.6 mg/kg, and to VX it was 0.10 mg/kg. To test the ability of the M291 SDK, either GD or VX was applied and removed 1 min later with the pads of the M291 SDK clasped in a pair of forceps and wiped across the flank of the animal. The MLDs for GD and VX removed with the M291 SDK pads were 76.9 mg/kg and 0.87 mg/kg, respectively. When neat GD or neat VX was applied and removed 1 min later in the same manner with gauze soaked in SANDIA foam (MDF-100), the MLDs were 412 mg/kg and 10.4 mg/kg respectively. These data demonstrate that GD and VX are significantly less potent when applied cutaneously than previously reported for subcutaneous injections and indicate that improvement is needed on the limited protective ratio provided by the M291 SDK.

- **Reference Type**: Journal Article
- **Record Number**: 6
- **Author**: D Schwartz, M, G Hurst, C, A Kirk, M, JD Reedy, S and H Braue, E
- **Year**: 2012
- **Title**: Reactive skin decontamination lotion (RSDL) for the decontamination of chemical warfare agent (CWA) dermal exposure
- **Journal**: Current Pharmaceutical Biotechnology
- **Volume**: 13
- **Issue**: 10
- **Pages**: 1971–1979
- **Short Title**: Reactive skin decontamination lotion (RSDL) for the decontamination of chemical warfare agent (CWA) dermal exposure
- **ISSN**: 1389-2010

Abstract: Rapid decontamination of the skin is the single most important action to prevent dermal absorption of chemical contaminants in persons exposed to chemical warfare agents (CWA) and toxic industrial chemicals (TICs) as a result of accidental or intentional release. Chemicals on the skin may be removed by mechanical means through the use of dry sorbents or water. Recent interest in decontamination systems which both partition contaminants away from the skin and actively neutralize the chemical has led to the development of several reactive decontamination solutions. This article will review the recently FDA-approved Reactive Skin Decontamination Lotion (RSDL) and will summarize the toxicity and efficacy studies conducted to date. Evidence of RSDL's superior performance against vesicant and organophosphorus chemical warfare agents compared to water, bleach, and dry sorbents, suggests that RSDL may have a role in mass human exposure chemical decontamination in both the military and civilian arenas.

- **Reference Type**: Journal Article
- **Record Number**: 4

- **Author**: Taysse, L, Dorandeu, F, Daulon, S, Foquin, A, Perrier, N, Lallement, G and Breton, P
- **Year**: 2011
- **Title**: Cutaneous challenge with chemical warfare agents in the SKH-1 hairless mouse (II): effects of some currently used skin decontaminants (RSDL and Fuller's earth) against liquid sulphur mustard and VX exposure
- **Journal**: Human & Experimental Toxicology
- **Volume**: 30
- **Issue**: 6
- **Pages**: 491–498
- **Short Title**: Cutaneous challenge with chemical warfare agents in the SKH-1 hairless mouse (II): effects of some currently used skin decontaminants (RSDL and Fuller's earth) against liquid sulphur mustard and VX exposure
- ISSN: 0960-3271

Abstract: Using the hairless mouse screening model presented in the companion paper1 the aim of this study was to assess two skin decontaminating systems: Fuller's earth (FE) and Reactive Skin Decontamination Lotion (RSDL) against two extremely toxic chemical warfare agents that represent a special percutaneous hazard, sulphur mustard (SM) and O-ethyl-S-(2[di-isopropylamino]ethyl)methylphosphonothioate (VX). Five minutes after being exposed on the back to either 2 μL of neat sulphur mustard or 50 μg.kg-1 of diluted VX, mice were decontaminated. Both systems were able to reduce blisters 3 days after SM exposure. However, RSDL was found to be more efficient than FE in reducing the necrosis of the epidermis and erosion. In the case of VX exposure, RSDL, whatever the ratio of decontaminant to toxicant used (RSDL 10, 20, 50), was not able to sufficiently prevent the inhibition of plasma cholinesterases taken as a surrogate marker of exposure and toxicity. Only FE reduced significantly the ChE inhibition. Some of these observations are different from our previous results obtained in domestic swine and these changes are thus discussed in the perspective of using SKH-1 hairless mice for the initial *in vivo* screening of decontaminants.

Mikler, J., et al. (2011). "Immobilization of Russian VX skin depots by localized cooling: Implications for decontamination and medical countermeasures." Toxicology Letters 206(1): 47–53.

Abstract: The chemical weapon nerve agent known as Russian VX (VR) is a potent organophosphorus (OP) compound that is much less studied than its VX analogue with respect to toxicity, as well as to the effectiveness of several known countermeasures against it. An anaesthetized domestic swine model was utilized to assess several approaches in mitigating its toxicity, including the utility of cooling VR treated skin to increase the therapeutic window for treatment. The 6 h LD_{50} for VR topically applied on the ear was 100 μg/kg. Treatment of VR exposed animals (5× LD_{50}) with pralidoxime (2PAM) very poorly regenerated inhibited blood cholinesterase activity, but was partially effective in preventing signs of OP poisoning and increasing survival. In contrast, treatment with the Hagedorn oxime

HI-6 reactivated cholinesterase, eliminated all signs of poisoning and prevented death. Decontamination with the Reactive Skin Decontaminant Lotion (RSDL) 15 min after VR exposure was completely effective in preventing death. Cooling of the VR exposure sites for 2 or 6 h prevented signs of OP poisoning and death during the cooling period. However, these animals died very quickly after the cessation of cooling, unless they were treated with oxime or decontaminated with RSDL. Blood analyses showed that cooling of agent exposure sites delayed the entry of VR into the bloodstream. Medical treatment with HI-6 and to a lesser extent 2PAM, or decontamination with RSDL are effective in protecting against the toxic effects of cutaneous exposure to VR. Immobilizing this agent (and related compounds) within the dermal reservoir by cooling the exposure sites, dramatically increases the therapeutic window in which these medical countermeasures are effective.

Braue Jr, E. H., et al. (2011). "Efficacy studies of Reactive Skin Decontamination Lotion, M291 Skin Decontamination Kit, 0.5% bleach, 1% soapy water, and Skin Exposure Reduction Paste against chemical warfare agents, part 1: guinea pigs challenged with VX." Cutaneous and Ocular Toxicology 30(1): 15–28.
Abstract:

Objective: This report, first in a series of five, directly compares the efficacy of 4 decontamination products and Skin Exposure Reduction Paste Against Chemical Warfare Agents (SERPACWA) in the haired guinea pig model following exposure to VX.

- **Reference Type**: Journal Article
- **Record Number**: 5
- **Author**: Bjarnason, S, Mikler, J, Hill, I, Tenn, C, Garrett, M, Caddy, N and Sawyer, TW
- **Year**: 2008
- **Title**: Comparison of selected skin decontaminant products and regimens against VX in domestic swine
- **Journal**: Human & Experimental Toxicology
- **Volume**: 27
- **Issue**: 3
- **Pages**: 253–261
- **Short Title**: Comparison of selected skin decontaminant products and regimens against VX in domestic swine
- ISSN: 0960-3271

Abstract: An anesthetized domestic swine model was used to compare the efficacy and cross-contamination potential of selected skin decontaminant products and regimens against the chemical warfare agent, VX. Animals topically exposed to 2×, 3× or 5× LD50 VX showed typical signs of organophosphate nerve agent poisoning, including miosis, salivation, mastication, dysrhythmias, and respiratory distress prior to death. Animals were exposed to 5× LD50 VX and then decontaminated 45 min later with the reactive skin decontamination lotion (RSDL®), Fuller's earth (FE), 0.5% hypochlorite, or soapy water. Survival was 100% when the reactive skin decontamination lotion or FE was utilized, although 50% of Fuller's earth-decontaminated animals exhibited serious signs of VX poisoning. Decontamination of VX-treated animals with 0.5% hypochlorite was less effective but also increased survival. Soapy water was ineffective in preventing lethality. Blood cholinesterase levels were not predictive of clinical outcome in decontaminated animals. The potential of "decontaminated" VX in open wounds to cause poisoning was assessed by vigorously mixing 5× LD50 VX with the test decontaminants for 5 min and then placing the mixture onto a full-thickness skin wound. Soapy water was ineffective in preventing lethality. Although treatment with dry Fuller's earth prevented death and all signs of organophosphate poisoning, a significant proportion of treated animals decontaminated with Fuller's earth in aqueous suspension exhibited serious signs of organophosphate poisoning, suggesting that live agent may be desorbed from Fuller's earth when it is exposed to a liquid environment. Animals treated with reactive skin decontamination lotion or 0.5% hypochlorite-VX mixtures showed no signs of organophosphate poisoning during the 6- h test period.

- **Reference Type**: Journal Article
- **Record Number**: 1
- **Author**: Lukey, BJ, Slife, HF, Clarkson, ED, Hurst, CG and Braue, EH
- **Year**: 2008
- **Title**: Chemical warfare agent decontamination from skin
- **Journal**: Chemical warfare agents chemistry, pharmacology, toxicology, and therapeutics, 2nd edn. Taylor & Francis Group, Boca Raton
- **Pages**: 611–625
- **Short Title**: Chemical warfare agent decontamination from skin

Abstract: N/A

Bartelt-Hunt, S. L., et al. (2008). "A review of chemical warfare agent simulants for the study of environmental behavior." Critical Reviews in Environmental Science and Technology 38(2): 112–136.

Abstract: There is renewed interest in the environmental fate of chemical warfare agents attributable to the intensified threat of chemical weapons use in a terrorist attack. Knowledge of processes that influence the fate of agents such as distilled mustard, lewisite, tabun, sarin, soman, and VX in the environment is important for development of disposal strategies and for risk and exposure assessments. However, it is often necessary to conduct studies examining chemical agent behavior using simulants due to the toxicity of the agents and usage restrictions. The objective of this study was to review the physical–chemical properties and mammalian toxicity of compounds that can be used to simulate chemical agents and to identify the most appropriate compounds to simulate specific environmental fate processes, including hydrolysis, sorption, bioavailability, and volatilization.

Ramaseshan, R. and S. Ramakrishna (2007). "Zinc titanate nanofibers for the detoxification of chemical warfare simulants." Journal of the American Ceramic Society 90(6): 1836–1842.

Abstract: Fabrication of a novel ceramic nanofiber system viz. zinc titanate using the well-known electrospinning technology with polyvinylpyrrolidone as a binder is reported. Use of zinc titanates as reactive sorbents to detoxify chemical warfare agents is hypothesized and proved. The zinc titanate nanofibers are tested against simulants of nerve and mustard agents and show satisfactory destructive activity. The extent of detoxification is measured using GC-MS analysis. The products of reaction of zinc titanate against the simulants are identified and are found to be relatively harmless. The possibility of replacement of conventional-activated carbon by electrospun ceramic nanofibers for face masks and protective clothing is proposed.

Romano Jr, J. A., et al. (2007). Chemical warfare agents: Chemistry, pharmacology, toxicology, and therapeutics, CRC Press.

Abstract: Edited By James A. Romano Jr., James A. Romano, Harry Salem, Brian J Lukey, Brian J. Lukey, Harry Salem

The first edition of this book, *Chemical Warfare Agents: Toxicity at Low Levels*, was published just prior to the terrorist attacks of September 11th, 2001. Reflecting a greater sense of urgency within the field of chemical defense since this event, research related to chemical warfare agents (CWAs) continues to expand at a remarkable pace.

- **Reference Type**: Journal Article
- **Record Number**: 79
- **Author**: Talmage, Sylvia Smith, Watson, Annetta Paule, Hauschild, Veronique, Munro, Nancy B and King, J
- **Year**: 2007
- **Title**: Chemical warfare agent degradation and decontamination
- **Journal**: Current Organic Chemistry
- **Volume**: 11
- **Issue**: 3
- **Pages**: 285–298
- **Short Title**: Chemical warfare agent degradation and decontamination
- **ISSN**: 1385-2728

Abstract: The decontamination of chemical warfare agents (CWA) from structures, environmental media, and even personnel has become an area of particular interest in recent years due to increased homeland security concerns. In addition to terrorist attacks, scenarios such as accidental releases of CWA from U.S. stockpile sites or from historic, buried munitions are also subjects for response planning. To facilitate rapid identification of practical and effective decontamination approaches, this paper reviews pathways of CWA degradation by natural means as well as those resulting from deliberately applied solutions and technologies; these pathways and technologies are compared and contrasted. We then review various technologies, both traditional and recent, with some emphasis on decontamination materials used for surfaces that are difficult to clean. Discussion is limited to the major threat CWA, namely sulfur mustard (HD, bis[2-chloroethyl]sulfide), VX (O-ethyl S-[2-diisopropylaminoethyl] methylphosphonothioate), and the G-series nerve agents. The principal G-agents are GA (tabun, ethyl N,N-dimethylphosphoramidocyanidate), GB (sarin, isopropyl methylphosphonofluoridate), and GD (soman, pinacolyl methylphosphonofluoridate). The chemical decontamination pathways of each agent are outlined, with some discussion of intermediate and final degradation product toxicity. In all cases, and regardless of the CWA degradation pathway chosen for decontamination, it will be necessary to collect and analyze pertinent environmental samples during the treatment phase to confirm attainment of clearance levels.

- **Reference Type**: Journal Article
- **Record Number**: 3
- **Author**: Taysse, L, Daulon, S, Delamanche, S, Bellier, B and Breton, P
- **Year**: 2007
- **Title**: Skin decontamination of mustards and organophosphates: comparative efficiency of RSDL and Fuller's earth in domestic swine
- **Journal**: Human & Experimental Toxicology
- **Volume**: 26
- **Issue**: 2
- **Pages**: 135–141
- **Short Title**: Skin decontamination of mustards and organophosphates: comparative efficiency of RSDL and Fuller's earth in domestic swine
- **ISSN**: 0960-3271

Abstract: Research in skin decontamination and therapy of chemical warfare agents has been a difficult problem due to the simultaneous requirement of rapid action and non-aggressive behaviour. The aim of this study was to compare the performance of two decontaminating systems: the Canadian Reactive Skin Decontaminant Lotion (RSDL) and the Fuller's Earth (FE). The experiment was conducted with domestic swine, as a good model for extrapolation to human skin. RSDL and FE were tested against sulphur mustard (SM), a powerful vesicant, and VX, a potent and persistent cholinesterase inhibitor. When used 5 min after contamination, the results clearly showed that both systems were active against SM (10.1 mg/cm2) and VX (0.06 mg/cm2). The potency of the RSDL/sponge was statistically better than FE against skin injury induced by SM, observed 3 days post-exposure. RSDL was rather more efficient than FE in reducing the formation of perinuclear vacuoles and inflammation processes in the epidermis and dermis. Against a severe inhibition (67%) of plasmatic cholinesterases induced by VX poisoning, the potencies of the RSDL/sponge and FE were similar. Both systems completely prevented cholinesterase inhibition, which indirectly indicates a prevention of toxic absorption through the skin. Human & Experimental Toxicology (2007) 26, 135–141

- **Reference Type**: Journal Article
- **Record Number**: 81
- **Author**: Hamilton, Murray G, Hill, Ira, Conley, John, Sawyer, Thomas W, Caneva, Duane C and Lundy, Paul M

- **Year**: 2004
- **Title**: Clinical aspects of percutaneous poisoning by the chemical warfare agent VX: effects of application site and decontamination
- **Journal**: Military Medicine
- **Volume**: 169
- **Issue**: 11
- **Pages**: 856–862
- **Short Title**: Clinical aspects of percutaneous poisoning by the chemical warfare agent VX: effects of application site and decontamination
- **ISSN**: 1930-613X

Abstract: O-ethyl S-(2-diisopropylaminoethyl) methylphosphonothioate (VX) is an extremely toxic organophosphate nerve agent that has been weaponized and stockpiled in a number of different countries, and it has been used in recent terrorist events. It differs from other well-known organophosphate nerve agents in that its primary use is as a contact poison rather than as an inhalation hazard. For this reason, we examined the effects of application site and skin decontamination on VX toxicity in anesthetized domestic swine after topical application. VX applied to the surface of the ear rapidly resulted in signs of toxicity consistent with the development of cholinergic crisis, including apnea and death. VX on the epigastrium resulted in a marked delayed development of toxic signs, reduced toxicity, and reduction in the rate of cholinesterase depression compared with animals exposed on the ear. Skin decontamination (15 minutes post-VX on the ear) arrested the development of clinical signs and prevented further cholinesterase inhibition and death. These results confirm earlier work that demonstrates the importance of exposure site on the resultant toxicity of this agent and they also show that decontamination postexposure has the potential to be an integral and extremely important component of medical countermeasures against this agent.

Chang, E., et al. (2003). Immobilized metalchelate complexes for catalysis and decontamination of pesticides and chemical warfare nerve-agents, Google Patents.

Abstract: The present invention relates to the preparation of metal chelate complexes immobilized on a support, immobilized metal chelate complexes and methods of using the supports and immobilized metal chelate complexes for the adsorption and/or hydrolysis of phosphate esters. More specifically, processes for the preparation of immobilized metal chelate complexes by attachment of metal chelate complexes to solids, polymers, micelles, liposomes, tubules and other self-organized polymolecular associations immobilized metal chelate complexes made by such processes and use of the supports and immobilized metal chelate complexes for the adsorption and/or hydrolysis of phosphate ester group containing compounds such as chemical warfare nerve agents and pesticides, are disclosed. The present invention provides the ability to efficiently decontaminate phosphate ester compounds under a wide range of conditions in a practical and cost-effective manner.

Miscellaneous (Misc)

- **Reference Type**: Journal Article
- **Record Number**: 17
- **Author**: Cao, Yachao, Hui, Xiaoying, Zhu, Hanjiang, Elmahdy, Akram and Maibach, Howard
- **Year**: 2018
- **Title**: *In vitro* human skin permeation and decontamination of 2-chloroethyl ethyl sulfide (CEES) using Dermal Decontamination Gel (DDGel) and Reactive Skin Decontamination Lotion (RSDL)
- **Journal**: Toxicology Letters
- **Volume**: 291
- **Pages**: 86–91
- **Short Title**: *In vitro* human skin permeation and decontamination of 2-chloroethyl ethyl sulfide (CEES) using Dermal Decontamination Gel (DDGel) and Reactive Skin Decontamination Lotion (RSDL)
- **ISSN**: 0378-4274

- **Reference Type**: Journal Article
- **Record Number**: 10
- **Author**: Kulkarni, Parag and Jeffery, Steven
- **Year**: 2018
- **Title**: The effects of the use of Diphoterine® solution on chemical burns in the Tarapur Industrial Complex, India
- **Journal**: Burns Open
- **Volume**: 2
- **Issue**: 2
- **Pages**: 104–107
- **Short Title**: The effects of the use of Diphoterine® solution on chemical burns in the Tarapur industrial complex, India
- **ISSN**: 2468-9122

Abstract: Tarapur is the biggest industrial complex in India. Chemical burns are relatively frequent due to the use of corrosive agents within these industries. Diphoterine®, a polyvalent hypertonic amphoteric first-aid solution has been adopted by some of the companies but not others. We decided to compare the cases of chemical injury which had been treated with Diphoterine® solution with those who had not.

- **Reference Type**: Journal Article
- **Record Number**: 62
- **Author**: Tazrart, A., Bolzinger, M.A., Lamart, S., Coudert, S., Angulo, J.F., Jandard, V., Briançon, S. and Griffiths, N.M.
- **Year**: 2018

- **Title**: Actinide-contaminated skin: comparing decontamination efficacy of water, cleansing gels, and DTPA gels
- **Journal**: Health Physics
- **Volume**: 115
- **Issue**: 1
- **Pages**: 12–20
- **Short Title**: Actinide-contaminated skin: comparing decontamination efficacy of water, cleansing gels, and DTPA gels
- **ISSN**: 0017-9078
- **DOI**: 10.1097/hp.0000000000000814
- **Accession Number**: 00004032-201807000-00003

Keywords: Actinides; Contamination, External; Decontamination; DTPA

Abstract: Skin contamination by alpha-emitting actinides is a risk to workers during nuclear fuel production and reactor decommissioning. Also, the list of items for potential use in radiological dispersal devices includes plutonium and americium. The actinide chemical form is important and solvents such as tributyl phosphate, used to extract plutonium, can influence plutonium behavior. This study investigated skin fixation and efficacy of decontamination products for these actinide forms using viable pig skin in the Franz cell diffusion system. Commonly used or recommended decontamination products such as water, cleansing gel, diethylenetriamine pentaacetic acid, or octadentate hydroxypyridinone compound 3,4,3-LI(1,2-HOPO), as well as diethylenetriamine pentaacetic acid hydrogel formulations, were tested after a 2-h contact time with the contaminant. Analysis of skin samples demonstrated that more plutonium nitrate is bound to skin as compared to plutonium-tributyl phosphate, and fixation of americium to skin was also significant. The data show that for plutonium-tributyl phosphate all the products are effective ranging from 80 to 90% removal of this contaminant. This may be associated with damage to the skin by this complex and suggests a mechanical/wash-out action rather than chelation. For removal of americium and plutonium, both Trait Rouge cleansing gel and diethylenetriamine pentaacetic acid are better than water, and diethylenetriamine pentaacetic acid hydrogel is better than Osmogel. The different treatments, however, did not significantly affect the activity in deeper skin layers, which suggests a need for further improvement of decontamination procedures. The new diethylenetriamine pentaacetic acid hydrogel preparation was effective in removing americium, plutonium, and plutonium-tributyl phosphate from skin; such a formulation offers advantages and thus merits further assessment.

URL: https://journals.lww.com/health-physics/Fulltext/2018/07000/Actinide_contaminated_Skin___Comparing.3.aspx

Lydon, H., et al. (2018). "The percutaneous toxicokinetics of VX in a damaged skin porcine model and the evaluation of WoundStat™ as a topical decontaminant." Journal of Applied Toxicology 38(3): 318–328.

Abstract: This study used a damaged skin, porcine model to evaluate the *in vivo* efficacy of WoundStat™ for the decontamination of superficial, nerve agent-contaminated wounds. Anaesthetized animals were randomly assigned to either control (n = 7), no decontamination (n = 12) or WoundStat™ (n = 12) treatment groups. Pigs were exposed to a 5× LD_{50} dose of neat, radiolabelled *S*-[2-(diisopropylamino)ethyl]-*O*-ethyl methyl-phosphonothioate (VX; or equivalent volume of sterile saline for the control group) via an area of superficially damaged skin on the ear. WoundStat™ was applied at 30 seconds post-exposure to assigned animals. The VX contaminant (or saline) and decontaminant remained in place for the duration of the study (up to 6 hours). Physiological parameters and signs of intoxication were recorded during the exposure period. Skin and organ samples were taken post mortem for ^{14}C–VX distribution analyses. Blood samples were taken periodically for toxicokinetic and whole-blood acetylcholinesterase (AChE) activity analyses. VX exposure was accompanied by a rapid decrease in AChE activity in all animals, regardless of decontamination. However, decontamination significantly improved survival rate and time and reduced the severity of signs of intoxication. In addition, the distribution of ^{14}C–VX in key internal organs and post mortem blood samples was significantly lower in the WoundStat™ treatment group. This study demonstrates that WoundStat™ may be a suitable medical countermeasure for increasing both survival rate and time following VX exposure. The results also suggest that AChE activity is not a useful prognostic indicator.

- **Reference Type**: Journal Article
- **Record Number**: 38
- **Author**: Pavlikova, Ruzena, Misik, Jan, Cabal, Jiri, Marek, Jan and Kuca, Kamil
- **Year**: 2018
- **Title**: *In vitro* skin decontamination of paraoxon – wet-type cleansing effect of selected detergents
- **Journal**: Cutaneous and Ocular Toxicology
- **Volume**: 37
- **Issue**: 1
- **Pages**: 77–83
- **Date**: 2018/01/02
- **Short Title**: *In vitro* skin decontamination of paraoxon – wet-type cleansing effect of selected detergents
- **ISSN**: 1556-9527
- **DOI**: 10.1080/15569527.2017.1354216

Abstract: The aim of this study was to determine optimal conditions for *in vitro* skin decontamination using water and detergents as decontamination agents and to test the cleansing efficiency of selected detergents. Experiments were performed using a peristaltic pump for showering of pig skin in modified static diffusion cells. Several conditions were tested including different flow rates (from 5 to 33 ml s−1), quantity of rinsing fluid (from 40 to 400 ml) and concentration of detergents (2; 5; 10%). Further, several types of detergents/commercial decontamination agents were evaluated under the selected conditions to find the most effective means of decontamination. The amount of paraoxon removed from the skin surface following wet-type decontamination was detected in the rinsing fluid spectrophotometrically after hydrolysis of paraoxon – a model contaminant. The efficacy of rinsing by water/Spolapon AES 253 increased with flow rate up to 25 ml s−1 and a rinsing volume of 200 ml. Lutensol AT 25 achieved maximum efficacy at the lowest tested concentration (2%). A flow rate of 16 ml s−1, rinsing volume of 100 ml (values from the middle part of the sigmoid curve) and 5% concentration of decontaminant solution were used for further evaluation of detergents as cleansing agents under the selected conditions. Cetylpyridinium bromide (cationic surfactant), carbethopendecinii bromidum (cationic surfactant) and polyoxyethylene-10-tridecyl ether (non-ionic surfactant), SDS (anionic surfactant), althosan MB (cationic surfactant), sodium dodecylbenzene sulphonate (anionic surfactant), neodekont (mixture), tergitol NPX (non-ionic surfactant), Korynt P (non-ionic surfactant) were found to be the most effective. These decontaminants were able to wash away more than 92% of paraoxon from the contaminated skin.

URL: https://doi.org/10.1080/15569527.2017.1354216

Bignon, C., et al. (2017). "Barrier cream based on CeO2 nanoparticles grafted polymer as an active compound against the penetration of organophosphates." Chemico-Biological Interactions 267: 17–24.

Abstract: Due to their small size, nanoparticles possess unique properties. Cerium oxide nanoparticles have been already studied for their capacity to adsorb and neutralize toxic compounds including organophosphates. By covalently grafting these nanoparticles to a thickening polymer, their potential aggregation resulting in a loss of surface area and their potential toxicity are avoided. Indeed, copolymers easily form gels in water at neutral pH thanks to low interactions occurring between polymeric chains; thus, gels can be spread on membrane supports to afford protective barriers. However, as we demonstrated previously, a formulation step of these hydride nanoparticle-polymeric compounds is necessary to overcome the cracking of the coating during drying. This work reports the impact of many factors on the efficiency of a new active Topical Skin Protectant (aTSP) including: (1) the presence of CeO_2 nanoparticles in the protective coating and their amount, (2) their grafting to a perfluorocarbon thickening polymer and (3) the formulation of the CeO_2 nanoparticle-grafted polymer. The combination of all the benefit parameters led to a very effective new aTSP against paraoxon penetration. The major *in vitro* diffusion studies were performed in Franz-type diffusion cells on two artificial membranes (silicone and Strat-M) and final validation on *ex vivo* human skin. The comparison of 24 h-exposure between membrane results indicated a difference in the behavior between the two artificial supports and the biological model; Strat-M membranes seeming closer to human skin results. Therefore, positive results regarding occlusive conditions should be confirmed with human skin.

Joosen, M., et al. (2017). "The impact of skin decontamination on the time window for effective treatment of percutaneous VX exposure." Chemico-Biological Interactions 267: 48–56.

Abstract: The main goal of the present study was to obtain insight into depot formation and penetration following percutaneous VX poisoning, in order to identify an appropriate decontamination window that can enhance or support medical countermeasures.

The study was executed in two phases, using the hairless guinea pig as an animal model. In the first phase the effect of various decontamination regimens on levels of free VX in skin and plasma were studied as well as on blood cholinesterase levels. Animals were exposed to 0.5 mg/kg VX and were not decontaminated (control), decontaminated with RSDL once at 15 or 90 min after exposure or three times at 15, 25 and 35 (10-min interval) or 15, 45 and 75 min after exposure (30-min interval).

There was no significant effect of any of the decontamination regimens on the 6-h survival rate of the animals. However, all animals that had been decontaminated 15 min after exposure, showed a survival rate of more than 90%, compared to 50–60% in animals that were not decontaminated or decontaminated at 90 min after exposure.

In the second phase of the study, hairless guinea pigs were exposed to 1 mg/kg VX on the shoulder, followed either by decontamination with RSDL (10 min interval), conventional treatment on indication of clinical signs or a combination thereof. It appeared that a thorough, repeated decontamination alone could not save the majority of the animals. A 100% survival rate was observed in the group that received a combination of decontamination and treatment.

In conclusion, the effects of VX exposure could be influenced by various RSDL decontamination regimens. The results in freely moving animals showed that skin decontamination, although not fully effective in removing all VX from the skin and skin depot is crucial to support pharmacological intervention.

- **Reference Type**: Journal Article
- **Record Number**: 20
- **Author**: Salerno, Alicia, Devers, Thierry, Bolzinger, Marie-Alexandrine, Pelletier, Jocelyne, Josse, Denis and Briançon, Stéphanie
- **Year**: 2017
- **Title**: *In vitro* skin decontamination of the organophosphorus pesticide Paraoxon with nanometric cerium oxide CeO2
- **Journal**: Chemico-Biological Interactions
- **Volume**: 267
- **Pages**: 57–66
- **Short Title**: *In vitro* skin decontamination of the organophosphorus pesticide Paraoxon with nanometric cerium oxide CeO2
- **ISSN**: 0009-2797
- **URL**: https://www.sciencedirect.com/science/article/pii/S000927971630165X?via%3Dihub

Abstract: Organophosphorus compounds (OP), which mainly penetrate via the percutaneous pathway, represent a threat for both military and civilians. Body surface decontamination is vital to prevent victims poisoning. The development of a cost-effective formulation, which could be efficient and easy to handle in case of mass contamination, is therefore crucial. Metal oxides nanoparticles, due their large surface areas and the large amount of highly reactive sites, present high reactivity towards OP. First, this study aimed at evaluating the reaction of CeO_2 nanoparticles, synthetized by microwave path and calcined at 500°C or 600°C, with Paraoxon (POX) in aqueous solution. Results showed that both nanoparticles degraded 60–70% of POX. CeO_2 calcined at 500°C, owing to its larger specific area, was the most effective. Moreover, the degradation was significantly increased under Ultra-Violet irradiation (initial degradation rate doubled). Then, skin decontamination was studied *in vitro* using the Franz cell method with pig-ear skin samples. CeO_2 powder and an aqueous suspension of CeO_2 (CeO_2-W) were applied 1 h after POX exposure. The efficiency of decontamination, including removal and/or degradation of POX, was compared to Fuller's earth (FE) and RSDL lotion which are, currently, the most efficient systems for skin decontamination. CeO_2-W and RSDL were the most efficient to remove POX from the skin surface and decrease skin absorption by 6.4 compared to the control not decontaminated. FE reduced significantly (twice) the absorbed fraction of POX, contrarily to CeO_2 powder. Considering only the degradation rate of POX, the products ranged in the order CeO_2 > RSDL > CeO_2-W > FE (no degradation). This study showed that CeO_2 nanoparticles are a promising material for skin decontamination of OP if formulated as a dispersion able to remove POX like CeO_2-W and to degrade it as CeO_2 powder.

- **Reference Type**: Journal Article
- **Record Number**: 23
- **Author**: Lu, Annie Xi, McEntee, Monica, Browe, Matthew A, Hall, Morgan G, DeCoste, Jared B and Peterson, Gregory W
- **Year**: 2017
- **Title**: MOFabric: electrospun nanofiber mats from PVDF/UiO-66-NH2 for chemical protection and decontamination
- **Journal**: ACS Applied Materials & Interfaces
- **Volume**: 9
- **Issue**: 15
- **Pages**: 13632–13636
- **Short Title**: MOFabric: electrospun nanofiber mats from PVDF/UiO-66-NH2 for chemical protection and decontamination
- **ISSN**: 1944-8244

Abstract: Textiles capable of capture and detoxification of toxic chemicals, such as chemical-warfare agents (CWAs), are of high interest. Some metal–organic frameworks (MOFs) exhibit superior reactivity toward CWAs. However, it remains a challenge to integrate powder MOFs into engineered materials like textiles, while retaining functionalities like crystallinity, adsorptivity, and reactivity. Here, we present a simple method of electrospinning UiO-66-NH_2, a zirconium MOF, with polyvinylidene fluoride (PVDF). The electrospun composite, which we refer to as "MOFabric", exhibits comparable crystal patterns, surface area, chlorine uptake, and simulant hydrolysis to powder UiO-66-NH_2. The MOFabric is also capable of breaking down GD (*O*-pinacolyl methylphosphonofluoridae) faster than powder UiO-66-NH_2. Half-life of GD monitored by solid-state NMR for MOFabric is 131 min versus 315 min on powder UiO-66-NH_2.

- **Reference Type**: Journal Article
- **Record Number**: 11
- **Author**: Roul, Annick, Le, Cong-Anh-Khanh, Gustin, Marie-Paule, Clavaud, Emmanuel, Verrier, Bernard, Pirot, Fabrice and Falson, Françoise
- **Year**: 2017
- **Title**: Comparison of four different fuller's earth formulations in skin decontamination
- **Journal**: Journal of Applied Toxicology
- **Volume**: 37
- **Issue**: 12
- **Pages**: 1527–1536
- **Short Title**: Comparison of four different fuller's earth formulations in skin decontamination
- **ISSN**: 1099-1263
- **URL**: https://onlinelibrary.wiley.com/doi/abs/10.1002/jat.3506

Abstract: Industrial accidents, wars and terrorist threats are potential sources of skin contamination by highly toxic chemical warfare agents and manufacturing compounds. We have compared the time-dependent adsorption capacity and decontamination efficiency of fuller's earth (FE) for four different formulations for the molecular tracer, 4-cyanophenol (4-CP), *in vitro* and ex vivo using water decontamination as standard. The adsorption capacity of FE was assessed *in vitro* for 4-CP aqueous solutions whereas decontamination efficiency was investigated ex vivo by tracking porcine skin 4-CP content using attenuated total reflectance Fourier transform infrared spectroscopy. Decontamination was performed on short time, exposed porcine skin to 4-CP by application of FE: (1) as free powder; (2) loaded on adhesive tape; (3) on powdered glove; or (4) in suspension. Removal rate of 4-CP from aqueous solutions correlates with the amount of FE and its contact time. Decontamination efficiency estimated by the percentage of 4-CP recovery from contaminated porcine skin, achieved 54% with water, ranged between ~60% and 70% with dry FE and reached ~90% with FE suspension. Successful decontamination of the FE suspension, enabling a dramatic reduction of skin contamination after a brief exposure scenario, appears to be rapid, reliable and should be formulated in a new device ready to use for self-application.

- **Reference Type**: Journal Article
- **Record Number**: 61
- **Author**: K., Ogai, M., Matsumoto, M., Aoki, R., Ota, K., Hashimoto, R., Wada, M., Kobayashi and J., Sugama
- **Year**: 2017

- **Title**: Wash or wipe? A comparative study of skin physiological changes between water washing and wiping after skin cleaning
- **Journal**: Skin Research and Technology
- **Volume**: 23
- **Issue**: 4
- **Pages**: 519–524
- **Short Title**: Wash or wipe? A comparative study of skin physiological changes between water washing and wiping after skin cleaning
- **DOI**: https://doi.org/10.1111/srt.12364

Abstract: Background/purpose Presently, skin-cleaning agents that claim to be removed by water or wiping alone are commercially available and have been used for the purpose of bed baths. However, there is a lack of knowledge on how water washing and wiping differently affect skin physiological functions or ceramide content. The aim of this study was to compare the effects of water washing and wiping on skin physiological functions and ceramide content. Methods Three kinds of the cleaning agents with different removal techniques (i.e., water washing and wiping) were used in this study. Skin physiological functions (i.e., transepidermal water loss, skin hydration, and skin pH) and skin ceramide content were measured before and after seven consecutive days of the application of each cleaning agent. Results No significant differences in skin physiological functions or ceramide content were observed between water washing and wiping. Conclusion Cleaning agents that claim to be removed by water washing or wiping do not affect skin physiological functions or ceramide content by either removal method.

URL: https://onlinelibrary.wiley.com/doi/abs/10.1111/srt.12364

- **Reference Type**: Journal Article
- **Record Number**: 22
- **Author**: Kim, Sohee, Ying, Wu Bin, Jung, Hyunsook, Ryu, Sam Gon, Lee, Bumjae and Lee, Kyung Jin
- **Year**: 2017
- **Title**: Zirconium hydroxide-coated nanofiber mats for nerve agent decontamination
- **Journal**: Chemistry – An Asian Journal
- **Volume**: 12
- **Issue**: 6
- **Pages**: 698–705
- **Short Title**: Zirconium hydroxide-coated nanofiber mats for nerve agent decontamination
- ISSN: 1861-471X

Abstract: Diverse innovative fabrics with specific functionalities have been developed for requirements such as self-decontamination of chemical/biological pollutants and toxic nerve agents. In this work, $Zr(OH)_4$-coated nylon-6,6 nanofiber mats were fabricated for the decontamination of nerve agents. Nylon-6,6 fabric was prepared via the electrospinning process, followed by coating with $Zr(OH)_4$, which was obtained by the hydrolysis of $Zr(OBu)_4$ by a sol–gel reaction on nanofiber surfaces. The reaction conditions were optimized by varying the amounts of $Zr(OBu)_4$,the reaction time, and the temperature of the sol–gel reaction. The composite nanofibers show high decontamination efficiency against diisopropylfluorophosphate, which is a nerve agent analogue, due to its high nucleophilicity that aids in the catalysis of the hydrolysis of the phosphonate ester bonds. Composite nanofiber mats have a large potential and can be applied in specific fields such as military and medical markets.

- **Reference Type**: Journal Article
- **Record Number**: 12
- **Author**: Lewinski, Nastassja A, Berthet, Aurélie, Maurizi, Lionel, Eisenbeis, Antoine and Hopf, Nancy B
- **Year**: 2017
- **Title**: Effectiveness of hand washing on the removal of iron oxide nanoparticles from human skin ex vivo
- **Journal**: Journal of Occupational and Environmental Hygiene
- **Volume**: 14
- **Issue**: 8
- **Pages**: D115–D119
- **Short Title**: Effectiveness of hand washing on the removal of iron oxide nanoparticles from human skin ex vivo
- **ISSN**: 1545-9624
- URL: https://www.tandfonline.com/doi/full/10.1080/15459624.2017.1296238

Abstract: In this study, the effectiveness of washing with soap and water in removing nanoparticles from exposed skin was investigated. Dry, nanoscale hematite (α-Fe_2O_3) or maghemite (γ-Fe_2O_3) powder, with primary particle diameters between 20–30 nm, were applied to two samples each of fresh and frozen *ex vivo* human skin in two independent experiments. The permeation of nanoparticles through skin, and the removal of nanoparticles after washing with soap and water were investigated. Bare iron oxide nanoparticles remained primarily on the surface of the skin, without penetrating beyond the stratum corneum. Skin exposed to iron oxide nanoparticles for 1 and 20 hr resulted in removal of 85% and 90%, respectively, of the original dose after washing. In the event of dermal exposure to chemicals, removal is essential to avoid potential local irritation or permeation across skin. Although manufactured at an industrial scale and used extensively in laboratory experiments, limited data are available on the removal of engineered nanoparticles after skin contact. Our finding raises questions about the potential consequences of nanoparticles remaining on the skin and whether alternative washing methods should be proposed. Further studies on skin decontamination beyond use of soap and water are needed to improve the understanding of the potential health consequences of dermal exposure to nanoparticles.

- **Reference Type**: Journal Article
- **Record Number**: 39
- **Author**: J., Kitsongsermthon, K., Duangweang, J., Kreepoke and A., Tansirikongkol
- **Year**: 2017
- **Title**: *In vivo* cleansing efficacy of biodegradable exfoliating beads assessed by skin bioengineering techniques
- **Journal**: Skin Research and Technology
- **Volume**: 23
- **Issue**: 4
- **Pages**: 525–530
- **Short Title**: *In vivo* cleansing efficacy of biodegradable exfoliating beads assessed by skin bioengineering techniques
- **DOI**: https://doi.org/10.1111/srt.12365

Abstract: Background/purpose The plastic microbeads, used in many cleansers, will be banned in cosmetic and personal care products within 2017 since they are non-degradable and can disturb the living organisms in water reservoirs. Various choices of biodegradable beads are commercially available, but their efficacy has not been proven yet. This study aimed to compare the cleansing efficacy in dirt and sebum removal aspects of three types of exfoliating beads. Methods The gel scrubs with polyethylene (PE) beads, mannan beads or wax beads, were formulated and evaluated for their stability. The *in vivo* evaluation was done in 38 healthy volunteers and the skin irritation, efficacy for dirt and sebum removal were measured by Mexameter®, Colorimeter®, and Sebumeter®, respectively. Results The selected gel scrubs did not cause an irritation in any volunteers. The differences in dirt residues between before and after scrubbing were not statistically significant among three gel scrubs and the similar result was also reported in the sebum removal study. Conclusion All gel scrubs demonstrated the comparable cleansing efficacy in term of dirt and sebum removal. Thus, mannan beads and wax beads may be replaced non-biodegradable PE beads to achieve the similar cleansing effect.

URL: https://onlinelibrary.wiley.com/doi/abs/10.1111/srt.12365

Thors, L., et al. (2017). "Comparison of skin decontamination efficacy of commercial decontamination products following exposure to VX on human skin." Chemico-Biological Interactions 273: 82–89.

Abstract: The decontamination efficacy of four commercially available skin decontamination products following exposure to the *nerve agent VX* was evaluated *in vitro* utilizing a diffusion cell and dermatomed human skin. The products included were Reactive Skin Decontamination Lotion (RSDL), the Swedish decontamination powder 104 (PS104), the absorbent *Fuller's Earth* and the *aqueous solution* alldecontMED. In addition, various decontamination procedures were assessed to further investigate important mechanisms involved in the specific products, *e.g.* decontamination removal from skin, physical removal by sponge swabbing and activation of degradation mechanisms. The efficacy of each decontamination product was evaluated 5 or 30 min after dermal application of *VX* (neat or diluted to 20% in water).

The RSDL-lotion was superior in reducing the penetration of VX through human skin, both when exposed as neat agent and when diluted to 20% in water. Swabbing with the RSDL-sponge during 2 min revealed decreased efficacy compared to applying the RSDL-lotion directly on the skin for 30 min. Decontamination with Fuller's Earth and alldecontMED significantly reduced the penetration of neat concentration of VX through human skin. PS104-powder was insufficient for decontamination of VX at both time-points, independently of the skin contact time of PS104. The PS104-slurry (a mixture of PS104-powder and water), slightly improved the decontamination efficacy. Comparing the time-points for initiated decontamination revealed less penetrated VX for RSDL and Fuller's Earth when decontamination was initiated after 5 min compared to 30 min post-exposure, while alldecontMED displayed similar efficacy at both time-points. Decontamination by washing with water only resulted in a significant reduction of penetrated VX when washing was performed 5 min after exposure, but not when decontamination was delayed to 30 min post-exposure of neat VX.

In conclusion, early initiated decontamination with the RSDL-lotion, containing both *absorption* and degrading properties, allowed to act on skin for 30 min was superior in preventing VX from penetrating human skin. Adding water during decontamination resulted in increased penetration of neat VX, however, water in the decontaminant removal process did not influence the decontamination efficacy. From our study on commercially available decontaminants, it is recommended that future *product developments* should include both strong absorbents and efficient nerve agent degrading components.

Dachir, S., et al. (2017). "Dermostyx (IB1) – High efficacy and safe topical skin protectant against percutaneous toxic agents." Chemico-Biological Interactions 267: 25–32.

Prevention of the penetration of toxic agents through the skin is crucial for both military troops and civilian populations.

We have developed a novel topical skin protectant (TSP), coded as IB1 and commercially available as Dermostyx protective solution (Rekah Pharm, Israel). The formulation afforded significant protection against chemical warfare agents such as sulfur mustard (SM) and VX (2LD50), pesticides such as parathion and irritants such as acrolein. The efficacy of the protectant was evaluated in the pig model using clinical, histological and biochemical monitoring.

A single topical application prior to exposure to the toxic agents reduced significantly the size and severity of skin lesions and ameliorated or prevented systemic clinical symptoms.

The barrier properties of IB1 are immediate upon application and remain effective for at least 12 h. It is absorbed into the stratum corneum of the skin and remains there until rinsing with water, yet the ingredients are not absorbed into the body.

The formulation is a hydrophilic water-based solution, composed of magnesium sulfate and glycerin that are widely used in cosmetic and medicine, and was shown to be safe in preclinical and in Phase I clinical studies. The suggested mode of action is based on the unique interaction of glycerin with the stratum corneum, changing its properties to hydrophilic and on the "salting out" effect of magnesium sulfate.

The expected use of the TSP is by application on exposed skin areas and sensitive skin sites (e.g. armpits, groin, waist), when necessary. A quantity of 10 ml is sufficient for one application covering approximately 20% of the body surface area.

The formulation was approved for human use by the Israel Ministry of Health and a CE mark certificate in Europe has been recently issued (Class I). Dermostyx has been adopted by the IDF and first responders as a skin protectant for special needs.

- **Reference Type**: Journal Article
- **Record Number**: 33
- **Author**: Fent, Kenneth W., Alexander, Barbara, Roberts, Jennifer, Robertson, Shirley, Toennis, Christine, Sammons, Deborah, Bertke, Stephen, Kerber, Steve, Smith, Denise and Horn, Gavin
- **Year**: 2017
- **Title**: Contamination of firefighter personal protective equipment and skin and the effectiveness of decontamination procedures
- **Journal**: Journal of Occupational and Environmental Hygiene
- **Volume**: 14
- **Issue**: 10
- **Pages**: 801–814
- **Date**: 2017/10/03
- **Short Title**: Contamination of firefighter personal protective equipment and skin and the effectiveness of decontamination procedures
- **ISSN**: 1545-9624
- **DOI**: https://doi.org/10.1080/15459624.2017.1334904

Abstract: Firefighters' skin may be exposed to chemicals via permeation/penetration of combustion byproducts through or around personal protective equipment (PPE) or from the cross-transfer of contaminants on PPE to the skin. Additionally, volatile contaminants can evaporate from PPE following a response and be inhaled by firefighters. Using polycyclic aromatic hydrocarbons (PAHs) and volatile organic compounds (VOCs) as respective markers for non-volatile and volatile substances, we investigated the contamination of firefighters' turnout gear and skin following controlled residential fire responses. Participants were grouped into three crews of twelve firefighters. Each crew was deployed to a fire scenario (one per day, four total) and then paired up to complete six fireground job assignments. Wipe sampling of the exterior of the turnout gear was conducted pre- and post-fire. Wipe samples were also collected from a subset of the gear after field decontamination. VOCs off-gassing from gear were also measured pre-fire, post-fire, and post-decon. Wipe sampling of the firefighters' hands and neck was conducted pre- and post-fire. Additional wipes were collected after cleaning neck skin. PAH levels on turnout gear increased after each response and were greatest for gear worn by firefighters assigned to fire attack and to search and rescue activities. Field decontamination using dish soap, water, and scrubbing was able to reduce PAH contamination on turnout jackets by a median of 85%. Off-gassing VOC levels increased post-fire and then decreased 17–36 min later regardless of whether field decontamination was performed. Median post-fire PAH levels on the neck were near or below the limit of detection (<24 micrograms per square meter [μg/m2]) for all positions. For firefighters assigned to attack, search, and outside ventilation, the 75th percentile values on the neck were 152 μg/m^2, 71.7 μg/m^2, and 39.3 μg/m^2, respectively. Firefighters assigned to attack and search had higher post-fire median hand contamination (135 μg/m^2 and 226 μg/m^2, respectively) than other positions (<10.5 μg/m^2). Cleansing wipes were able to reduce PAH contamination on neck skin by a median of 54%.

URL: https://doi.org/10.1080/15459624.2017.1334904

Jacquet, P., et al. (2016). "Current and emerging strategies for organophosphate decontamination: Special focus on hyperstable enzymes." Environmental Science and Pollution Research 23(9): 8200–8218.

Abstract: Organophosphorus chemicals are highly toxic molecules mainly used as pesticides. Some of them are banned warfare nerve agents. These compounds are covalent inhibitors of acetylcholinesterase, a key enzyme in central and peripheral nervous systems. Numerous approaches, including chemical, physical, and biological decontamination, have been considered for developing decontamination methods against organophosphates (OPs). This work is an overview of both validated and emerging strategies for the protection against OP pollution with special attention to the use of decontaminating enzymes. Considerable efforts have been dedicated during the past decades to the development of efficient OP degrading biocatalysts. Among these, the promising biocatalyst *Sso*Pox isolated from the archaeon *Sulfolobus solfataricus* is emphasized in the light of recently published results. This hyperthermostable enzyme appears to be particularly attractive for external decontamination purposes with regard to both its catalytic and stability properties.

Tewari-Singh, N. and R. Agarwal (2016). "Mustard vesicating agent-induced toxicity in the skin tissue and silibinin as a potential countermeasure." Annals of the New York Academy of Sciences 1374(1): 184–192.

Abstract: Exposure to the vesicating agents sulfur mustard (SM) and nitrogen mustard (NM) causes severe skin injury with delayed blistering. Depending upon the dose and time of their exposure, edema and erythema develop into blisters, ulceration, necrosis, desquamation, and pigmentation changes, which persist weeks and even years after exposure. Research advances have generated data that have started to explain the probable mechanism of action of vesicant-induced skin toxicity; however, despite these advances, effective and targeted therapies are still deficient. This review highlights studies on two SM analogs, 2-chloroethyl ethyl sulfide (CEES) and NM, and CEES- and NM-induced skin injury mouse models that have substantially added to the knowledge on the complex pathways involved in mustard vesicating agent–induced skin injury. Furthermore, employing these mouse models, studies under the National Institutes of Health Countermeasures Against Chemical Threats program have identified the flavanone silibinin as a novel therapeutic intervention with the potential to be developed as an effective countermeasure against skin injury following exposure to mustard vesicating agents.

Koplovitz, I., et al. (2016). Evaluation of Veriox as a skin decontamination product after dermal exposure to the nerve agent VX, US Army Medical Research Institute of Chemical Defense Aberdeen Proving Ground United States.

Abstract: Veriox (R) is a topical antimicrobial anti-infective/disinfectant, which is under development for various uses to include medical device sterilization, advanced wound care, surface disinfection, a coating on medical products, hand sanitization, and veterinary wound care. The purpose of these experiments was to determine whether Veriox had efficacy as a decontamination product (DC) after skin exposure to the chemical warfare agent VX. This study compared the effectiveness of Veriox to Reactive Skin Decontamination Lotion (RSDL) when each was used as a DC product 2 min after dermal exposure to VX in hair-clipped, unanesthetized guinea pigs. Efficacy was established by generating VX dose-lethality curves for each DC product based on 24 survival/lethality responses and calculating the VX dose at which 50% (LD50) of animals died. The dermal LD50 of VX in Veriox-treated animals was 5959 micro g/kg, which was 1.8 fold higher than the VX LD50 of 3380 micro g/kg in RSDL-treated animals. Veriox was significantly ($p < 0.005$) more effective than RSDL. Further studies with Veriox are needed to determine its ultimate usefulness as a skin DC product for military use.

- **Reference Type**: Journal Article
- **Record Number**: 7
- **Author**: Phuong, Christina and Maibach, Howard I
- **Year**: 2016
- **Title**: Effect of massage on percutaneous penetration and skin decontamination: man and animal
- **Journal**: Cutaneous and Ocular Toxicology
- **Volume**: 35
- **Issue**: 2
- **Pages**: 153–156
- **Short Title**: Effect of massage on percutaneous penetration and skin decontamination: man and animal
- **ISSN**: 1556-9527

- **Reference Type**: Journal Article
- **Record Number**: 15
- **Author**: Noury, Barbara, Coman, Garrett, Blickenstaff, Nicholas and Maibach, Howard
- **Year**: 2015
- **Title**: *In vitro* skin decontamination model: comparison of salicylic acid and aminophylline

- **Journal**: Cutaneous and Ocular Toxicology
- **Volume**: 34
- **Issue**: 2
- **Pages**: 124–131
- **Short Title**: *In vitro* skin decontamination model: comparison of salicylic acid and aminophylline
- **ISSN**: 1556-9527

- **Reference Type**: Journal Article
- **Record Number**: 10
- **Author**: Stratilo, Chad W, Crichton, Melissa KF and Sawyer, Thomas W
- **Year**: 2015
- **Title**: Decontamination efficacy and skin toxicity of two decontaminants against *Bacillus anthracis*
- **Journal**: PloS One
- **Volume**: 10
- **Issue**: 9
- **Pages**: e0138491
- **Short Title**: Decontamination efficacy and skin toxicity of two decontaminants against *Bacillus anthracis*
- **ISSN**: 1932-6203

Abstract: Decontamination of bacterial endospores such as *Bacillus anthracis* has traditionally required the use of harsh or caustic chemicals. The aim of this study was to evaluate the efficacy of a chlorine dioxide decontaminant in killing *Bacillus anthracis* spores in solution and on a human skin simulant (porcine cadaver skin), compared to that of commonly used sodium hypochlorite or soapy water decontamination procedures. In addition, the relative toxicities of these decontaminants were compared in human skin keratinocyte primary cultures. The chlorine dioxide decontaminant was similarly effective to sodium hypochlorite in reducing spore numbers of *Bacillus anthracis* Ames in liquid suspension after a 10 minute exposure. After five minutes, the chlorine dioxide product was significantly more efficacious. Decontamination of isolated swine skin contaminated with *Bacillus anthracis* Sterne with the chlorine dioxide product resulted in no viable spores sampled. The toxicity of the chlorine dioxide decontaminant was up to two orders of magnitude less than that of sodium hypochlorite in human skin keratinocyte cultures. In summary, the chlorine dioxide based decontaminant efficiently killed *Bacillus anthracis* spores in liquid suspension, as well as on isolated swine skin, and was less toxic than sodium hypochlorite in cultures of human skin keratinocytes.

- **Reference Type**: Journal Article
- **Record Number**: 8
- **Author**: Dennerlein, Kathrin, Jaeger, Thomas, Goeen, Thomas, Kilo, Sonja, Schaller, Karl Heinz, Drexler, Hans and Korinth, Gintautas

- **Year**: 2015
- **Title**: Evaluation of the effect of skin cleaning procedures on the dermal absorption of chemicals
- **Journal**: Toxicology *In Vitro*
- **Volume**: 29
- **Issue**: 5
- **Pages**: 828–833
- **Short Title**: Evaluation of the effect of skin cleaning procedures on the dermal absorption of chemicals
- **ISSN**: 0887-2333

Abstract: To reduce the internal exposure, skin decontamination is the most important measure after dermal contact to chemicals. However, no harmonized skin cleaning procedure for experimental ex vivo studies is published. In our study, the impact of two skin cleaning techniques on dermal penetration kinetics and intradermal deposition of 1,4-dioxane, 5% hydrofluoric acid (HF, detected in terms of fluoride ions), and anisole was evaluated to develop a reliable ex vivo skin cleaning method using the diffusion cell technique. After exposure (duration: 3 min (HF); 1 h (1,4-dioxane and anisole)) of excised human skin ($n = 6–8$) decontamination was performed by (I) water–soaked cotton swabs or (II) direct application of water on the exposure area. The effect of skin cleaning was investigated by analysing the concentration time course of chemicals in the receptor fluid of diffusion cells and by determining the deposition in skin. Both skin cleaning procedures reduced the amount of fluoride in the skin compartments ($p < 0.05$) and the receptor fluid ($p < 0.1$). However, the effect of cleaning on the dermal absorption of the organic test compounds was not significant. The results demonstrate the suitability of the applied ex vivo protocol for investigating the effectiveness of skin cleaning measures following dermal exposure. In addition, data reveal that the determination of test compounds in both, skin compartments as well as receptor fluid as equivalent for the systemic uptake needs to be considered in studies assessing the effectiveness of skin decontamination procedures.

- **Reference Type**: Journal Article
- **Record Number**: 60
- **Author**: Dennerlein, Kathrin, Jäger, Thomas, Göen, Thomas, Kilo, Sonja, Schaller, Karl Heinz, Drexler, Hans and Korinth, Gintautas
- **Year**: 2015
- **Title**: Evaluation of the effect of skin cleaning procedures on the dermal absorption of chemicals
- **Journal**: Toxicology *In Vitro*
- **Volume**: 29
- **Issue**: 5
- **Pages**: 828–833

- **Date**: 2015/08/01/
- **Short Title**: Evaluation of the effect of skin cleaning procedures on the dermal absorption of chemicals
- **ISSN**: 0887-2333
- **DOI**: https://doi.org/10.1016/j.tiv.2015.03.001

Keywords: Skin decontamination; Percutaneous absorption; Diffusion cell studies; 1,4-Dioxane

Hydrofluoric acid; Anisole

Abstract: To reduce the internal exposure, skin decontamination is the most important measure after dermal contact to chemicals. However, no harmonized skin cleaning procedure for experimental ex vivo studies is published. In our study, the impact of two skin cleaning techniques on dermal penetration kinetics and intradermal deposition of 1,4-dioxane, 5% hydrofluoric acid (HF, detected in terms of fluoride ions), and anisole was evaluated to develop a reliable ex vivo skin cleaning method using the diffusion cell technique. After exposure (duration: 3 min (HF); 1 h (1,4-dioxane and anisole)) of excised human skin ($n = 6–8$) decontamination was performed by (I) water–soaked cotton swabs or (II) direct application of water on the exposure area. The effect of skin cleaning was investigated by analysing the concentration time course of chemicals in the receptor fluid of diffusion cells and by determining the deposition in skin. Both skin cleaning procedures reduced the amount of fluoride in the skin compartments ($p < 0.05$) and the receptor fluid ($p < 0.1$). However, the effect of cleaning on the dermal absorption of the organic test compounds was not significant. The results demonstrate the suitability of the applied ex vivo protocol for investigating the effectiveness of skin cleaning measures following dermal exposure. In addition, data reveal that the determination of test compounds in both, skin compartments as well as receptor fluid as equivalent for the systemic uptake needs to be considered in studies assessing the effectiveness of skin decontamination procedures.

URL: http://www.sciencedirect.com/science/article/pii/S0887233315000429

Valle, A. K. (2014). Microporous polymer beads for chemical decontamination of organophosphorus nerve agents, Norwegian University of Life Sciences, Ås.

Abstract: The objective of the work presented in this thesis was the development of reactive polymer beads for use as decontaminants of organophosphorus nerve agents. The physiological mode of action of nerve agents, which is the cause of their high toxicity, is the ability to bind and inhibit the enzyme acetylcholinesterase (AChE). As organophosphorus nerve agents easily reach the active site of AChE and inhibit the enzyme, it was hoped that effective polymeric decontaminants could be prepared by mimicking the structural and functional characteristics of AChE.

In the present study, a suspension polymerization method suitable for polymerization of water-soluble monomers was developed for copolymerization of methyl acrylate and styrene. This method was used for the synthesis of cross-linked poly(methyl acrylate-co-styrene) beads. The established suspension polymerization technique was developed further by incorporation of acid-scavenging monomers into the polymer structure, more specifically 4-vinylpyridine and N-[3-(dimethylamino)propyl]methacrylamide (DMAPMA), entities which were believed to be capable of binding toxic byproducts formed during decontamination. Synthesized polymer products containing these monomers included cross-linked poly(methyl acrylate-co-4-vinylpyridine) and poly(methyl acrylate-co-styrene-co¬-DMAPMA) beads. However, due to low incorporation of DMAPMA and low yields, only cross-linked poly(methyl acrylate-co-styrene) and poly(methyl acrylate-co-4-vinylpyridine) beads were used in further studies as these gave both high incorporation of monomers and consistent, high yields.

The cross-linked poly(methyl acrylate-co-styrene) and poly(methyl acrylate-co-4-vinylpyridine) products were further functionalized with hydroxylamine to convert methyl acrylate moieties to the corresponding hydroxamate anion of hydroxamic acid. In the functionalized product, styrene constitutes the hydrophobic part of the polymer network, contributing to increased affinity of the reactive polymer beads towards the hydrophobic, organophosphorus nerve agents. The converted hydroxamate anions facilitate solvation of the polymer network in aqueous environments, in addition to providing nucleophilic functionalities capable of hydrolyzing the organophosphorus nerve agents. Successful conversion was confirmed by CHN analysis and IR spectroscopy.

- **Reference Type**: Journal Article
- **Record Number**: 19
- **Author**: Castellani, Romain, Poulesquen, Arnaud, Goettmann, Frédéric, Marchal, Philippe and Choplin, Lionel
- **Year**: 2014
- **Title**: Efficiency enhancement of decontamination gels by a superabsorbent polymer
- **Journal**: Colloids and Surfaces A: Physicochemical and Engineering Aspects
- **Volume**: 454
- **Pages**: 89–95
- **Short Title**: Efficiency enhancement of decontamination gels by a superabsorbent polymer
- **ISSN**: 0927-7757

Abstract: Physical gels have been studied as an advantageous alternative to traditional decontamination techniques, which most often rely on the use of surfactant solutions. Such physical gels consist of colloidal particles suspended in a decontaminating solution. They can be sprayed over the surfaces to be treated, where they dry and form solid disposable residues. In order to improve their efficiency, the formulation of gels containing superabsorbents (such as sodium polyacrylate) has recently been suggested. But the mechanism accounting for the observed efficiency increase has not yet been investigated. These additives have a large swelling potential in aqueous media and the amount of adsorbed water depends on the presence of salts in the medium. We anticipated that specific ion effects on the swelling behavior of superabsorbent polymers were the driving force of efficiency enhancement and confirmed this assumption by rheology and *in situ* tests.

- **Reference Type**: Journal Article
- **Record Number**: 34
- **Author**: Peter, Elsner, Florian, Seyfarth, Flora, Sonsmann, Swen-Malte, John, Thomas, Diepgen and Sibylle, Schliemann
- **Year**: 2014
- **Title**: Development of a standardized procedure for testing the efficacy of workplace cleansers
- **Journal**: Contact Dermatitis
- **Volume**: 70
- **Issue**: 1
- **Pages**: 35–43
- **Short Title**: Development of a standardized procedure for testing the efficacy of workplace cleansers
- **DOI**: https://doi.org/10.1111/cod.12121

Abstract: Background – Occupational skin cleansing is a risk factor for cumulative irritant dermatitis. Standardized methods are required to assess the cleaning efficacy of occupational skin cleansers, allowing us to choose the optimal cleanser with minimal irritation for specific workplaces. Objectives – To develop a standardized procedure for testing the cleaning efficacy of occupational skin cleansers. Methods – In this single-blind, randomized, monocentric clinical trial in 24 healthy volunteers, the cleaning efficacy of generic reference cleansers was assessed against standardized test dirts. The test procedure included standardized dirt application, standardized washing with an automated skin cleaning device, and quantification of the cleaning efficacy by chromametry. For two cleansers, reproducibility of the cleaning efficacy assessment was studied. Furthermore, the performance of two cleansers was compared with that of commercial skin cleansers. Results – Cleaning factors ranged from 12% up to 97% for the respective model dirts. A high reproducibility of the washing and the assessment procedure could be shown. The comparison of the washing efficacies for two reference cleansers with those of commercial cleansers showed partly similar performances, but also a higher cleaning efficacy for some dirts of the reference cleansers. Conclusions – The testing procedure proved to be applicable to a wide spectrum of cleansers and model dirts.

URL: https://onlinelibrary.wiley.com/doi/abs/10.1111/cod.12121

- **Reference Type**: Journal Article
- **Record Number**: 3
- **Author**: Chan, Heidi P, Zhai, Hongbo, Hui, Xiaoying and Maibach, Howard I
- **Year**: 2013
- **Title**: Skin decontamination: principles and perspectives
- **Journal**: Toxicology and Industrial Health

- **Volume**: 29
- **Issue**: 10
- **Pages**: 955–968
- **Short Title**: Skin decontamination: principles and perspectives
- **ISSN**: 0748-2337

- **Reference Type**: Journal Article
- **Record Number**: 29
- **Author**: Zhang, Ming and Gao, Bin
- **Year**: 2013
- **Title**: Removal of arsenic, methylene blue, and phosphate by biochar/AlOOH nanocomposite
- **Journal**: Chemical Engineering Journal
- **Volume**: 226
- **Pages**: 286–292
- **Date**: 2013/06/15/
- **Short Title**: Removal of arsenic, methylene blue, and phosphate by biochar/AlOOH nanocomposite
- **ISSN**: 1385-8947
- **DOI**: https://doi.org/10.1016/j.cej.2013.04.077

Keywords: Biochar; AlOOH; Nanocomposite; Adsorbent; Contaminants

Abstract: In this work, a biochar based composite material with AlOOH nanoflakes was fabricated from AlCl3 pretreated biomass through slow pyrolysis in a N2 environment at 600 °C. Physicochemical properties of the biochar/AlOOH nanocomposite were studied systematically with several commonly used material characterization instruments, including electron microscopes and X-ray techniques. Structure and morphology analysis of the sample showed that the AlOOH particles/flakes are nanosized and uniformly grow on the carbon surface within the pores of the biochar. Laboratory batch sorption experiments were conducted to evaluate the sorption ability of the biochar/AlOOH nanocomposite to three representative aqueous contaminants: arsenic, methylene blue, and phosphate. The adsorption isotherm and adsorption kinetics data suggested that the biochar/AlOOH nanocomposite is an excellent multifunctional adsorbent that can effectively remove all these contaminants from aqueous solutions.

URL: http://www.sciencedirect.com/science/article/pii/S138589471300555X

Misík, J., et al. (2013). "Percutaneous toxicity and decontamination of soman, Vx, and paraoxon in rats using detergents." Archives of Industrial Hygiene and Toxicology 64(2): 211–217.
Abstract: N/A

Brent, J. (2013). "Water-based solutions are the best decontaminating fluids for dermal corrosive exposures: a mini review." Clinical Toxicology 51(8): 731–736.
Abstract: The intention is to assess whether the fundamental principle ("the solution to pollution is dilution") should be the guide for the initial medical management

of corrosive dermal exposures. *Methods.* The US National Library of Medicine PubMed database was searched utilizing all combinations of the search terms "decontamination", "corrosive", and "dermal". A separate search was done specifically related to hydrofluoric acid. These searches found 69 relevant papers. *Results.* Only four controlled clinical studies comparing early and intensive water decontamination with no or less dilution treatment have been published on human corrosive dermal exposures. Although the authors' conclusion in the first study of 273 patients was that those that had more intensive water irrigation tended to have less time to skin grafting and shorter periods of hospitalization, the results were not statistically significant. In the second study of 51 patients, those who had "adequate" decontamination (immediate dilution or neutralization therapy) had shortened length of stay (7.2 vs. 16.2 days), lower mortality (9.5% vs. 21%), and fewer skin grafts (19% vs. 36%) despite having slightly greater burn surface area (19.7% vs. 17.2%). However, no statistical analysis was provided. The third and fourth studies were conducted in the same center. In the third study of 35 patients, those who had "immediate" water lavage (done within 10 min of exposure and continued for at least 15 min) had significantly fewer burns that progressed to full thickness (12.5% vs. 63%; $p < 0.01$) and significantly shorter mean hospital stays (7.7 days vs. 20.5 days; $p < 0.01$) than those who did not, despite the mean total burn surface area being twice as large in the adequate water decontamination group (12% vs. 6%; $p < 0.05$). In the fourth study of 83 patients (35 of whom had been reported in the previous study), those who had copious water lavage within 3 min of injury were less likely to progress to full thickness burns (13.5% vs. 60.8%; $p < 0.01$), had fewer delayed complications (5.4% vs. 30.4%; $p < 0.01$) and shorter lengths of stay (6.2 vs. 22 days; $p < 0.01$), compared with those who did not. In a further study, water was compared to the proprietary agent Diphoterine® in a controlled prospective cohort study of 180 dermal alkali exposures. The Diphoterine® first group was decontaminated significantly faster than the water first group (median times to irrigation 1 vs. 5 min; $p < 0.001$). No analysis adjusted for time to decontamination was provided, so the study demonstrated that only those individuals who decontaminated early did better than those who decontaminated later. *Conclusions.* The data support water as the best decontaminating solution. It has been shown to be efficacious in clinical trials, is widely available, and inexpensive.

- **Reference Type**: Journal Article
- **Record Number**: 6
- **Author**: Hui, Xiaoying, Domoradzki, Jeanne Y and Maibach, Howard C
- **Year**: 2012
- **Title**: *In vitro* study to determine decontamination of 3, 5-dichloro-2, 4, 6-trifluoropyridine (DCTFP) from human skin
- **Journal**: Food and Chemical Toxicology
- **Volume**: 50
- **Issue**: 7
- **Pages**: 2496–2502

- **Short Title**: *In vitro* study to determine decontamination of 3, 5-dichloro-2, 4, 6-trifluoropyridine (DCTFP) from human skin
- **ISSN**: 0278-6915

- **Reference Type**: Conference Proceedings
- **Record Number**: 18
- **Author**: Mathieu, Laurence, Belliard, Berengere, Wang, Hui-fei, Zhang, Fan, Burgher, Francois, Fosse, Celine, Coudouel, Herve, Blomet, Joel, Lati, Elain and Peno-Mazzarino, Laurent
- **Year of Conference**: 2011
- **Title**: Corrosive acid (sulfuric acid; H2SO4) and base (sodium hydroxide; NaOH) skin injury and decontamination: *in vitro*, experimental animal, and human skin explant ex vivo studies, and illustrative case report
- **Conference Name**: Abstracts of Papers of the American Chemical Society
- **Publisher**: Amer Chemical Soc, 1155 16th St, NW, Washington, DC 20036 USA
- **Volume**: 241
- **Short Title**: Corrosive acid (sulfuric acid; H2SO4) and base (sodium hydroxide; NaOH) skin injury and decontamination: *In vitro*, experimental animal, and human skin explant ex vivo studies, and illustrative case report
- **ISBN**: 0065-7727

- **Reference Type**: Journal Article
- **Record Number**: 18
- **Author**: Wagner, George W, Procell, Lawrence R, Sorrick, David C, Lawson, Glenn E, Wells, Claire M, Reynolds, Charles M, Ringelberg, David B, Foley, Karen L, Lumetta, Gregg J and Blanchard Jr, David L
- **Year**: 2010
- **Title**: All-weather hydrogen peroxide-based decontamination of CBRN contaminants
- **Journal**: Industrial & Engineering Chemistry Research
- **Volume**: 49
- **Issue**: 7
- **Pages**: 3099–3105
- **Short Title**: All-weather hydrogen peroxide-based decontamination of CBRN contaminants
- **ISSN**: 0888-5885

Abstract: A hydrogen peroxide-based decontaminant, Decon Green, is efficacious for the decontamination of chemical agents VX (*S*-2-(diisopropylamino)ethyl *O*-ethyl methylphosphonothioate), GD (Soman, pinacolyl methylphosphonofluoridate), and HD (mustard, bis(2-chloroethyl) sulfide); the biological agent anthrax (*Bacillus anthracis*); and radiological isotopes ^{137}Cs and ^{60}Co; thus demonstrating the ability of this decontamination approach to ameliorate the aftermath of all three types of weapons of mass destruction (WMD). Reaction mechanisms afforded for the chemical agents are discussed as are rationales for the enhanced removal efficacy of recalcitrant ^{60}Co on certain surfaces. Decontaminants of this nature can be deployed, and are effective, at very low temperatures (−32 °C), as shown for studies done with VX and HD simulants, without the need for external heat sources. Finally, the efficacy of a lower-logistics, dry decontaminant powder concentrate (utilizing the solid active-oxygen compounds peracetyl borate and Peroxydone) which can be reconstituted with water in the field prior to use, is presented.

- **Reference Type**: Journal Article
- **Record Number**: 11
- **Author**: Amlôt, Richard, Larner, Joanne, Matar, Hazem, Jones, David R, Carter, Holly, Turner, Elizabeth A, Price, Shirley C and Chilcott, Robert P
- **Year**: 2010
- **Title**: Comparative analysis of showering protocols for mass-casualty decontamination
- **Journal**: Prehospital and Disaster Medicine
- **Volume**: 25
- **Issue**: 5
- **Pages**: 435–439
- **Short Title**: Comparative analysis of showering protocols for mass-casualty decontamination
- **ISSN**: 1945-1938

Abstract: A well-established provision for mass-casualty decontamination that incorporates the use of mobile showering units has been developed in the UK. The effectiveness of such decontamination procedures will be critical in minimizing or preventing the contamination of emergency responders and hospital infrastructure. The purpose of this study was to evaluate three empirical strategies designed to optimize existing decontamination procedures: (1) instructions in the form of a pictorial aid prior to decontamination; (2) provision of a washcloth within the showering facility; and (3) an extended showering period. The study was a three-factor, between-participants (or "independent") design with 90 volunteers. The three factors each had two levels: use of washcloths (washcloth/no washcloth), washing instructions (instructions/no instructions), and shower cycle duration (three minutes/six minutes). The effectiveness of these strategies was quantified by whole-body fluorescence imaging following application of a red fluorophore to multiple, discrete areas of the skin. All five showering procedures were relatively effective in removing the fluorophore "contaminant", but the use of a cloth (in the absence of instructions) led to a significant (~20%) improvement in the effectiveness of decontamination over the standard protocol ($p < 0.05$). Current mass-casualty decontamination effectiveness, especially in children, can be optimized by the provision of a washcloth. This simple but effective approach indicates the value of performing controlled volunteer trials for optimizing existing decontamination procedures.

Prasad, G., et al. (2008). "Decontamination of sulfur mustard and sarin on titania nanotubes." AIChE Journal 54(11): 2957–2963.

Abstract: Decontamination reactions of sulfur mustard and sarin were studied on the surface of titania nanotubes and the data were compared with that of bulk titania. Before the reaction studies, titania nanotube samples were made by using hydrothermal method and were characterized by scanning electron microscopy, N_2 BET, X-ray diffractometry, and thermogravimetry. Soon after that, titania nanotube samples were exposed to sulfur mustard and sarin separately at room temperature (30°C) and the reactions were monitored by gas chromatography, whereas the reaction products were characterized by GC-MS. The data explore the role of hydrolysis reactions and surface reactions for the decontamination of both sulfur mustard and sarin. © 2008 American Institute of Chemical Engineers AIChE J, 2008

- **Reference Type**: Journal Article
- **Record Number**: 5
- **Author**: Zhai, HONGBO, Barbadillo, S, Hui, X and Maibach, HI
- **Year**: 2007
- **Title**: *In vitro* model for decontamination of human skin: formaldehyde
- **Journal**: Food and Chemical Toxicology
- **Volume**: 45
- **Issue**: 4
- **Pages**: 618–621
- **Short Title**: *In vitro* model for decontamination of human skin: formaldehyde
- **ISSN**: 0278-6915
- **Reference Type**: Journal Article
- **Record Number**: 1
- **Author**: Hall, Alan H and Maibach, Howard I
- **Year**: 2006
- **Title**: Water decontamination of chemical skin/eye splashes: a critical review
- **Journal**: Cutaneous and Ocular Toxicology
- **Volume**: 25
- **Issue**: 2
- **Pages**: 67–83
- **Short Title**: Water decontamination of chemical skin/eye splashes: a critical review
- **ISSN**: 1556-9527

- **Reference Type**: Journal Article
- **Record Number**: 19
- **Author**: Moody, Richard P and Maibach, Howard I
- **Year**: 2006
- **Title**: Skin decontamination: importance of the wash-in effect
- **Journal**: Food and Chemical Toxicology

- **Volume**: 44
- **Issue**: 11
- **Pages**: 1783–1788
- **Short Title**: Skin decontamination: importance of the wash-in effect
- **ISSN**: 0278-6915

- **Reference Type**: Journal Article
- **Record Number**: 82
- **Author**: Filon, Francesca Larese, Boeniger, Mark, Maina, Giovanni, Adami, Gianpiero, Spinelli, Paolo and Damian, Adriano
- **Year**: 2006
- **Title**: Skin absorption of inorganic lead (PbO) and the effect of skin cleansers
- **Journal**: Journal of Occupational and Environmental Medicine
- **Volume**: 48
- **Issue**: 7
- **Pages**: 692–699
- **Short Title**: Skin absorption of inorganic lead (PbO) and the effect of skin cleansers
- **ISSN**: 1076-2752

Abstract:

Objective: The aim of this study was to investigate the percutaneous penetration of lead oxide (PbO) powder and the effect of rapid skin decontamination with two different detergents.

Methods: Franz cells were used to study *in vitro* PbO skin penetration through human skin during a 24-hour period. The tests were performed without or with decontamination using either Ivory Liquid soap or a new experimental cleanser 30 minutes after the start of exposure.

Results: We confirm that PbO can pass through the skin with a median penetration of 2.9 ng/cm^2 (25–75th percentiles 0.35–6). The cleaning procedure using Ivory Liquid soap significantly increased skin penetration with a median value of 23.6 ng/cm^2 (25–75th percentiles 12–47.1; Mann-Whitney U test, $P = 0.0002$), whereas the new experimental cleanser only marginally increased penetration (7.1 ng/cm^2).

Conclusions: Our results indicate that it is necessary to prevent skin contamination from occurring because a short contact can increase skin content and penetration even if quickly followed by washing. This study demonstrated that PbO powder can pass through the skin and that skin decontamination done after 30 minutes of exposure did not decrease skin absorption occurring over 24 hours and stresses the need to prevent skin contamination when using toxic substances.

Saboori, A. M. and R. K. Gordon (2005). Selective binding of organophosphate pesticides using molecular imprinted polymers, Walter Reed Army Inst of Research, Silver Spring, MD.

Abstract: Molecular Imprinted Polymers (MIPs) have been used for recognition and binding of different compounds. We are developing MIPs to selectively bind organophosphate pesticides and toxic chemical warfare nerve agents. MIPs were made to the pesticide Dichlorvos. Control MIPs were made without the template. Dichlorvos-MIPs bound more Dichlorvos in comparison to control-MIPs. The Dichlorvos-MIPs can be regenerated after binding the pesticide and reused at least three times by repeating the washing procedure. Dichlorvos-MIPs demonstrated specificity for its template since these MIPs did not bind Methamidophos, Phosdrin, and Metasystox I, compounds with similar chemical structures to that of Dichlorvos.

- **Reference Type**: Journal Article
- **Record Number**: 11
- **Author**: Wester, RM, Maibach, HI and Wester, RC
- **Year**: 2005
- **Title**: Chemical warfare agent VX penetration through military uniform and human skin: risk assessment and decontamination
- **Journal**: Drugs and the Pharmaceutical Sciences
- **Volume**: 155
- **Pages**: 481
- **Short Title**: Chemical warfare agent VX penetration through military uniform and human skin: risk assessment and decontamination
- **ISSN**: 0360-2583

- **Reference Type**: Journal Article
- **Record Number**: 80
- **Author**: Soderberg, Kjell, Kuusinen, Petri, Mathieu, Laurence and Hall, Alan H
- **Year**: 2004
- **Title**: An improved method for emergent decontamination of ocular and dermal hydrofluoric acid splashes
- **Journal**: Veterinary and Human Toxicology
- **Volume**: 46
- **Issue**: 4
- **Pages**: 216–218
- **Short Title**: An improved method for emergent decontamination of ocular and dermal hydrofluoric acid splashes
- **ISSN**: 0145-6296

Abstract: Accidental hydrofluoric acid (HF) splashes often occur in industrial settings. HF easily penetrates into tissues by initial acid action allowing fluoride ions to penetrate deeply, chelating calcium and magnesium. Resultant hypocalcemia and hypomagnesemia can be fatal. This report describes the utilization of Hexafluorine—a hypertonic, amphoteric, chelating decontamination solution—in workplaces where water decontamination followed by calcium gluconate inunction failed to prevent HF burns and systemic toxicity. Between 1998 and 1999, 16 cases of ocular and dermal HF splashes with either 70% HF or 6% HF/15% nitric acid (HNO3) were decontaminated with Hexafluorine at the worksite. HF burns did not develop and medical treatment other than initial decontamination was not required in 12/16

(75%). In 7/16 (44%) cases, lost work time corresponded to duration of hospital observation (mean < 1 d).

- **Reference Type**: Journal Article
- **Record Number**: 26
- **Author**: Morton, Jackie, Carolan, Vikki A. and Gardiner, Philip H. E.
- **Year**: 2002
- **Title**: Removal of exogenously bound elements from human hair by various washing procedures and determination by inductively coupled plasma mass spectrometry
- **Journal**: Analytica Chimica Acta
- **Volume**: 455
- **Issue**: 1
- **Pages**: 23–34
- **Date**: 2002/03/18
- **Short Title**: Removal of exogenously bound elements from human hair by various washing procedures and determination by inductively coupled plasma mass spectrometry
- **ISSN**: 0003-2670
- **DOI**: https://doi.org/10.1016/S0003-2670(01)01578-1

Keywords: Hair analysis; Washing; ICP-MS; Metals; Exogenous

Abstract: A review of the literature shows that a variety of washing procedures to remove external contamination from hair have been proposed, but as yet no standardised procedures are available. In this study, methods for the pre-treatment and determination of antimony, arsenic, cadmium, chromium, lead, mercury and selenium in human hair by inductively coupled plasma mass spectrometry (ICP-MS) are developed.

Investigations of various washing procedures to remove external contaminants show that in unexposed hair samples cadmium, lead and mercury are significantly removed from hair using a 0.1 M HCl wash, with 87%, 73% and 5%, respectively being washed-off. The removal of antimony, arsenic and chromium from unexposed hair is, however, more efficient with 1% (v/v) sodium lauryl sulphate (SLS), with 43%, 40% and 13% of each element, respectively being washed-off. Selenium is not removed from the hair by any of the washing methods studied. For the digestion of hair samples a digestion mixture of nitric acid and hydrogen peroxide is used.

Experiments with simulated sweat spiked with each of these elements show that exogenously bound chromium, cadmium and lead are removed after washing with 0.1 M HCl. In contrast, antimony, arsenic, selenium and mercury irreversibly bind and, thus, are not removed with any of the washing solutions investigated. This work also compares hair levels of these elements in an unexposed and exposed group using the method developed.

URL: http://www.sciencedirect.com/science/article/pii/S0003267001015781

- **Reference Type**: Journal Article
- **Record Number**: 78
- **Author**: Mathieu, L, Nehles, J, Blomet, J and Hall, AH
- **Year**: 2001
- **Title**: Efficacy of hexafluorine for emergent decontamination of hydrofluoric acid eye and skin splashes
- **Journal**: Veterinary and Human Toxicology
- **Volume**: 43
- **Issue**: 5
- **Pages**: 263–265
- **Short Title**: Efficacy of hexafluorine for emergent decontamination of hydrofluoric acid eye and skin splashes

Abstract: Hexafluorine is an amphoteric, hypertonic, polyvalent compound for decontaminating hydrofluoric acid (HF) eye and skin splashes. In a German metallurgy facility during the period of 1994–1998, all eye or skin splashes with 40% HF alone or with a 6% HF/15% HNO3 mixture were initially decontaminated with Hexafluorine within 2 min following the splash at the accident site by the victims themselves or co-workers who witnessed the accident. Eleven workers using 40% HF or a 6% HF/15% HNO3 mixture sustained eye (2 cases) or skin (10 cases) splashes (1 combined) during 1994–1998. Hexafluorine was used within 2 min, and a second Hexafluorine decontamination was done on arrival at the plant infirmary. No further medical or surgical treatment was needed, no workers developed chemical burns, and none lost work time. These II cases demonstrate the efficacy of Hexafluorine in decontaminating HF or combined HF/HNO3 splashes.

- **Reference Type**: Journal Article
- **Record Number**: 9
- **Author**: Stibich, Adam S, Yagan, Mark, Sharma, Vidya, Herndon, Betty and Montgomery, Christopher
- **Year**: 2000
- **Title**: Cost-effective post-exposure prevention of poison ivy dermatitis
- **Journal**: International Journal of Dermatology
- **Volume**: 39
- **Issue**: 7
- **Pages**: 515–518
- **Short Title**: Cost-effective post-exposure prevention of poison ivy dermatitis
- **ISSN**: 1365-4632
- **URL**: https://onlinelibrary.wiley.com/doi/abs/10.1046/j.1365-4362.2000.00003.x

Abstract: Poison ivy (toxicodendron) dermatitis is the most common allergic contact dermatitis in the USA. No studies have shown an effect of washing after a short period of time for the prevention of binding of urushiol to the skin.

- **Reference Type**: Journal Article
- **Record Number**: 27
- **Author**: Brouwer, Derk H., Boeniger, Mark F. and van Hemmen, Joop
- **Year**: 2000
- **Title**: Hand wash and manual skin wipes
- **Journal**: The Annals of Occupational Hygiene
- **Volume**: 44
- **Issue**: 7
- **Pages**: 501–510
- **Short Title**: Hand wash and manual skin wipes
- **ISSN**: 0003-4878
- **DOI**: https://doi.org/10.1093/annhyg/44.7.501

Abstract: Hand wash and skin wipes are major techniques that have been used for dermal exposure sampling. Both techniques remove chemicals either deposited on or transferred to the skin contaminant layer by a combination of chemical and mechanical actions. The paper overviews identified methods and techniques, with emphasis on sampling parameters and sampling efficiency. It is concluded that identified sampling protocols, including sampling techniques, deviate at possible key issues, which hampers comparisons of study results. It is recommended to conduct sampling efficiency studies prior to field sampling, under conditions that are quite similar to conditions of exposure regarding exposure process, levels of skin loading, and time of residence of the compound on the skin. Harmonization of sampling protocols will be a first step in creating a database for better understanding the influence of sampling parameters on the performance of removal techniques to assess dermal exposure.

Notes: https://doi.org/10.1093/annhyg/44.7.501
URL: https://doi.org/10.1093/annhyg/44.7.501

- **Reference Type**: Journal Article
- **Record Number**: 2
- **Author**: Wester, Ronald C, Hui, Xiaoying, Landry, Timothy and Maibach, Howard I
- **Year**: 1999
- **Title**: *In vivo* skin decontamination of methylene bisphenyl isocyanate (MDI): soap and water ineffective compared to polypropylene glycol, polyglycol-based cleanser, and corn oil
- **Journal**: Toxicological Sciences: An Official Journal of the Society of Toxicology
- **Volume**: 48
- **Issue**: 1
- **Pages**: 1–4
- **Short Title**: *In vivo* skin decontamination of methylene bisphenyl isocyanate (MDI): soap and water ineffective compared to polypropylene glycol, polyglycol-based cleanser, and corn oil
- **ISSN**: 1096-0929

- **Reference Type**: Journal Article
- **Record Number**: 13
- **Author**: Wester, Ronald C, Hui, Xiaoying, Landry, Timothy and Maibach, Howard I
- **Year**: 1999
- **Title**: Biotransformation and Toxicokinetics-*In Vivo* Skin Decontamination of Methylene Bisphenyl Isocyanate (MDI): Soap and Water Ineffective Compared to Polypropylene Glycol, Polyglycol-Based Cleanser
- **Journal**: Toxicological Sciences
- **Volume**: 48
- **Issue**: 1
- **Pages**: 1–4
- **Short Title**: Biotransformation and Toxicokinetics-*In Vivo* Skin Decontamination of Methylene Bisphenyl Isocyanate (MDI): Soap and Water Ineffective Compared to Polypropylene Glycol, Polyglycol-Based Cleanser
- **ISSN**: 1096-6080

- **Reference Type**: Journal Article
- **Record Number**: 76
- **Author**: Gordon, Richard K., Feaster, Shawn R., Russell, Alan J., LeJeune, Keith E., Maxwell, Donald M., Lenz, David E., Ross, Michelle and Doctor, Bhupendra P.
- **Year**: 1999
- **Title**: Organophosphate skin decontamination using immobilized enzymes
- **Journal**: Chemico-Biological Interactions
- **Volume**: 119–120
- **Pages**: 463–470
- **Date**: 1999/05/14/
- **Short Title**: Organophosphate skin decontamination using immobilized enzymes
- **ISSN**: 0009-2797
- **DOI**: https://doi.org/10.1016/S0009-2797(99)00059-9

Keywords: Acetylcholinesterase; Cholinesterases; Organophosphorus; Bioscavenger; Oxime reactivation; Polyurethane foam sponge; Decontamination

Abstract: We previously demonstrated that a combination of cholinesterase (ChE) pre-treatment with an oxime is an effective measure against soman and sarin. We describe here a novel approach for the preparation of covalently linked ChEs which are immobilized to a polyurethane matrix. Such preparation of ChE-sponges enhances the stability and usefulness of the enzymes in non-physiological environments. The ChE-sponges, which can be molded to any form, can effectively be used to remove and decontaminate organophosphates (OPs) from surfaces, biological (skin or wounds) or otherwise (clothing or sensitive medical equipment), or the environment. The ChE-sponges retained their catalytic activity under conditions of temperature, time, and drying where the native soluble enzyme would rapidly denature, and can be reused in conjunction with oximes many times. The ChE-sponge in the presence of oxime repeatedly detoxified OPs such as DFP or MEPQ. These developments in ChE technology have extended the applicability of OP scavengers from *in vivo* protection, to a variety of external detoxification and decontamination schemes. In addition to treatment of OP-contaminated soldiers, the ChE-sponge could protect medical personnel from secondary contamination while attending chemical casualties, and civilians exposed to pesticides or highly toxic nerve agents such as sarin.

URL: http://www.sciencedirect.com/science/article/pii/S0009279799000599

Gold, M. B., et al. (1994). "Hypochlorite solution as a decontaminant in sulfur mustard contaminated skin defects in the euthymic hairless guinea pig." Drug and Chemical Toxicology 17(4): 499–527.

Abstract: Hypochlorite solutions are thought to be efficacious when used to topically decontaminate intact skin. However, few studies have examined the efficacy of decontamination of chemically contaminated wounds. Therefore, we compared the decontamination efficacy of sodium hypochlorite (0.5% and 2.5% solutions), calcium hypochlorite (0.5% and 2.5% solutions) and sterile water to untreated controls in wounds exposed to sulfur mustard (HD). Anesthetized euthymic hairless guinea pigs (EHGP) ($n = 6$) were exposed to 20 mg/kg (approximately 0.4 LD_{50}) HD in a full-thickness 8 mm surgical biopsy skin defect (i.e., wound). Each animal was subsequently decontaminated, after a two-minute intra-wound exposure to liquid HD, with nothing or one of the decontamination solutions. Decontamination efficacy was determined by the visual grading of the HD-traumatized wound lesion and by comparison of the expected HD-induced leukocyte suppression. Leukocyte suppression was inconsistent in all animals; therefore, the visual grading was the only viable evaluation method. No significant differences were observed among wounds decontaminated with any of the solutions. However, the skin surrounding non-decontaminated (but exposed) control animals showed the least visual pathology. The lesions induced following decontamination are presumed to be due to the mechanical flushing of HD onto the peri-lesional skin, or by chemical damage induced by the solution, or HD-solution interaction. Further studies are required to best delineate the optimal decontamination process for HD contaminated wounds.

- **Reference Type**: Journal Article
- **Record Number**: 83
- **Author**: Fenske, Richard A and Lu, Chensheng
- **Year**: 1994
- **Title**: Determination of handwash removal efficiency: incomplete removal of the pesticide chlorpyrifos from skin by standard handwash techniques
- **Journal**: American Industrial Hygiene Association Journal
- **Volume**: 55
- **Issue**: 5
- **Pages**: 425–432
- **Short Title**: Determination of handwash removal efficiency: incomplete removal of the pesticide chlorpyrifos from skin by standard handwash techniques
- **ISSN**: 0002-8894

Abstract: This study was designed to develop standard procedures whereby the removal efficiency of handwash techniques can be determined. A known amount of the insecticide chlorpyrifos (Dursban™), was transferred to the hands of volunteers, which were washed by a standard technique. The following experimental variables were studied: time between exposure and washing, washing solvent, and skill loading. Ethanol removed only 30% of the chlorpyrifos on skin at loadings of approximately 7 μg/cm^2, with residence time on skin having no effect. Prewashing with ethanol increased removal efficiency. A 10% isopropanol/distilled-water wash removed 43% immediately following exposure, and 23% one hour post-exposure, with skin loadings of approximately 12μg/cm^2. Removal efficiency immediately following contact decreased for lower skin loading levels (21–23% for loadings of 0.1–1 μg/cm^2). These findings indicate that substantial amounts of the insecticide were either absorbed through or adsorbed to the skin, and that pesticide residue levels recovered by standard handwashing techniques are unlikely to represent accurate estimates of dermal exposure. Approximately two-fold to five-fold underestimations of exposure can occur for pesticides with handwash procedures similar to those tested. All experimental variables studied can each alter significantly the fraction of total pesticide on skin that handwashing removes. If handwashing is to be used to estimate dermal exposure in the workplace, appropriate laboratory-based removal efficiency studies should be conducted prior to field investigations. Further efforts should be made to develop accurate and reproducible hand measurement techniques.

- **Reference Type**: Book Section
- **Record Number**: 8
- **Author**: Wester, Ronald C and Maibach, Howard I
- **Year**: 1993
- **Title**: *In vivo* topical bioavailability and skin decontamination
- **Book Title**: Topical drug bioavailability, bioequivalence, and penetration
- **Publisher**: Springer
- **Pages**: 197–207
- **Short Title**: *In vivo* topical bioavailability and skin decontamination

- **Reference Type**: Journal Article
- **Record Number**: 84
- **Author**: Weber, Lutz WD, Zesch, Achim and Rozman, Karl
- **Year**: 1992
- **Title**: Decontamination of human skin exposed to 2, 3, 7, 8-tetrachlorodibenzo-p-dioxin (TCDD) *in vitro*
- **Journal**: Archives of Environmental Health: An International Journal
- **Volume**: 47
- **Issue**: 4
- **Pages**: 302–308
- **Short Title**: Decontamination of human skin exposed to 2, 3, 7, 8-tetrachlorodibenzo-p-dioxin (TCDD) *in vitro*
- **ISSN**: 0003-9896

Abstract: Human post-mortem skin was exposed *in vitro* to 2,3,7,8-tetrachlorodi benzo-p-dioxin (TCDD) at 32 °C, under controlled humidity. In one-half of the samples, damage to the surface of the skin was simulated by stripping of the stratum corneum. After incubation with TCDD for 100 min, four different decontamination protocols were performed: (1) the sample was wiped with dry, adsorbent material (cotton balls); (2) a 10-min topical treatment with mineral oil was followed by dry wiping with cotton balls; (3) a 10-min topical treatment with mineral oil was followed by wiping with acetone-soaked cotton balls; and (4) the sample was washed with water and soap. After decontamination, skin samples were incubated (up to 300 min) again at 32 °C. One set of both intact and stripped TCDD-exposed skin samples was incubated for 300 min—absent decontamination—and was used as a control. Mineral oil treatment and acetone wipes, or water and soap, were effective in reducing (i.e., about two-fold) the amount of TCDD in the stratum corneum of intact skin. Mineral oil plus dry wipes reduced the amount of TCDD in the stratum corneum by about one-third, whereas dry wiping alone was ineffective. All protocols, however, were similarly effective in reducing the amount of TCDD in the epidermis and upper dermis; TCDD concentrations were decreased locally by factors of up to ten. In the lower dermis, a minimal effect of the decontamination procedures was observed. After artificial removal of the stratum corneum, dry wiping with adsorbent material had a deleterious effect, i.e., TCDD was rubbed into the skin, which lead to increased concentrations in various layers of the skin. Mineral oil treatment, followed either by dry wipes or by acetone wipes, and washing with water and soap were quite effective in the decontamination of damaged skin. These data, the availability of agents, and the ease of handling the different protocols led the authors to the conclusion that washing with water and soap is the method of choice to decontaminate intact or damaged skin exposed to TCDD.

Wester, R. C., et al. (1992). "*In vivo* percutaneous absorption and skin decontamination of alachlor in rhesus monkey." Journal of Toxicology and Environmental Health, Part A Current Issues 36(1): 1–12.
Abstract: The objectives of this study were to determine the percutaneous absorption of alachlor relative to formulation dilution with water, and to determine the ability of soap and water, and of water only, to remove alachlor from skin, relative to time. Alachlor is a preemergence herbicide. The *in vivo* percutaneous absorption of alachlor in rhesus monkeys was 17.3 ± 3.3, 15.3 ± 3.9, and 21.4 ± 14.2% for 24-h skin exposure to Lasso formulation diluted 1:20, 1: 40, and 1: 80, respectively. *In vivo*, there was no support for increased alachlor skin absorption with water dilution, as previously reported for *in vitro* absorption. The average *in vivo* absorption of 18% applied dose over 24 h (0.75%/h) was similar to the maximum *in vitro* rate of 0.8%/h using human skin and human plasma as receptor fluid. Dose accountability *in vivo* was 80.6–95.2%. [^{14}CJAlachlor in Lasso diluted 1:20 with water was placed on rhesus monkeys at concentrations of 23 μg/10 μl/cm^2. Skin decontamination at 0 h with soap and water (50% Ivory liquid 1:1 v/v with water) removed 73 ± 15.8% (*n* – 4) of the applied dose with the first wash; this increased to a total of 82.3 ± 14.8% with two additional washes. Decontamination after 1 h removed 87.5 ±

12.4% with three successive washes. After 3 h decontamination ability decreased, and after 24 h only 51.9 ± 12.2% could be recovered with three successive washes. Using water only, at 0 h 36.6 ± 12.3% alachlor was removed with the first wash and the total increased to 56.0 ± 14.0% with two additional washes. At 24 h the total amount decreased to 28.7 ± 72.2% for three successive washes.

Alachlor as Lasso in field-use rate (11 μg/cm^2) and undiluted (217 and 300 μg/cm^2) proportions were left on rhesus monkey skin for 12 h and decontaminated with soap and water (10% Ivory liquid v/v with water). Continual successive washes (6–8 in sequence) recovered 80–90% of the skin-applied alachlor. These results suggest that simple washing with soap and water is appropriate for removing some chemicals from skin. Decontamination with only water was less effective than with soap and water.

Wester, R. C., et al. (1992). "Percutaneous absorption of [14C] chlordane from soil." Journal of Toxicology and Environmental Health, Part A Current Issues 35(4): 269–277.

Abstract: The objective was to determine percutaneous absorption of chlordane *in vitro* and *in vivo* from soil into and through skin. The data are needed to calculate the absorbed dose of chlordane from soil, which is then used to assess the toxicity risk. Chlordane, an insecticide for which residues exist in soil, is restricted currently to use for termite control. Chlordane is highly lipophilic with little or no movement out of soil. Soil (Yolo County 65-California-57–8; 26% sand, 26% clay, 48% silt, 0.9% organic) was passed through 10-, 20-, and 48-mesh sieves. Soil then retained by 80-mesh was mixed with ^{14}C-labeled chemical at 67 ppm. Acetone solutions were prepared for comparative analysis. Human cadaver skin was dermatomed to 500 pm and used in glass diffusion cells with human plasma as the receptor fluid (3 ml/h flow rate) for a 24-h skin application time. Chlordane concentration within skin from *in vitro* studies was 0.34 ± 0.31% from soil and 10.8 ± 8.2% from acetone vehicle ($p < .01$). Individual variation from human skin sources was evident ($p < .008$). Chlordane accumulation in human plasma receptor fluid was the same for soil (0.04 ± 0.05%) and acetone (0.07% ± 0.06%) formulations. Most of the remaining chlordane was recovered in the soap and water skin surface wash. In contrast, *in vivo* percutaneous absorption of chlordane in the rhesus monkey was the same for soil (4.2 ± 1.8%) and acetone (6.0 ± 2.8%) formulations ($p = .29$, nonsignificant). Multiple soap and water washings were necessary to remove chlordane from skin, suggesting that a single wash may not adequately remove all the chlordane.

Wester, R. C., et al. (1991). "Glyphosate skin binding, absorption, residual tissue distribution, and skin decontamination." Toxicological Sciences 16(4): 725–732.

Abstract: Glyphosate Skin Binding, Absorption, Residual Tissue Distribution, and Skin Decontamination. Wester, R. C., Melendres, J., Sarason, R., McMaster, J., and Maibach, H. I. (1991). *Fundam. Appl. Toxicol.* **16**, 725–732. Glyphosate is a broad-spectrum postemergence translocated herbicide. Its interactions with skin and potential systemic availability through percutaneous absorption was studied by skin binding, skin absorption, residual tissue distribution, and skin decontamination. Glyphosate in a final formulation (Roundup) undiluted and diluted with water 1:20 and 1:32, would not partition into powdered human stratum corneum (<1%). *In* *vitro* percutaneous absorption through human skin into human plasma as receptor fluid was no more than 2% over a concentration range of 0.5–154 μg/cm^2 and a topical volume range of 0.014–0.14 ml/cm^2. Disposition of glyphosate following iv administration of 93 and 9 μg doses to rhesus monkeys was mainly through urine excretion, 95 ± 8 and 99 ± 4% in 7 days, respectively. Percutaneous absorption *in vivo* in rhesus monkey was 0.8 ± 0.6% for the low dose (25 μg/cm^2) and 2.2 ± 0.8% for the high dose (270 μg/cm^2). No residual ^{14}C was found in organs of the monkeys euthanized 7 days after the topical application. Washing the skin application site with soap and water removed 90 ± 4% of applied dose, and washing with water only removed 84 ± 3% of applied dose. Both soap and water and water only were equal in ability to remove glyphosate from skin over a 24 hr skin application period. About 50% of the initially applied dose could be recovered after 24 hr. Glyphosate is very soluble in water and insoluble in most organics (octanol/water log $P = -1.70$) and therefore not compatible with the lipid-laden stratum corneum. This is consistent with the low skin binding and skin absorption and also consistent with the efficient removal from skin with soap and water or water-only wash.

Wester, R. C., et al. (1990). "Percutaneous absorption and skin decontamination of PCBs: *in vitro* studies with human skin and *in vivo* studies in the rhesus monkey." Journal of Toxicology and Environmental Health, Part A Current Issues 31(4): 235–246.

Abstract: Knowledge of the entry of polychlorinated biphenyls through the skin into the body and subsequent disposition aids estimation of potential for human health hazard. [^{14}C]Aroclor 1242 and [^{14}C]Aroclor 1254 were separately administered intravenously and topically to rhesus monkeys. Following iv administration, 30-d excretion was 39.4% ± 5.9% urine and 16.1% ± 0.8% feces (total 55.5% ± 5.1%) for Aroclor 1242, and 7.0% ± 2.2% urine and 19.7% ± 5.8% feces (total 26.7% ± 7.5%) for Aroclor 1254. Mineral oil and trichlorobenzene are common PCB cosolvents in transformers. Skin absorption of Aroclor 1242 was 20.4% ± 8.5% formulated in mineral oil and 18.0% ± 3.8% in trichlorobenzene ($p > .05$). Absorption of Aroclor 1254 was 20.8% ± 8.3% in mineral oil and 14.6% ± 3.6% in trichlorobenzene ($p > .05$). PCBs are thus absorbed through skin, and excretion from the body is slow. Vehicle (trichlorobenzene or mineral oil) did not affect percutaneous absorption.

In vitro skin absorption in human cadaver skin did not correlate with *in vivo* findings. This was due to lack of PCB partition from skin into the water receptor fluid, even with addition of 6% Oleth 20 (Volpo 20) solubilizer.

Skin decontamination of PCBs showed soap and water to be as effective as or better than the solvent ethanol, mineral oil, and trichlorobenzene in removing PCBs from skin. There is a dynamic time lapse for PCBs between initial skin contact and skin absorption (irreversible removal). Thus initially most PCBs could be removed from skin, but this ability decreased with time to the point where at 24 h only about 25% of the initial PCB skin dose could be recovered with skin washing.

- **Reference Type**: Journal Article
- **Record Number**: 58
- **Author**: L., Rigano, S., Savonelli and L., Bencini P.

- **Year**: 1989
- **Title**: Use and properties of perfluoropolymethyl-isopropylethers in skin and hair cleaning; system stabilization and interference with sebum redistribution on skin and hair
- **Journal**: International Journal of Cosmetic Science
- **Volume**: 11
- **Issue**: 6
- **Pages**: 259–282
- **Short Title**: Use and properties of perfluoropolymethyl-isopropylethers in skin and hair cleaning; system stabilization and interference with sebum redistribution on skin and hair
- **DOI**: https://doi.org/10.1111/j.1467-2494.1989.tb00516.x

Abstract: Synopsis Perfluoro-polymethyl-isopropyl ethers (PPIE) are known for their low surface tension and spreading characteristics. Their use in detergent systems was difficult because of their insolubility in most fluids (except fluorinated ones), but microdispersions have been obtained with surfactant blends, the compositions of which minimize the interfacial tension. Thickeners have been tried in order to improve suspension stability during shelf life. Spreading of PPIE has been studied by using *in vivo* and *in vitro* evaluations, both on hair and on skin. Results are discussed, as these systems could improve greasy skin conditions and decrease the rebound effect.

URL: https://onlinelibrary.wiley.com/doi/abs/10.1111/j.1467-2494.1989.tb00516.x

Wester, R. C. and H. I. Maibach (1985). "*In vivo* percutaneous absorption and decontamination of pesticides in humans." Journal of Toxicology and Environmental Health, Part A Current Issues 16(1): 25–37.

Abstract: Regulators today face complex problems in assessing the health hazards associated with the use of pesticides. Pesticide exposure occurs at manufacturing, application, work area, and consumption situations, and in the air, water, and soil of our daily lives. The skin is the largest organ of the body and thus has become a major environmental port for pesticides to enter the body. In this paper, we review the principles of percutaneous absorption—the rate and extent that chemicals enter the body through the skin—using data currently available for pesticides.

Reifenrath, W. G., et al. (1984). "Evaluation of diethyl malonate as a simulant for 1, 2, 2-trimethylpropyl methylphosphonofluoridate (soman) in shower decontamination of the skin." Journal of Pharmaceutical Sciences 73(10): 1388–1392.

Abstract: A shower decontamination bench model has been used to assess quantitatively the importance of several variables (water pressure and temperature, surfactant concentration in the decontamination fluid, nozzle type, and shower time) on decontamination of nontoxic chemical warfare-agent simulants diethyl malonate and thickened diethyl malonate from pig skin *in vitro*. Diethyl malonate was validated as a simulant for 1,2,2-trimethylpropyl methylphosphonofluoridate (soman) by comparison of the skin penetration and decontamination of radiolabeled diethyl malonate to the radiolabeled phosphonofluoridate in shower decontamination trials of pig skin *in vitro*. Percutaneous penetration of diethyl malonate was significantly greater than that of the phosphonofluoridate during the 15-min period after application. However, both were <0.1% of the applied dose. Showering or thickener had no significant effect on the percutaneous penetration of diethyl malonate or the phosphonofluoridate. Most of the phosphonofluoridate removed by showering or scrubbing the skin was inactivated. The quantity of intact 1,2,2-trimethylpropyl methylphosphonofluoridate that penetrated through the skin was below the detection limit of the enzymatic analysis. There was no statistically significant difference between the phosphonofluoridate and diethyl malonate in efficacy of shower decontamination. The presence of thickener did not have a significant effect on decontamination efficacy.

Scheufler, E. and K. K. Rozman (1984). "Comparative decontamination of hexachlorobenzene-exposed rats and rabbits by hexadecane." Journal of Toxicology and Environmental Health, Part A Current Issues 14(2–3): 353–362.

Abstract: The effect of 8 wk of hexadecane (Hex; 5% w/w) in the diet on the disposition of [^{14} C]hexachlorobenzene (HCB) was examined under Identical conditions in rats and rabbits. Urine and feces were collected daily. Blood was obtained periodically. HCB was determined in serum, erythrocytes, heart, muscle, lungs, liver, kidney, spleen, fat, skin, and brain, as well as in excreta. The half-life of HCB was similar in the two species examined (rat 24 d; rabbit 32 d). Hex treatment increased by 4–5-fold the daily fecal excretion of HCB, resulting in correspondingly reduced half-lives of HCB in both species (rat 8 d, rabbits 12 d). As a result of Hex treatment, HCB concentrations in fat (major tissue of storage) of rabbits were about 5 times and in rats about 13 times lower than in corresponding controls. In general, the decrease of HCB in other tissues paralleled that in fat. Data indicate that the effect of Hex on the disposition of HCB is very similar in rats and rabbits.

- **Reference Type**: Journal Article
- **Record Number**: 52
- **Author**: Andreeva, NA, Sit'ko, RIa and Khodyreva, MA
- **Year**: 1982
- **Title**: Evaluation of the effectiveness of cleansing the skin of beryllium compounds
- **Journal**: Gigiena i sanitariia
- **Issue**: 3
- **Pages**: 87
- **Short Title**: Evaluation of the effectiveness of cleansing the skin of beryllium compounds
- **ISSN**: 0016-9900

- **Reference Type**: Journal Article
- **Record Number**: 53
- **Author**: Sul'zhenko, AI and Levin, MM

- **Year**: 1979
- **Title**: Agent for cleansing skin of a binding substance based on phenol formaldehyde resins
- **Journal**: Gigiena truda i professional'nye zabolevaniia
- **Issue**: 6
- **Pages**: 47–47
- **Short Title**: Agent for cleansing skin of a binding substance based on phenol formaldehyde resins
- **ISSN**: 0016-9919

- **Reference Type**: Journal Article
- **Record Number**: 77
- **Author**: Brown, Vernon K. H., Box, Valerie L. and Simpson, Barry J.
- **Year**: 1975
- **Title**: Decontamination procedures for skin exposed to phenolic substances
- **Journal**: Archives of Environmental Health: An International Journal
- **Volume**: 30
- **Issue**: 1
- **Pages**: 1–6
- **Date**: 1975/01/01
- **Short Title**: Decontamination procedures for skin exposed to phenolic substances
- **ISSN**: 0003-9896
- **DOI**: https://doi.org/10.1080/00039896.1975.10666623

Abstract:

Spraying or swabbing with a mixture of polyethylene glycol 300/industrial methylated spirits (PEG-300/IMS) (2:1 by volume) has been shown to substantially reduce mortality, systemic effects, and skin burns resulting from skin contamination by phenol, cumene hydroperoxide, or phenol/acetone cleavage product.

The skin-damaging potentials of sodium hydroxide and sulfuric acid have also been investigated. PEG-300/IMS (2:1 by volume) mixture was found, in rats, to be slightly less effective than water as means of decontamination.

The PEG-300/IMS mixture has been shown not to cause eye irritation, and so should not present a hazard where this mixture is used as a decontaminant spray.

URL: https://doi.org/10.1080/00039896.1975.10666623

- **Reference Type**: Journal Article
- **Record Number**: 25
- **Author**: Bate, L.C.
- **Year**: 1965
- **Title**: The use of activation analysis in procedures for the removal and characterization of the surface contaminants of hair
- **Journal**: Journal of Forensic Sciences (U.S.)
- **Pages**: Medium: X; Size: Pages: 60-72

- **Short Title**: The use of activation analysis in procedures for the removal and characterization of the surface contaminants of hair
- **Accession Number**: 0022-1198

Keywords: Chemistry; Analytical procedures; Activation analysis; Aluminum; Antimony; Arsenic; Bromine; Chlorine; Chromium; Cobalt; Contamination; Gold; Hair; Man; Manganese; Mercury; Quantitative analysis; Selenium; Sodium; Surfaces; Uses; Zinc

Marshall Jr, E., et al. (1919). "On dichlorethylsulphide (mustard gas) II. Variations in susceptibility of the skin to dichlorethylsulphide." Journal of Pharmacology and Experimental Therapeutics 12: 291–301.
Abstract: N/A

Sollmann, T. (1919). "Dichloroethylsulphid ("mustard gas") II. The question of induced hypersusceptibility of the skin." Journal of Pharmacology and Experimental Therapeutics 12: 319–332.
Abstract: N/A

Lynch, V., et al. (1918). "On dichlorethylsulphide (mustard gas). I. The systemic effects and mechanism of action." Journal of Pharmacology and Experimental Therapeutics 12: 265–290.
Abstract: N/A

Warthin, A. S. and C. V. Weller (1918). "The pathology of the skin lesions produced by mustard gas (dichlorethylsulphide)." Translational Research 3(8): 447–479.
Abstract:

- 1.1 Dichlorethylsulphide (mustard gas) is an escharotic, specific in its action upon the epidermis and tissues of corium, particularly upon the endothelium of the vessels.
- 2.2. The lesion is a chemical burn unlike that produced by heat, electricity, or the ordinary corrosives such as sulphuric, nitric, and hydrochloric acids or strong alkalies. Of all these agents, the effects are most closely allied to those of hydrochloric acid, but are much greater in intensity. It differs from a heat burn in the absence of thrombosis, in the greater degree of fluid exudation, in the greater moistness of the affected area and in the fact that the necrosis as shown by the loss of nuclei requires hours, or even days, for its complete development. The coagulated, shrunken and cooked appearance of the tissues in heat burns is not apparent in the tissues of mustard gas burns.
- 3.3. The vessels in the affected area are severely damaged and collapsed and there is a local anemia in the earlier stages, with a marked fluid exudation and leucocyte migration. The process is nonhemorrhagic and nonthrombosing.
- 4.4. In man the necrosis of the epidermis is usually evident in two hours through the hydropic change in the epithelium and early vesicle formation. There is no deep edema. It is confined to the epidermis and to the papillary layer in the early stages.

- 5.5. In animals the intense and deep edema is most striking and altogether different from that seen in man. Vesicle formation was not noted by us in animals.
- 6.6. The deep penetration of the smallest quantities applied to the surface is a most striking feature. There is an undoubted entrance through the hair follicles, sebaceous and sweat glands.
- 7.7. The slowly progressive character of the necrosis is a specific characteristic, the height of the necrosis being reached five to ten days after application. This may, in part, be explained by contraction and death of the vessels with resulting anemia in the affected area.
- 8.8. The painlessness of the lesion is also a marked characteristic. This may be explained by the edema and degeneration of the nerve endings in the affected portion.
- 9.9. In none of our animals was there any conjunctivitis or irritation of the respiratory tract produced by the cutaneous applications. We conclude that there is no evidence of metastasis from the local lesion as claimed by both Meyer and Haldane. We believe that the conjunctival and respiratory lesions are due alone to the direct action of mustard gas and when animals are protected from the vapor no lesions in these organs will result, no matter how severe the skin burn.
- 10.10. Contrary to the statements of certain English and French observers, the admixture of water does not increase the escharotic action, but if the oil is immediately washed away, the lesion is greatly reduced in intensity. Washing within two minutes with tincture of green soap may entirely prevent the lesion or result in only a slight hyperemia.
- 11.11. We believe that the lesions observed in the axilla, between the fingers and toes, around the genitals and between the thighs of men gassed in action are probably due to the greater moisture of these parts from perspiration and the resulting re-solution of the gas.
- 12.12. The slow healing is probably chiefly due to the vessel injury and the relatively slight leucocytic demarcating infiltration. In this respect the lesion is strikingly like an x-ray burn of the skin.

Patents

Process for removing or lightening stains caused by skin coloring agents

- Isabelle Hansenne Paula Reis Angelike Galdi
- https://patents.google.com/patent/US20070258917A1/en

Abstract: A process for removing or lightening a stain from human skin caused by a sunless tanning product involving contacting the stain with a stain removing composition containing at least one skin-abrading metal oxide to form a clean or lightened skin surface.

Selective removal of contaminants from a surface using articles having magnets

- David W. Koenig Brenda M. Nelson Beth Anne Lange
- https://patents.google.com/patent/US6503761B1/en

Abstract: A system and method for removing contaminants from a surface. The system is designed to use particles having means thereon which are capable of selectively binding to a contaminant or contaminants of interest. The particles are applied to the surface whereupon the contaminants bind to the particle. When the particle is removed, the desired contaminants are also removed. Preferably, the present invention utilizes magnetic particles having iron therein. The particles may then be readily removed using magnets. The means for binding the contaminant to the particle preferably comprise a ligand or a charge specifically designed to remove the contaminant of interest. The particles may be included in a carrier to facilitate their application to the surface. The invention is especially useful for the removal of contaminants from skin.

Index

H. Zhu, H. I. Maibach (eds.), *Skin Decontamination*,
https://doi.org/10.1007/978-3-030-24009-7

The manufacturer's authorised representative in the EU is Springer
Nature Customer Service Centre GmbH, Europaplatz 3, 69115 Heidelberg,
Germany. If you have any concerns regarding our products, please
contact ProductSafety@springernature.com

Printed and bound by CPI Group (UK) Ltd, Croydon, CR0 4YY
24/07/2026
02175954-0001